MEDICINAL PLANTS:
Phytochemistry, Pharmacology and Therapeutics

MEDICINAL PLANTS: *Phytochemistry, Pharmacology and Therapeutics*

– Volume 2 –

Editor-in-Chief
V.K. Gupta
Deputy Director & Head,
Central Animal Facility

Editors
G.D. Singh
Senior Scientist,
PK-PD-Toxicology Division

Surjeet Singh
Scientist
Department of Pharmacology

A. Kaul
Scientist,
Department of Pharmacology

Indian Institute of Integrative Medicine (CSIR),
Canal Road, Jammu – 180 001,
India

2012
DAYA PUBLISHING HOUSE®
New Delhi – 110 002

ISBN 978-81-7035-767-4 (Series)
ISBN 978-81-7035-768-1 (Volume 2)

Published by : **Daya Publishing House®**
4760-61/23, Ansari Road, Darya Ganj,
New Delhi - 110 002
Phone: 23245578, 23244987
Fax: (011) 23260116
e-mail : dayabooks@vsnl.com
website : www.dayabooks.com

Laser Typesetting : **Classic Computer Services**
Delhi - 110 035

Printed at : **Salasar Imaging Systems**
Delhi-110035 (India)

— *Dedication* —

This book is dedicated
to my beloved parents

NATURAL PRODUCT RESEARCH CENTER
FACULTY OF SCIENCE
PRINCE OF SONGKLA UNIVERSITY, THAILAND

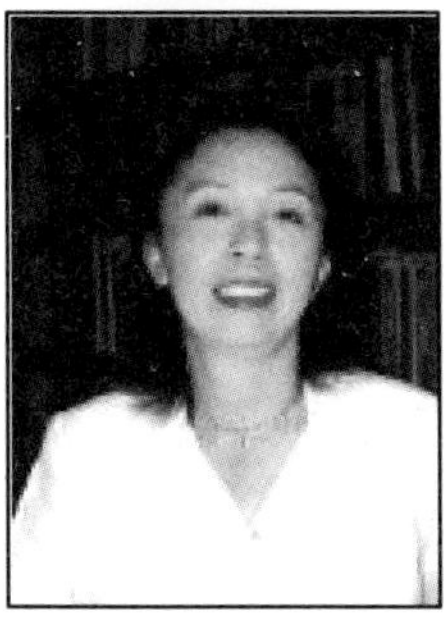

Foreword

Plants are an integral part of a number of alternative therapies such as herbalism, ayurveda, homeopathy, naturopathy, aromapathy, Unani, and other folklore systems of medicine. Day-by-day interest in gaining knowledge about medicinal plants has been considerably increasing worldwide due to sharp rise in problems as a result of adverse/side effects of modern medical science treatments. According to World Health Organization, 80% of world population is turning towards natural products based, mainly plant based medications for their primary health care needs. Currently plants, which have been documented as traditional medicines, are being examined in the hope of finding new or improved medications or therapeutics. Present volume of this book *"Medicinal Plants: Phytochemistry, Pharmacology and Therapeutics"*, contain validated scientific data on quality, safety, and efficacy and application of various medicinal plants in many countries including India, Mexico, Brazil, Norway, Nigeria, Iran, South-Africa, Thailand, and Malaysia. It comprises 25 research/review articles, contributed by eminent scientists in detecting the efficacy of various medicinal plants and its active principles as potent antioxidants, anti-diabetic, antibacterial, anti-inflammatory, and anti-ulcerogenic agents. It also describes current research methodologies in view of phytochemistry and pharmacology for developing safe and effective plant based drugs.

I can promise that this book will serve as an excellent data base of medicinal plants towards developing safer, cost effective and potent therapeutics. To my delight, I found that it contain a lot of information that would create great interest to general readers, especially graduates, researchers, pharmacists, phytochemists, medical.

I feel, it is a great honor to have the opportunity to write foreword of this book and I appreciate the painstaking effort of the editors, Dr. V.K. Gupta, Dr. G.D. Singh, Dr. Surjeet Singh, and Dr. A. Kaul to compile a knowledge bank of medicinal plants, phytochemicals and their therapeutic effects.

It is hoped that this book would be extensively read and it benefits the mankind for their prosperity in health aspects.

Professor Dr. S.P. Voravuthikunchai

Director of Natural Products Research Center,
Faculty of Science, Prince of Songkla University,
Thailand

Preface

Plants have been the eternal source of food and medicine since antiquity in all traditions and cultures. The exponents of Ayurvedic medicine in Indian and traditional systems of different countries developed great theoretical insights into the subject with comprehensive concepts of plant medicines. Historically, in last 100 years, the majority of new drugs have been discovered from organic natural products isolated from plants and microbial species. Large numbers of US-FDA approved drugs are natural products or their semi-synthetic derivatives/analogues. Despite this consistent track record of success, the pharmaceutical industrial research on natural products has declined in last 15 years due to the promise of combinatorial chemistry and high throughput screening. However, this shift in strategy led to dramatic decline in number of new drug approvals in last 10 years. Hence, the focus is bound to shift back to natural product based drug discovery keeping phytochemistry, pharmacology and their therapeutics in consideration. Furthermore, the World Health Organization estimated that 80% of people worldwide rely on herbal medicines for some aspect of their primary healthcare. This is observed that the upsurge in the use of herbal remedies in developed countries is due to consumer's preference for products of natural origin. In developing countries on the other hand, inspite of the fact that some people regard phytomedicines as primitive medicine, they still rely on it for the treatment of many illnesses (minor or major) or when orthodox medicines fail to produce the desired results.

Progress in medicinal plant research has undergone phenomenal growth in last few decades. Day by day medicinal plant research is gaining popularity because of its lesser side effects, lesser price, broad spectrum activity and non narcotic nature. Being immense value to the mankind it is the need of the time to increase the safety, effectiveness and efficacy of novel as well as current medicinal plants. Vigorous research on medicinal plants is going on to divulge the secret treasure present in plants as pharmacologically and therapeutically active phytochemicals.

Herbal treatments are the most popular form of traditional medicine, and are highly lucrative in the international market place. Annual revenues in Western Europe reached US$ 5 billion in 2003-2004. In China sales of products totaled US$ 14 billion in 2005. Herbal medicine revenue in Brazil was US$ 160 million in 2007. Traditional use of medicines is recognized as a way to learn about potential future medicines. In 2001, researchers identified 122 compounds used in mainstream medicine which were derived from ethnomedical plant sources; 80% of these compounds were used in the same or related manner as the traditional ethnomedical use.

The presentation of details of closely interdependent area of sciences is the cumbersome to understand the full potential of a medicinal plant. So authors have put their all sorts of effort to broadly integrate information over diverse group of sciences like phytochemistry, pharmacology, and therapeutics to achieve the over reaching goals. Materials presented in this book is completely updated, it is an outcome of thoroughly involved expertise and has the ability to save others time and effort they need to gather and arrange it in systematic and moreover in a scientific manner. We hope that this book helps in enhancing interest in the study of medicinal plants, against a proper cultural and scientific perspective, as medicinal plants cannot be studied, understood, evaluated and utilized in isolation.

It is owing to a world wide and sustained effort of scientists that an enormous information is being generated and there has been a series of publicatiions on medicinal plant research. Based on this rational, the present volume, *"Medicinal Plants: Phytochemistry, Pharmacology and Therapeutics Vol. 2"* presents edited information on 25 research and review communications received from eminent scientists from India and abroad. Data topics include: The Importance of Dietary Plant Lectins; Hepatoprotective and Antioxidant Effects of *Rosmarinus officinalis*; Antiulcerogenic Activity of Citrus lemon Essential Oil; Therapeutic Potential of Saptaparna, *Alstonia scholaris* in Treatment of Cancer; Jeju Seaweeds Inhibit Proinflammatory Cytokines, iNOS and COX-2 Expression in Macrophage RAW Cells;Mining of Novel Antifungal Proteins from Medicinal Plants; Role of Herbal Medicines Use in HIV / AIDS Treatment; Effect of *Alternanthera brasiliana* (L.) Kuntze on Modified Swim Test in Rats; Growth Characteristics, Phytochemicals and Mineral Composition of *Ocimun gratissimum* Applied with Albit® Biosubstance; Effect of Mulberry (*Morus inica* L.) Leaves on Blood Glucose, Glycosylated Hemoglobin and Serum Glucogenic Enzymes in NIDDM Patients; Treating Diabetes Mellitus with Natural Products;*In vitro* and *In vivo* Efficacy of Some Ethno-Medicinal Plant Species Against *Xanthomonas oryzae*; Effects of *Hypericum scabrum* Plant Extract on Signs of Morphine Withdrawal Syndrome in Rats; Importance of *Labisia pumila* (Kacip Fatimah), a Malaysian Medicine Herb etc. will definitely be eye-catching chapters and shall provide useful information regarding the uses of medicinal plants in combating a number of diseases and for their excellence over the modern medicine.

The first volume of this book series has already been submitted to general perusal in 2010. It was a big success. We hope that the volume II of the series will also become a boom for the researchers of this area. In this volume experts may rationally endeavor to impart more updated and fruitful information on the topics, hence accomplishment of this book is expected.

V.K. Gupta

Contents

Medicinal Plants: Phytochemistry, Pharmacology and Therapeutics Vol. 2 (2012) *Pages* **1–17**
Editor-in-Chief: **V.K. Gupta**
Published by: **DAYA PUBLISHING HOUSE, NEW DELHI**

1

Hepatoprotective and Antioxidant Effects of *Rosmarinus officinalis* in Nimesulide-induced Liver Damage in Rat

Patricia Yahuaca-Mendoza[1]*, Rosalinda Gutiérrez-Hernández[1] and José L. Alvarado-Acosta[1]

ABSTRACT

The non-steroidal anti-inflammatory drugs (NSAID), extensively used in the therapeutic of pain and inflammatory diseases, have caused liver damage in some patients. One of these NSAID is Nimesulide, a more selective inhibitor for COX-2 than COX-1, whose administration has been associated to some cases of acute hepatitis in humans. There is no reported data for characterizing of toxicity by nimesulide, and this knowledge is necessary to establish security basis in the use of analgesic and anti-inflammatory therapy. In this work, we considered convenient to study the extent of damage by Nimesulide and also try a hepatoprotective therapy with Rosemary (Rosmarinus officinalis, L.), which has shown beneficial antioxidant effect in experimental liver damage. It was raised an acute model, in adult Wistar male rats (weighing 200 g) separated into 5 groups of administration (during 5, 10 and 15 days): (1) vehicle, (2) Nimesulide, (3) Nimesulide plus R. officinalis and (4) R. officinalis alone (10 mg/kg weight); group 5 received carbon tetrachloride (CCl_4) to compare against our model. After treatments, liver damage was evaluated measuring markers oxidatives, metabolic, enzymatic and histological. Results showed abnormalities confirming liver damage; Nimesulide increased the degree of lipoperoxidation (> 4 times against control), gradually over the time, in the same

1 Programa Doctorado en Farmacología Médica y Molecular, Unidad Académica de Medicina Humana, Universidad Autónoma de Zacatecas. Zacatecas, Zac., 98160, México.

* *Corresponding author*: Campus UAZ Siglo XXI, Edificio Laboratorios, 3er nivel, Sección Investigación y Posgrado, Carretera Zacatecas-Guadalajara, km 6, C.P. 98160, Zacatecas, Zac., México.

E-mail: yahuacap@uaz.edu.mx, Tel: +52 (492) 925-6690 ext 6033.

way compared to CCl_4 which increased up to 6 times. Serum level of total lipid peroxide increased in a similar way, as well as enzymatic activities of alanine aminotransferase and gamma-glutamyl transpeptidase. Histological pattern showed massive necrosis and periportal inflammation among others. R. officinalis avoided partially the extent of liver damage Nimesulide-induced, thus preventing observed alterations, suggesting a probable oxidative mechanism of damage and a suitable antioxidant effect of R. officinalis. Findings let us suggest the use of R. officinalis as a potential therapy to modify the course of hepatotoxicity caused by Nimesulide.

Keywords: Acute Hepatotoxicity, Antioxidative hepatoprotection, Lipoperoxidation, Nimesulide, *Rosmarinus officinalis*.

Introduction

Today, the pharmaceutical industry continues constantly seeking new drugs and optimizes the use of existing ones, in order to make life easier for people. For that reason has developed a diversity of drugs, among them, nonsteroidal anti-inflammatory drugs (NSAID), which are widely used in Europe and the Western world for its anti-inflammatory, analgesic and antipyretic effects. In the last decades the use of some NSAIDs has been associated with some degree of hepatocellular damage, as the much known case of acetaminophen, which produces major hepatotoxicity (Makin *et al.*, 1995; Bessone and Tanno, 2000; Tajiri and Shimizu, 2008; Albertson *et al.*,2010). Therapeutic dose of acetaminophen induce a progressive hepatotoxicity which increases with the time of exposure, whereas an overdose can cause fatal liver damage (Larrey and Pageaux, 2005; Naiki-Ito *et al.*, 2010). Other NSAIDs associated with serious liver damage are indomethacin, sulindac, diclofenac, ibuprofen, naproxen, piroxicam and in recent years there were reports that involve Nimesulide (Bessone and Tanno, 2000; Traversa *et al.*, 2003; Licata *et al.*, 2010).

Nimesulide is a potent NSAID which selectively inhibits cyclooxygenase type 2, initially with a few adverse effects reported, like gastrointestinal irritation. In México it was introduced in 1999 and then, as in throughout the world, its clinical use was associated with hepatotoxicity, including fatal cases which have been reported due fulminant hepatic failure (Schattner *et al.*, 2000; Merlani *et al.*, 2001; Gallego-Rojo *et al.*, 2002; Traversa *et al.*, 2003; Tan *et al.*, 2007; Walker *et al.*, 2008). To date is not known the exact mechanism by which Nimesulide produces liver damage; however it was suggested that likely caused by an idiosyncratic reaction-type (Bessone and Tanno, 2000; Ferreiro *et al.*, 2000; Russmann *et al.*, 2009). In the liver, Nimesulide is biotransformed into various metabolites, with 4-hydroxy-Nimesulide, as the most abundant; such reductive biotransformation in aromatic nitro group can cause oxidative stress and induce covalent binding of reactive intermediaries to proteins. These conjugates, which are considered genetic and environmental factors for individual susceptibility, are rapidly inactivated and excreted in urine and feces (Boelsterli, 2002; Russmann *et al.*, 2009).

Because the liver is a vital organ in the body, for the multiplicity of roles that develops, it is important to keep it in optimal conditions. Thus, in cases of drug-induced liver injury (DILI), by any drug (Chalasani and Bjornsson, 2010; Daly, 2010; Fontana, 2010), it becomes essential to provide the fact patient treatment that can restore liver function that has been damaged.

Previous studies in experimental models have provided evidence for hepatoprotective effect of some drugs (Yahuaca *et al.*, 1985; Yahuaca and Mourelle, 1991; Yahuaca-Mendoza *et al.*, 2005), even some of them used in the treatment of liver damage in humans (Yahuaca and Alvarado, 1993). An important source for obtaining compounds, active principles with hepatoprotective effect are from natural plants such as Rosemary (*Rosmarinus officinalis*) (Al-Sereiti *et al.*, 1999; Gutierrez *et al.*, 2010), *Rosmarinus tomentosus* (Galisteo *et al.*, 2006), *Origanum vulgare* and *Origanum majorana* (Nakatani, 2000), besides the *Silybum marianum* and *Picrorrhiza kurroa* (Abenavoli *et al.*, 2010; Ferrucci *et al.*, 2010), among others.

As regards the specific case of *Rosmarinus officinalis*, several authors, as well as our research group, reported that the plant has active substances that induce hepatoprotective effect in experimental models of liver damage, and it has been suggested that this effects are due to its antioxidant properties (Sotelo-Félix *et al.*, 2002; Amin and Hamza, 2005; Thring *et al.*, 2009; Gutiérrez *et al.*, 2010; Luo *et al.*, 2010).

The possibility of a drug with hepatoprotective properties, that can be used to modify the course of acute liver injury caused by any drug, like new NSAIDs, such as Nimesulide, opens an important therapeutic perspective because this type of research could propose new alternative therapy in patients with hepatic injury. Therefore, in this work we studied the effect of *Rosmarinus officinalis* in an experimental model of Nimesulide-induced hepatotoxicity in rat, in order to assess the antioxidant effect and the hepatoprotective therapy.

Materials and Methods

Chemicals

Nimesulide, thiobarbituric acid (TBA), bovine serum albumin, anthrone, activated charcoal, were obtained from Sigma Chemical Co. (St. Louis, MO); carbon tetrachloride (CCl_4) and general chemicals from J.T. Baker (Xalostoc, Estado de México, México); solvents for spectrophotometry and high performance liquid chromatography (HPLC) were from J. T. Baker, Div. of Mallinckrodt Baker (Phillipsburg, NJ, USA). Enzymatic determinations were measured by Kit´s from commercial sources (Diagnostica Merck-México, S.A., ALT cat. 3364). The *R. officinalis* standard extract (Herbalox) and Carnosol, were a kindly gift by Dr. Don Berdahl from Research Department, Kalsec Industries, Inc. (Kalamazoo, MI, USA).

Preparation of Methanol Extract from Rosmarinus officinalis Ground Leaves

Rosmarinus officinalis (Lamiaceae) leaves were collected from cultivated plants in Zacatecas, México, and its taxonomy was authenticated by Jesús Balleza Cadengo, M. in Sc., at the Department of Botany, Unidad Académica de Agronomía, Universidad Autónoma de Zacatecas, México. Leaves were shade-dried and the plant extract was obtained by a modification to the method reported by Wu *et al.*, in 1982. Briefly, 1 kg dried leaves was powdered, macerated and extracted with 6 liters of methanol at 60 °C for 2 h. After extraction, the mixture was filtered and the filtrate was bleached three times with 180 g activated charcoal then filtered to yield a light-brown filtrate. Methanolic solution was concentrated to a final volume of 600 mL on a vacuum rotatory evaporator (Yamato) and then filtered again. One liter of distilled water was added to the filtrate to form a precipitate that was filtered and air-dried to yield the *Rosmarinus officinalis* extract used for animal administration. This extract was suspended in distilled water to 200 mg/mL. The extract was compared to Herbalox by HPLC and by spectrophotometric scan analysis.

High Performance Liquid Chromatography Analysis

A sample of *Rosmarinus officinalis* extract dissolved in methanol (4 µg/mL) was analyzed by reverse phase high performance liquid chromatography (HPLC) analysis with gradient separation and ultraviolet detection (UV) as described by Cuvelier *et al.* (1996). The separation was carried out in Agilent equipment (Model 1100) on a 5-µm Zorbax Ultrasphere column C8 (4.6 mm x 150 mm), a 5-µL loop (adapted with auto sampler) and a multi-wavelength detector (Agilent Model G1365B, MWD DE40502601). The mobile phase was solvent A (acetonitrile/1 per cent acetic acid in water; 15/85) and solvent B (methanol) according to the step gradient, lasting 100 min, from 0 per cent to 100 per cent solvent B with a flow rate of 1 mL/min. The absorbance was monitored at 284 nm. Standard Herbalox and carnosol, one of the main active compounds of *Rosmarinus officinalis*, were used in order to quantify its content in our extract.

Animal Treatments and Liver Damage Induction

Male Wistar rats (weighting 200-250 g at the onset of experiment) breed in our facilities were used. They were maintained under standard conditions (temperature of 24 °C, light/darkness cycles of 12 h) with free access to food (Harlan Teklad Global Diets) and water *ad libitum*. All procedures were in accordance with the 'Guide for the Care and Use of Laboratory Animals' of the Mexican Council for Animal Care (based in Mexican Official Norm, NOM-062-ZOO-1999) as approved by our Animal Care Committee (UAZ). Acute liver injury was induced by Nimesulide (10 mg/kg, body weight, in an oral daily dose); comparatively a reference hepatotoxicity model was induced with CCl_4 (4 $g{\cdot}kg^{-1}$ body weight, single dose; by oral route) dissolved in mineral oil (EHC, 1999). Nimesulide-induced hepatotoxicity group was treated with *R. officinalis* extract (10 mg/kg body weight, daily; outdated 4 hours post-Nimesulide). *R. officinalis* extract was suspended in water and administered through an esophageal cannula to assure the dose of 10 mg/kg of body weight, according to the extract's HPLC analysis (Sotelo-Félix *et al.*, 2002). Control groups (no treatment, vehicles or *R. officinalis* alone) were included, to compare with injured groups. The acute study was carried out for 15 days, sampling every 5 days. After the last administration, animals (n=10, each group) were anesthetized in an ether chamber and slaughtered. Blood was collected by cardiac puncture and the serum obtained by centrifugation at 1500 *x* g for 10 min, at 4°C on Avanti Beckman centrifuge. After liver perfusion with sodium phosphate buffer (0.2 M, pH 7.4, at 4 °C) we obtained the tissue to measure damage markers.

Enzymatic Activities

Alanine aminotransferase (ALT) activity in serum was measured as specified by commercial source (Diagnostica Merck-México, S.A., ALT cat. 3364). Gamma-glutamyl transpeptidase (γ-GTP) activity in serum was determined as described by Szasz (1976). Briefly, a reaction mixture of 3 mL containing Tris-HCl buffer 200 mM pH 8.2, $MgCl_2$ 20 μmol, glycil-glycine 4 μmol, γ-glutamyl p-nitroanilide 2 μmol and 100 μL of serum, was allowed to react for 30 minutes at 37°C; the reaction was stopped by acetic acid addition (1.5 M, cooled). P-nitroanilide production was measured by spectrophotometric analysis at 410 nm. Activity was reported in $\mu molL^{-1}min^{-1}$.

Determination of Hepatic Glycogen Content

Glycogen content in liver was determined by the anthrone method (Fong *et al.*, 1953). Briefly, 3 mL KOH 30 per cent (v/v in distilled water) was added to 1 g of liver tissue mixed and heated in boiling water during 30 min. The hydrolyzate was diluted in distilled water (1:250) and 20 μL of this dilution were added to 2 mL of anthrone reagent (2 mg/mL in sulfuric acid). The resultant mixture was heated in boiling water for 10 min. The samples were allowed to reach room temperature to determine the absorbance at 620 nm and the results were expressed as μg/g of liver.

Lipid Peroxidation: Hepatic and Total from Serum

MDA in liver homogenate was determined by the reaction with TBA and used as a lipid peroxidation index (Uchiyama and Mihara, 1978). Briefly, 1 g of liver was homogenized in 10 mL KCl 1.15 per cent (w/v); the homogenate was filtered through 4-folded gauze and 0.5 mL aliquots were mixed with 3 mL of H_3PO_4 1 per cent (v/v) and 1 mL of TBA 0.67 per cent (w/v), and boiling heated for 45 min. Samples were allowed to reach room temperature and 3 mL of 1-butanol was added. After shaking, the butanolic phase was obtained by centrifugation at 4000 x g for 10 min, and absorbance at 535 nm determined. Values were reported as MDA μg/g of liver. Total lipid peroxides were also measured according to Yagi (1998), based on serum thiobarbituric acid reactive substances (TBARS) and reported on μmol/mL.

Rat Red Blood Cells (RRBC) Membrane Stabilization

The percentage of RRBC membrane stabilization or membrane erythrocyte protection was measured according to Mounnissamy *et al.* (2007). This measurement is based on that increased lipid peroxidation occurs greater loss of plasma membrane stability in rat erythrocyte. The method includes hypotonicity and high temperature conditions and showing the degree of lability of plasma membrane as free hemoglobin. A portion of blood collected was mixed with an equal volume of Alsever solution (dextrose 10 per cent, sodium citrate 0.8 per cent, citric acid 0.05 per cent, sodium chloride 0.42 per cent). The mixture was centrifuged at 2000 *x* g and package cell washed with sterile isotonic saline (0.85 per cent, pH 7.2) and centrifuged again. This operation is repeated as many times as necessary to eliminate remnants of free hemoglobin. A 10 per cent RRBC suspension v/v in isotonic saline was prepared, and aliquots of 0.5 mL were mixed with 1 mL of sodium phosphate-buffered solution 0.2 M, pH 7.4 and 2 mL of distilled water and incubated at 50° C for 30 minutes. After incubation the tubes were centrifuged to obtain the supernatant and the hemoglobin content was estimated using spectrophotometric analysis at 532 nm. Results are expressed as a percentage of protection compared to control. The percentage hemolysis was calculated by assuming the hemolysis produced in the presence of distilled water as 100 per cent.

Histological Study

Liver slides were processed for histological observation, stained with Hematoxylin-Eosine. A microscope Carl Zeiss Axiostar pluz model 440950 CP ACHROMAT coupled with digital camera Olympus, model C'7070 Wide Zoom was used.

Statistical Analysis

All values are the mean ± SEM obtained from ten different animals. For statistical analysis, ANOVA with the Bonferroni test were used to compare the groups. In all cases, a difference was considered significant when p value was < 0.05.

Results

The *R. officinalis* extract obtained was a light yellow powder very aromatic, and the recovery was around 12 per cent. HPLC analysis of *Rosmarinus officinalis* extract revealed the presence of chromatographic peaks with the pattern shown by Herbalox as a standard, showing in both cases a major peak at a retention time of 67.8 min, which corresponds to carnosol, one of the most active constituent, finding a 3.02 per cent (w:w) of carnosol content in the *Rosmarinus officinalis* extract.

Evaluation of the Effectiveness of Rosmarinus officinalis in the Normalization of Biochemical Parameters in Hepatotoxicity Nimesulide-induced

To confirm the Nimesulide-induced liver damage, enzymatic serum activities (ALT and γ-GTP), metabolic (liver glycogen content) and structural changes were measured. The amount of damage was compared with that seen in the CCl_4-hepatotoxicity model. In both liver damage cases, Nimesulide and CCl_4, was observed an increased enzymatic activity in ALT (Figure 1.1), almost double compared to the control, from the beginning to the end of the study. Likewise, γ-GTP (Figure 1.2) increased in intoxicated rats by Nimesulide, although there is some difference against CCl_4 group it is not significant, but significantly different from control ($p<0.05$). When rats were treated with the extract of *R. officinalis*, the alteration in both enzyme markers of hepatotoxicity was prevented, suggesting a protective effect.

Nimesulide reduced the liver glycogen, up to 78 per cent on day 15 (compared to control). *Rosmarinus officinalis* extract prevented the Nimesulide-induced hepatotoxicity, avoiding lost of glycogen deposit, which also suggests protective effect. Figure 1.3 shows the comparative data for liver glycogen content, during intoxication time, showing deposit lost during liver damage (for CCl_4 and Nimesulide) and the protection afforded by *R. officinalis*.

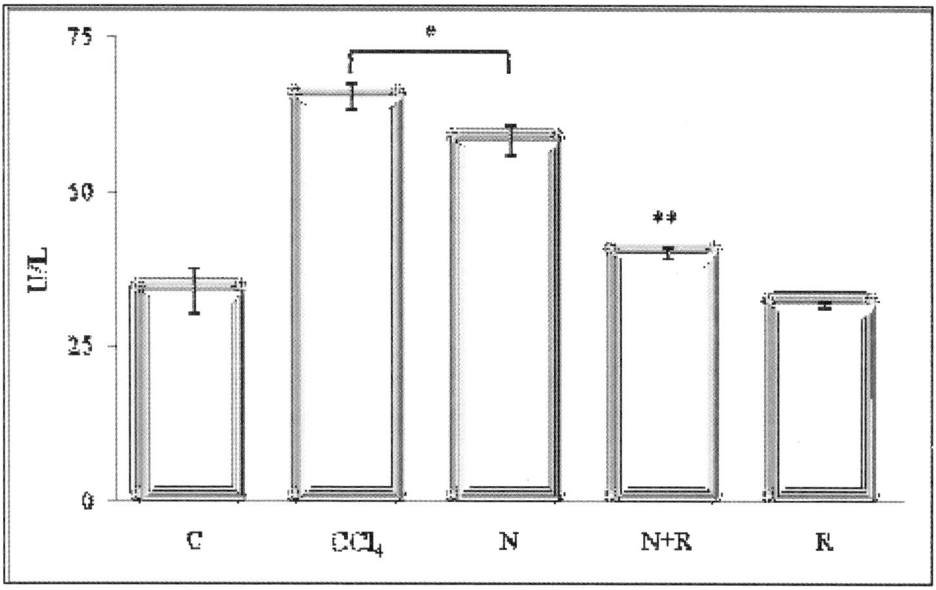

Figure 1.1. Alanine amino-transferase serum activity in rat. Each bar represents the mean value ± SEM of ten animals. C = Control; CCl_4 = Carbon tetrachloride; N = Nimesulide, N+R = Nimesulide plus *R. officinalis*; R = *R. officinalis*. (*) = significantly different from control group; (**) = significantly different from Nimesulide group; $p<0.05$.

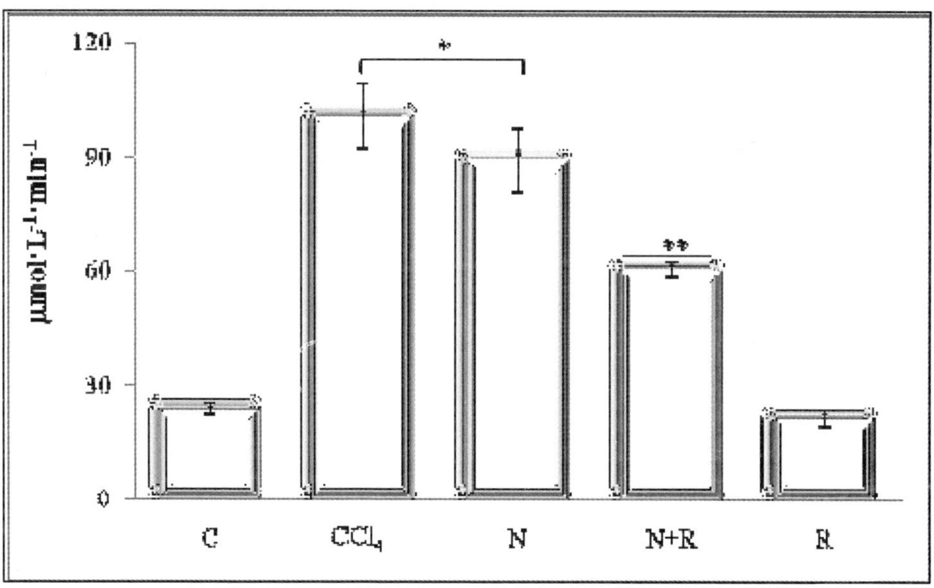

Figure 1.2. Gamma-glutamyl transpeptidase serum activity in rat. Each bar represents the mean value ± SEM of ten animals. C = Control; CCl_4 = Carbon tetrachloride; N = Nimesulide, N+R = Nimesulide plus *R. officinalis*; R = *R. officinalis*. (*) = significantly different from control group; (**) = significantly different from Nimesulide group; $p<0.05$.

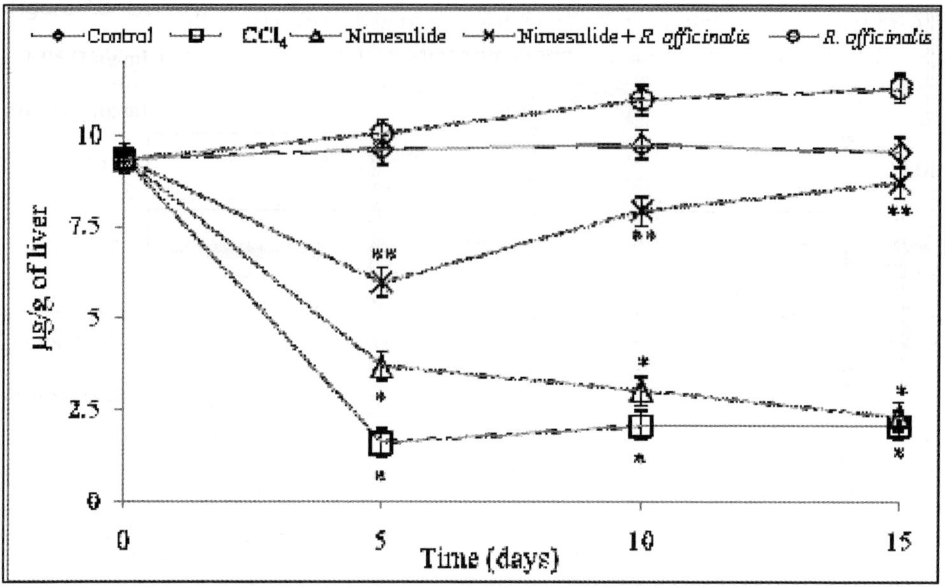

Figure 1.3. Preventive effect of *Rosmarinus officinalis* on hepatic glycogen content over the time course of Nimesulide-induced hepatotoxicity. Each point represents the mean value ± SEM of ten animals. Samples were assayed in duplicate. (*) = significantly different from control group; (**) = significantly different from Nimesulide-induced hepatotoxicity group; $p<0.05$.

Evaluation of the Effectiveness of Rosmarinus officinalis in the Normalization of Nimesulide-induced Oxidative Stress

When the oxidative stress was analysed during hepatotoxicity by Nimesulide, we found the lipoperoxidation level gradually increased above the control. Figure 1.4 shows hepatic levels of MDA as the main measured TBARS, which increased 413 per cent when animals received Nimesulide. Instead, in the CCl_4 group, the determined quantity of MDA reached up to 590 per cent (178 per cent over Nimesulide group), compared to the control. The antioxidant effect of *R. officinalis,* in hepatotoxicity induced by Nimesulide, was evident, because the *Rosmarinus* extract could avoid the extent of lipoperoxidation degree, reducing MDA level near to control. These results confirm the antioxidant action of *R. officinalis,* because there was difference statistically no significant between the control animals and those with hepatotoxicity treated with Rosemary, which suggests a positive effect antioxidant. *R. officinalis* alone did not changed the MDA content, even slightly diminished the control value.

Serum total lipid peroxides increased both in CCl_4 liver damaged animals and in Nimesulide-induced hepatotoxicity (Figure 1.5) to about 12-fold and 6-fold over the control value, respectively. *R. officinalis* treatment reduced this rise to only 0.17-fold. Administration of the vehicles to untreated animals did not modify total lipid peroxides basal levels in serum, but when animals were administered with*Rosmarinus officinalis* alone, the levels were again lower than for the control group, suggesting a free radical scavenging effect (Figure 1.5).

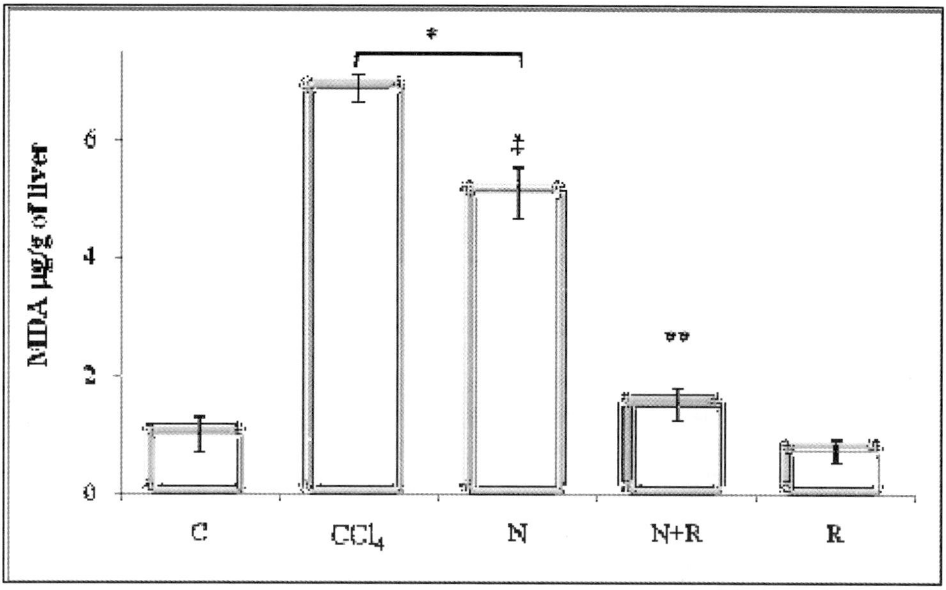

Figure 1.4. Effect of *Rosmarinus officinalis* on Nimesulide-induced lipid peroxidation on liver homogenates. Each bar represents the mean ± SEM of ten animals. C = Control; CCl_4 = Carbon tetrachloride; N = Nimesulide, N+R = Nimesulide plus *R. officinalis*; R = *R. officinalis*. (*) = significantly different from control group; (**) = significantly different from Nimesulide group; (‡) = significantly different from CCl_4 group. $p<0.05$.

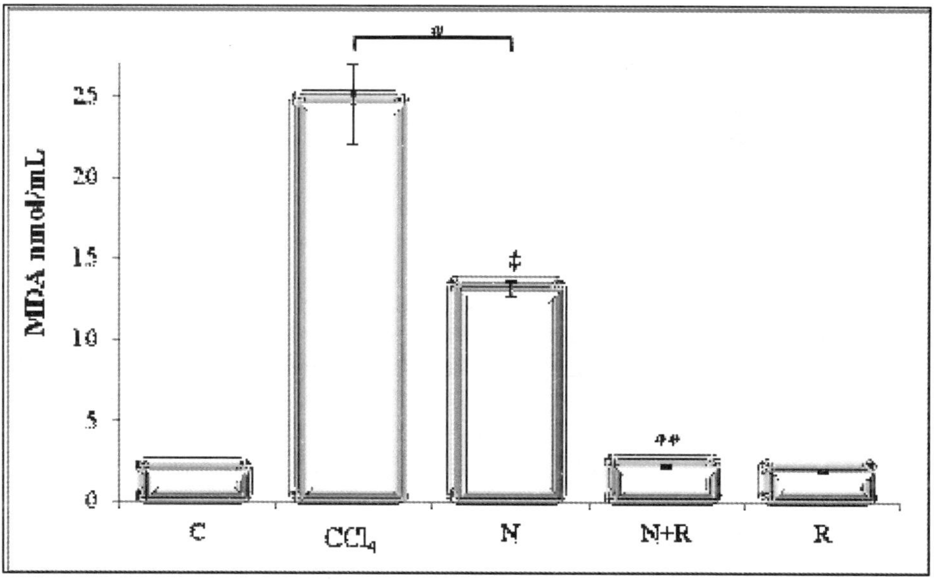

Figure 1.5. Effect of *Rosmarinus officinalis* on Nimesulide-induced serum total lipid peroxides. Each bar represents the mean ± SEM of ten animals. C = Control; CCl_4 = Carbon tetrachloride; N = Nimesulide, N+R = Nimesulide plus *R. officinalis*; R = *R. officinalis*. (*) = significantly different from control group; (**) = significantly different from Nimesulide group; (‡) = significantly different from CCl_4 group. $p<0.05$.

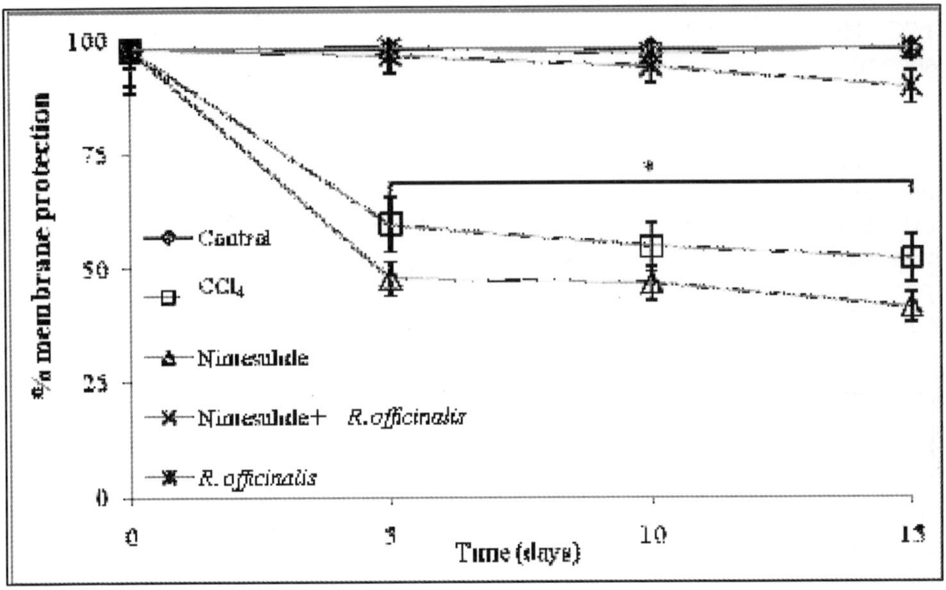

Figure 1.6. Effect of *Rosmarinus officinalis* on Nimesulide-induced erythrocyte plasma membrane instability. Each point represents the mean value ± SEM of ten animals. Samples were assayed in duplicate. (*) = significantly different from control group; (**) = significantly different from Nimesulide-induced hepatotoxicity group; p<0.05.

Erythrocyte plasma membrane stability was grossly impaired by Nimesulide administration, producing a labile membrane which was easier to lyse, and the instability was measured as an increase in hemoglobin release. Because the erythrocyte plasma membrane stability protection was very low on the intoxicated animals compared to control (untreated) group, membrane instability values are in accordance with other oxidative and damage indicators measured (metabolic, histological and enzymatic). *R. officinalis* treatment increased the erythrocyte plasma membrane stability in the treated animals and this effect was maintained over the experimental course from 15 days (p<0.05).

Evaluation of the Effectiveness of Rosmarinus officinalis in the Normalization of Nimesulide-induced Histological Alterations

Nimesulide administration produced intense periportal necrotic zones, edema, acute inflammatory infiltration, and hepatocyte degeneration characterized by cytoplasmic swelling and nuclear pyknosis (Figure 1.7B). As well as, we found periportal congestion and sinusoidal and Kuppfer cells hyperplasia. These changes in the hepatic architecture were not observed in any of the control rats (Figure 1.7A) or animals treated with*Rosmarinus officinalis* alone (Figure 1.7D). *Rosmarinusofficinalis* treatment partially prevented Nimesulide-induced morphological changes.

In some zones, edematous hepatocytes but with less cytoplasmatic degeneration were observed along with less inflammatory infiltration and no necrosis (Figure

1.7C). However, hepatic architecture was well conserved in other zones (data not shown).

Discussion

Our results show that the administration of *Rosmarinus officinalis* partially normalized the altered biochemical parameters in acute liver injury and limited the extent of histological changes. *Rosmarinus officinalis* modified those parameters in two ways. On the one hand, the treatment prevented Nimesulide effects on lipid peroxidation, ALT and γ-GTP activities. These results suggest that *Rosmarinus officinalis*, acting as an antioxidant or as a free radical scavenger, was able to stabilize

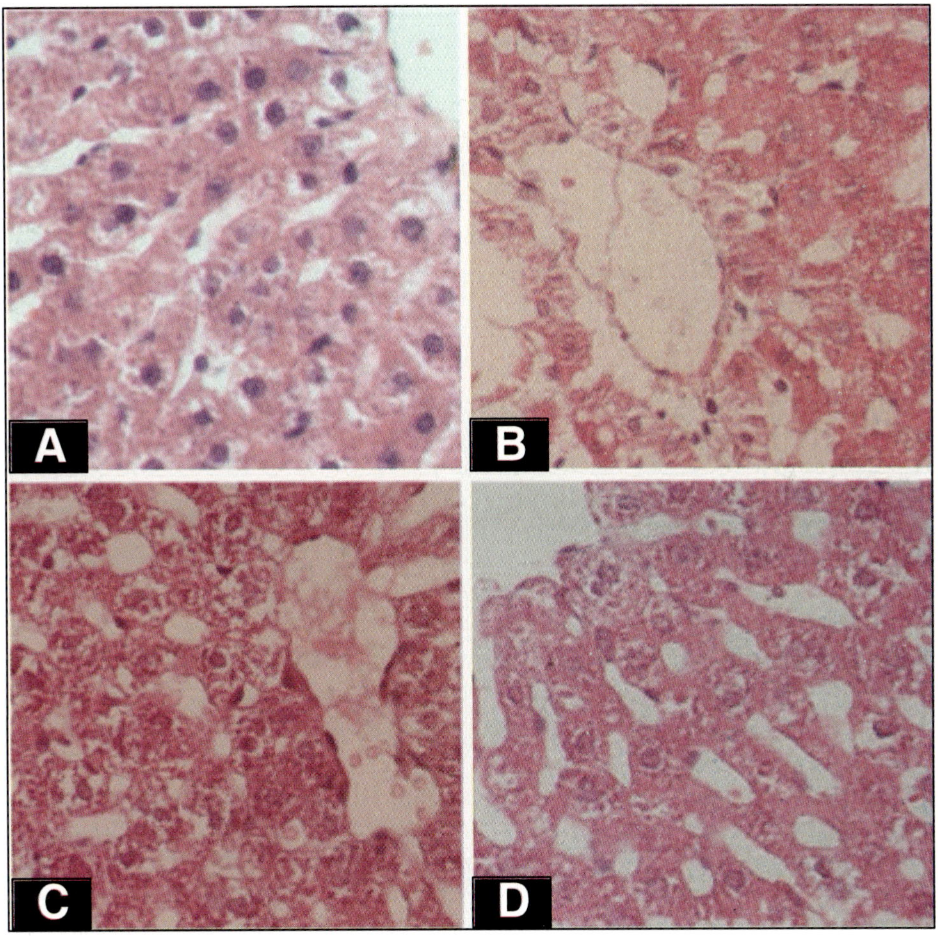

Figure 1.7. Photomicrographs of the liver, 15 days after *Rosmarinus officinalis* administration in Nimesulide-induced acute hepatotoxicity and control rats. Sections from control (A) and from animals administered with Nimesulide alone (B) or co-administered with *Rosmarinus officinalis* (C), and sections from *Rosmarinus officinalis*-treated animals (D) were stained with Hematoxylin-Eosine (final magnification 125X).

membrane structures, thus, to preserve the cellular integrity and to restrain the severity of Nimesulide-induced injury. On the other hand, *Rosmarinus officinalis* accelerated recuperation of glycogen stores in the liver. Based on these results, it is reasonable to suggest that *Rosmarinus officinalis* might exert other mechanism different from its antioxidant action or free radical scavenger activity.

Although it is not known precisely the mechanism by which Nimesulide produces liver damage and even though it is suggested to be due to reaction-type idiosyncratic (Bessone and Tanno, 2000; Ferreiro *et al.*, 2000; Russmann *et al.*, 2009), it is known that can cause oxidative stress and induce histopathological changes (Boelsterli, 2002). Our results suggest that Nimesulide induces a kind of oxidative damage, similar in all individuals studied, and almost compared to that produced by CCl_4. This is it, the degree of lipoperoxidation increased more than 4 times on the control value; a similar event occurred in major extent when total lipid peroxides were measured; damage in plasma membranes of red blood cells was magnified by lipid peroxidation, marker that could be used as a non-invasive routine test, even in humans. These data support the possibility of a mechanism probably by oxidative free radicals in the induction of hepatotoxicity with Nimesulide (Boelsterli, 2006; Chakraborty *et al.*, 2007).

Other appropriate indicators for liver damage are the enzymes ALT and γ-GTP, from cytosolic and membranal location, respectively, which were greatly increased, helping in diagnosis of liver damage by Nimesulide (Tajiri and Shimizu, 2008). In addition, lost of liver glycogen content serves as a metabolic biomarker to confirm the damage and structural alterations found in liver. That means, there was massive necrosis as well as destruction of Kupffer cells, with negative consequences for liver functionality, in agreement with the observed in human cases (Daly, 2010; Fontana, 2010; Licata *et al.*, 2010). Because the important role of the liver, in cases of hepatotoxicity, it becomes essential to provide to the patient a treatment that can restore alterated liver function (Abenavoli *et al.*, 2010; Ferrucci *et al.*, 2010; Luo *et al.*, 2010). The possibility that a drug can be used, with hepatoprotective properties (Galisteo *et al.*, 2006; Gutiérrez *et al.*, 2010), to alter the course of acute liver injury caused by Nimesulide, opens a new therapeutic perspective because this kind of research could be offering new pharmacological alternatives for patients in this condition.

It is essential to emphasize that in line with other authors (Caparroz-Asseff *et al.*, 1998; Mingato *et al.*, 2002; Boelsterli, 2002; Traversa *et al.*, 2003), Nimesulide is able to generate an oxidative damage, which can be modified with the use of antioxidant compounds from *Rosmarinus officinalis* commonly named Rosemary (Galisteo *et al.*, 2006; Gutiérrez *et al.*, 2010). These results suggest a beneficial therapy as a substance trapping of free radicals, among other effects (Hoefler *et al.*, 1987; Jones, 1998; Nakatani, 2000; Sotelo-Félix *et al.*, 2002; Yahuaca-Mendoza *et al.*, 2005; Thring *et al.*, 2009; Dias *et al.*, 2000). Our results are related to those reported by other authors, since in some work describes the involvement of oxygen radicals in carcinogenesis and there is a relationship between action as scavenger of free radicals and anticarcinogenic action (Minnunni, 1992; Huang *et al.*, 1994; Ho *et al.*, 1994; Jones, 1998).

Moreover, it is important to note that, in certain pathological processes liver damage involves free radicals, and even experimental models have been described (Recknagel and Glende, 1973). It is relevant to count with experimental models for the study of future medications that are implemented in such pathological processes. In this work, we compare against the model of carbon tetrachloride, which is already well established that generate free radicals which attack biomolecules especially phospholipids of biological membranes, inducing the cited lipoperoxidation. The decrease of glycogen in liver damage was consistent with that described in other reports (Mourelle *et al.*, 1989; Perez-Alvarez *et al.*, 1990; Muriel, 1998), and in terms of Nimesulide, still no scientific experiments that match the results that we have found. However, reduction in liver glycogen associated to metabolic changes by Nimesulide, may be due to glycogenolysis, in turn by increase in glycogen phosphorylase activity which is induced by cAMP and Ca^{2+}.

In summary, the results of this study allows us to conclude about the importance of alternative phytotherapeutic with *Rosmarinus officinalis* which showed hepatoprotective effect in the experimental model of liver injury, improving the structural integrity of the hepatocyte through the scavenging activity of the free radicals induced by Nimesulide and, consequently, avoid the propagation of lipid peroxide. Particularly, it is relevant the administration of *R. officinalis* in a hepatotoxicity condition by Nimesulide, whose toxic properties, in some cases, could lead to fatal liver failure. It was clearly obvious the presence of oxidative stress in Nimesulide-induced hepatotoxicity, which was prevented by the action of *Rosmarinus officinalis*, confirming its antioxidant effect.

Acknowledgements

The authors thank to Dr. Manuel Presno-Bernal for their invaluable experimental support in the histopathological diagnosis. Financial support came from *Programa de Fortalecimiento al Postgrado, Secretaría de Educación Pública, México* (code PIFOP-2002-33-04).

References

Abenavoli, L., Capasso, R., Milic, N., and Capasso, F. (2010). Milk thistle in liver diseases: past, present, future. *Phytothe. Res.*, **24(10)**: 1423-1432.

Albertson, T.E., Walker, V.M., Stebbins, M.R., Ashton, E.W., Owen, K.P., and Sutter, M.E. (2010). A population study of the frequency of high dose acetaminophen prescribing and dispensing. *Ann Pharmacother.*, **44**: 1191-1195.

Al-Sereiti, M.R., Abu-Amer, K.M., and Sen, P. (1999). Pharmacology of rosemary (*Rosmarinus officinalis Linn.*) and its therapeutic potentials. *Indian J Exp Biol.*, **37(2)**: 124-130.

Amin, A., and Hamza, A.A. (2005). Hepatoprotective effects of *Hibiscus, Rosmarinus* and *Salvia* on azathioprine-induced toxicity in rats. *Life Sci.*, **77**: 266-278.

Bessone, F., and Tanno, H. (2000). Hepatotoxicity induced by non-steroidal antiinflammatory drugs. *Gastroenterol Hepatol.*, **23(4)**: 200-205.

Boelsterli, U.A., Ho, H.K., Zhou, S., and Leow, K.Y. (2006). Bioactivation and hepatotoxicity of nitroaromatic drugs. *Curr Drug Metab.*, **7**: 715-727.

Boelsterli, U.A. (2002). Nimesulide and hepatic adverse effects; roles of reactive metabolites and host factors. *Int. J. Clin. Pract.*, **128**: 30-36.

Carson, J.L., Strom, B.L., Duff, A., Gupta, A., and Das, K. (1993). Safety of nonsteroidal anti-inflammatory drugs with respect to acute liver disease. *Arch Intern Med.*, **153(11)**: 1331-1336.

Chakraborty, S., Roy, K., and Sengupta, Ch. (2007). Exploring effects of different nonsteroidal antiinflammatory drugs on lipid peroxidation. Part II. 4-HNE profile. *Acta Pol Pharm.*, **64**: 211-216.

Chalasani, N., and Bjornsson, E. (2010). Risk factors for idiosyncratic drug-induced liver injury. *Gastroenterology*, **138**: 2246-2259.

Cuvelier, M.E., Richard, H., and Berset, C. (1996). Antioxidative activity and phenolic composition of pilot-plant and commercial extracts of sage and rosemary. *J. Amer. Oil Chem. Soc.*, **73**: 645-652.

Daly, A.K. (2010). Drug-induced liver injury: past, present and future. *Pharmacogenomics*, **11**: 607-611.

Días, P.C., Foglio, M.A., Possenti, A., and de Carvalho, J.E. (2000). Antiulcerogenic activity of crude hydroalcoholic extract of *Rosmarinus officinalis L. J Ethnopharmacol.*, **69(1)**: 57-62.

EHC (Environmental Health Criteria) 208. (1999). Carbon Tetrachloride. World Health Organization, Geneva, Switzerland.

Ferreiro, C., Vivas, S., Jorquera, F., Dominguez, A.B., Espinel, J., Munoz, F., Herrera, A., Fernandez, M.J., Olcoz, J.L., and Ortiz de Urbina, J. (2000). Toxic hepatitis caused by Nimesulide, presentation of a new case and review of the literature. *Gastroenterol Hepatol.*, **23(9)**: 428-430.

Ferrucci, L.M., Bell, B.P., Dhotre, K.B., Manos, M.M., Terrault, N.A., Zaman, A., Murphy, R.C., Vanness, G.R., Thomas, A.R., Bialek, S.R., Desai, M.M., and Sofair, A.N. (2010). Complementary and alternative medicine used in chronic liver disease patients. *J. Clin. Gastroenterol.*, **44**: 40-45.

Fong, I., Schoffner, F.C., and Kirk, P. (1953). The ultramicrodetermination of glycogen in liver. A comparison of the anthrone and reducing sugar methods. *Arch. Biochem. Biophys.*, **45(2)**: 319-326.

Fontana, R.J. (2010). Approaches to the study of drug-induced liver injury. *Clin. Pharmacol. Ther.*, **88**: 416-419.

Galisteo, M., Suárez, A., Montilla, M.P., Torres, M.I., Fernandez, M.I., Gil, A., and Navarro, M.C. (2006). Protective effects of *Rosmarinus tomentosus* ethanol extract on thioacetamide-induced liver cirrhosis in rats. *Phytomedicine*, **13**: 101-108.

Gallego-Rojo, F.J., Fernández-Pérez, F., Fernández-Pérez, R., Parcel, A., Blas, J.M., and Diez, F. (2002). Nimesulide-induced hepatotoxicity. *Rev. Esp. Enferm Dig.*, **94(1)**: 41-42.

Gutiérrez, R., Presno, M., Serrano, C.J., Pérez-Veyna, O., Alvarado, J.L., and Yahuaca, P. (2010). Oxidative stress modulation by phytotherapy with *Rosmarinus officinalis* in CCl_4-induced liver cirrhosis. *Phytotherapy Research*, **24**(4): 595-601.

Ho, C.-T., Ferraro, T., Chen, Q., Rosen, R.T., and Huang, M.-T. (1994). Phytochemicals in tea and Rosemary and their cancer-preventive properties. *In*: Ho, C-T., Osawa, T., Huang, M.-T. and Rosen, R.T. (eds) *Food Phytochemical for Cancer Prevention* 2. American Chemical Society Symposium Series, **547**, American Chemical Society, Washington D.C., USA, pp. 2-19.

Hoefler, C., Fleurentin, J., Mortier, F., Pelt, J.M., and Guillemain, J. (1987). Comparative choleretic and hepatoprotective properties of young sprouts and total plant extracts of *Rosmarinus officinalis* in rats. *J. Ethnopharmaco.*, **19(2)**: 133-143.

Huang, T.L., Villalobos, S.A., and Hammock, B.D. (1994). Effect of hepatotoxic doses of paracetamol and carbon tetrachloride on the serum and hepatic carboxylesterase activity in mice. *J. Pharm. Pharmacol.*, **45**: 458-465.

Jones, C.L.A. (1998). Rosemary has anti-Carcinogenic properties. *Nutrition Science News*, **10**: 1-2

Larrey, D., and Pageaux, G-P. (2005). Drug-induced acute liver failure. *Eur J Gastroenterol Hepatol.*, **17**: 141-143.

Licata, A., Calvaruso, V., Cappello, M., Craxì, A. and Almasio, P.L. (2010). Clinical course and outcomes of drug-induced liver injury: Nimesulide as the first implicated medication. *Dig. Liv. Dis.*, **42(2)**: 143-148.

Luo, Y., Pan, J., Pan, Y., Han, Z., and Zhong, R. (2010). Evaluation of the protective effects of Chinese herbs against biomolecule damage induced by peroxynitrite. *Biosci. Biotechnol. Biochem.*, **74**: 1350-1354.

Makin, A.J., Wendon, J., and Williams, R. (1995). 7-year experience of severe acetaminophen-induced hepatotoxicity (1987-1993). *Gastroentrol.*, **109(6)**: 1907-1916.

Merlani, G., Fox, M., Oehen, H.P., Cathomas, G., Renner, E.L., Fattinger, K., Schneemann, M., and Kullak-Ublick, G.A. (2001). Fatal hepatoxicity secondary to Nimesulide. *Eur J Clin Pharmacol.*, **57(4)**: 321-326.

Mingatto, F.E., Rodrigues, T., Pigoso, A.A., Uyemura, S.A., Curti, C., and Santos, A.C. (2002). The critical role of mitochondrial energetic impairment in the toxicity of Nimesulide to hepatocytes. *J Pharmacol Exp Ther.*, **303(2)**: 601-607.

Minnunni, M., Wolleb, U., Mueller, O., Pferfer, A., and Aeschbacher, H.U. (1992). Natural antioxidant as inhibitor of oxigen species induced mutagenicity. *Mut. Res.*, **269(2)**: 193-200.

Mounnissamy, V.M., Kavimani, S., Balu, V., and Darlin-Quine, S. (2007). Evaluation of Anti-inflammatory and Membrane stabilizing property of Ethanol Extract of *Cansjera rheedii* J. Gmelin (*Opiliaceae*). *Iranian J. Pharmacol. Ther.*, **6(2)**: 235–237.

Mourelle, M., Muriel, P., Favari, L., and Franco, T. (1989). Prevention of CCl_4-induced liver cirrhosis by silymarin. *Fundam. Clin. Pharmacol.*, **3(3)**: 183-91.

Muriel, P. (1998). Nitric oxide protection of rat liver from lipid peroxidation, collagen accumulation and liver damage induced by carbon tetrachloride. *Biochem. Pharmacol.*, **56**: 773-779.

Naiki-Ito, A., Asamoto, M., Naiki, T., Ogawa, K., Takahashi, S., Sato, S., and Shirai, T. (2010). Gap junction dysfunction reduces acetaminophen hepatotoxicity with impact on apoptotic signaling and connexin 43 protein induction in rat. *Toxicol. Pathol.*, **38**: 280-286.

Nakatani, N. (2000). Phenolic antioxidants from herbs and spices. *Biofactors*, **13(1-4)**: 141-146.

Pérez-Alvarez, V., Bobadilla-Lugo, R.A., Muriel, P., Favari, L., and Villanueva-López, C. (1990). Effects of leukotrienes sintesis inhibition on acute liver damage induced by carbon tetrachloride. *Pharmacol.*, **47**: 330-336.

Recknagel, R.O., and Glende, E.A.Jr. (1973). Carbon tetrachloride hepatotoxicity: an example of lethal cleavage. *Crit. Rev. Toxicol.*, , **2**: 263-279.

Russmann, S., Kullak-Ublick, G.A., and Grattagliano, I. (2009). Current Concepts of Mechanisms in Drug-Induced Hepatotoxicity. *Curr. Med. Chem.*, **6**: 3041-3053.

Schattner, A., Sokolovskaya, N., Cohen, J. (2000). Fatal hepatitis and renal failure during treatment with Nimesulide. *J. Int. Med.*, **247(1)**: 153-157.

Sotelo-Felix, J.I., Martinez-Fong, D., Muriel, P., Santillan, R.L., Castillo, D., and Yahuaca, P. (2002). Evaluation of the efectiveness of *Rosmarinus officinalis* (*Lamiaceae*) in the alleviation of carbon tetrachloride-induced acute hepatotoxicity in the rat. *J Ethnopharmacol.*, **81(2)**: 145-154.

Szasz, G. (1976). Reaction-rate method for gamma-glutamyl transferase activity in serum. *Clin. Chem.*, **22**: 2051–2055.

Tajiri, K., and Shimizu, Y. (2008). Practical guidelines for diagnosis and early management of drug-induced liver injury. *World J. Gastroenterol.*, **14(44)**: 6774-6785.

Tan, H.H., Ong, W.M.C., Lai, S.H., and Chow, W.C. (2007). Nimesulide-induced hepatotoxicity and fatal hepatic failure. *Singapore Med. J.*, **48(6)**: 582-585.

Thring, T.S.A., Hili, P., and Naughton, D.P. (2009). Anti-collagenase, anti-elastase and anti-oxidant activities of extracts from 21 plants. *BMC Complementary and Altern. Med.*, **9**: 27-37.

Traversa, G., Bianchi, C., Da Cas, R., Abraha, I., Menniti-Ippolito, F., and Venegoni, M. (2003). Cohort study of hepatotoxicity associated with Nimesulide and other non-inflammatory drugs. *Brit. Med. J.*, **327(7405)**: 18-22.

Uchiyama, M., and Mihara, M. (1978). Determination of malonaldehide precursor in tisues by thiobarbituric acid test. *Anal. Biochem.*, **86**: 271-278.

Walker, S.L., Kennedy, F., Niamh, N., and McCormick, P.A. (2008). Nimesulide associated fulminant hepatic failure. *Pharmacoepidemiol. Drug Saf.*, **17(11)**: 1108-1112.

Wu, J.W., Lee, M.-H., Ho, C.-T., and Chang, S.S. (1982). Elucidation of the chemical structures of natural antioxidants isolated from rosemary. *J. Am. Oil Chem. Soc.*, **59**: 339-345.

Yagi, K. (1998). Simple assay for the level of total lipid peroxides in serum or plasma. *In:* Methods in molecular biology, Vol.108: *Free radicals and antioxidant protocols*, Armstrong D. (ed.). Humana Press Inc, Totowa NJ, USA, pp. 101–106.

Yahuaca, P., Amaya, A., Rojkind, M., and Mourelle, M. (1985). Cryptic ATPase activities in plasma membrane of CCl_4 cirrhotic rats. Its modulation by changes in cholesterol/phospholipids ratios. *Lab. Invest.*, **53(5)**: 541-545.

Yahuaca-Mendoza, P., and Alvarado-Acosta, J.L. (1993). Uso clínico de colchicina y propranolol en la cirrosis hepática alcohólica. *Inves. Cientif.*, **1(4)**: 52-58.

Yahuaca-Mendoza, P., and Mourelle-Mancini, M. (1991). Efecto del propranolol y la colchicina en la cirrosis hepática experimental. *Rev. Méd. ISSSTE Zac.*, **2(3)**: 53-56.

Yahuaca-Mendoza, P., Alvarez-Amezcua, M.C., Gutiérrez-Hernández, R., and Alvarado-Acosta, J.L. (2005). Efecto del extracto acuoso del Romero (*Rosmarinus officinalis*) en la cirrosis hepática experimental inducida con tetracloruro de carbono. *Rev. Méd. del Centro*, **1(1)**: 33-41.

Medicinal Plants: Phytochemistry, Pharmacology and Therapeutics Vol. 2 (2012) *Pages* **19–40**
Editor-in-Chief: **V.K. Gupta**
Published by: **DAYA PUBLISHING HOUSE, NEW DELHI**

2

Indian Gooseberry (*Phyllanthus emblica* L.): Phytochemistry, Pharmacology and Therapeutics

Vadde Ramakrishna[1], Sriram Gopi[2] and Oruganti H. Setty[2*]

ABSTRACT

Indian gooseberry (Phyllanthus emblica L.) is one of the most celebrating plants in Indian traditional medicine, Ayurveda. It commonly known as amla, has long been used in Indian folk medicine to treat broad spectrum of diseases, such as liver diseases, stomach ulcers, inflammatory diseases, metabolic disorders, geriatric complains, skin disorders, etc. Amla acts as a strong rejuvenating agent and is considered as the best in preventing aging. This also exhibits significant adaptogenic, anti-bacterial, anti-viral, anti-stress, immunopotentiating, antianaemic, antiemetic, astringent, antihaemorrhagic, antidiarrhoeal, diuretic, antidiabetic, carminative, antioxidant and memory-facilitating effects. Amla is highly nutritious and is an important dietary source of vitamin C, minerals and amino acids. Amla fruits have long been endowed with many pharmacological properties, which are attributable to their rich vitamin C content. Although fruits contain high amounts of vitamin C, but the overall antioxidant potential of amla can be attributed to the high content of tannins and other polyphenols. The fruit also contains flavonoids, kaempferol, ellagic acid and gallic acid. It nourishes all the body tissues and accelerates the cell regeneration process. It is an important component in Rasayana drugs which is used against a plethora of seemingly diverse disorders with no pathophysiological connections according to modern medicine. Amla has enjoyed a long

1 Department of Biotechnology and Bioinformatics, Yogi Vemana University, Kadapa – 516 003, India

2 Department of Biochemistry, School of Life Sciences, University of Hyderabad, Hyderabad – 500 046, India

* *Corresponding author*: E-mail: ohssl@uohyd.ernet.in, Tel: 91-40-23134561; Fax: +91-40-23010120; +91-40-23010145.

history of safe use and was not shown to have any adverse effects in clinical practice. In this review, we have made an attempt to bring together recent work and current trends in the field of modern phytomedicine from different parts of the world about Indian gooseberry's (Phyllanthus emblica L.) phytochemistry, pharmacology and therapeutics.

Keywords: Amla, *Emblica*, *Emblica officinalis*, Phytochemistry, Pharmacology, Therapeutics.

Introduction

Herbal medicines are also referred as herbal remedies, herbal products, herbal medicinal products, phytomedicines, phytotherapeutic agents and phytopharmaceuticals. The use of herbal medicines in an evidence or science-based approach for the treatment and prevention of disease is known as phytotherapy. Herbal medicines have been in widespread use since time immemorial. Ancient texts of India and China contain detailed depictions of the use of a variety of plant-derived medications. Even in present days, plants remain the main source of medicines for a large proportion of the world's population, particularly in the developing world, despite the advent of the pharmaceutical chemistry. Over the years, synthetic drugs have been plagued by unwanted side-effects, toxicity, and inefficiency, among other problems. In addition, the search for new drugs against a variety of illnesses through chemical synthesis and other modern approaches has not been encouraging. These factors, as well as the emergence of new infectious diseases, the proliferation of disorders such as cancer, and growing multidrug resistance in pathogenic microorganisms, have prompted renewed interest in the discovery of potential drug molecules from medicinal plants. Herbal medicine is now globally accepted as a valid alternative system of therapy in the form of pharmaceuticals, functional foods, etc., a trend recognized and advocated by the World Health Organization (WHO). Though ancient medical treatises have documented a large number of medicinal plants, most have remained undocumented and uncharacterized, the knowledge of their use being passed down from generation to generation by word of mouth (Khare, 2007; Barnes *et al.*, 2007; Yang, 2010). Here we have made an attempt to bring together recent work and current trends in the field of modern phytomedicine from different parts of the world about Indian gooseberry's phytochemistry, pharmacology and therepeutics.

Indian gooseberry is one of the most important plants of Ayurveda and Siddha, the traditional Indian medicine. *Emblica officinalis* Gaertn. (*Phyllanthus emblica* L.; *Dichelactina nodicaulis* Hance; *Emblica arborea* Raf.; *Phyllanthus glomeratus* Wall.; *Cicca emblica* Kurz.; *Diasperus emblica* Kuntze) is a small to medium deciduous tree belonging to a small sub-genus of trees of the Euphorbiaceae growing in India, Sri Lanka, Pakistan, Uzbekistan, South East Asia, and China. The plant is 8-18 meters height with thin light grey bark exfoliating in small thin irregular flakes, leaves are simple, subsessile, closely set along the branchlets, light green having the appearance of pinnate leaves; flowers are greenish yellow. The fruits are globose, fleshy, pale yellow with six obscure vertical furrows enclosing six trigonous seeds in 2-seeded 3 crustaceous cocci. The name, *Phyllanthus emblica* L. was attributed by Linneaus with reference to a peculiar characteristic of this plant. The branches of this tree are oddly flattened in the manner of a leaf; the flowers bloom from the edges of these leaf-like branches, thus the name *Phyllanthus*, from the Greek words *"phyllon"* (leaf) and *"anth`os"* (flower). In Sanskrit, *Emblica* has many synonyms: Amalaki (pure, clean), Dhatriphala (nurse fruit), Amritaphala (fruit of immortality), and others. All of these synonyms show how important this plant is in traditional Indian medicine. The fruits of *Emblica* are widely consumed as raw, cooked, or pickled. They are also principal constituents of many Ayurvedic preparations (Scartezzini and Speroni, 2000; Khatoon *et al.*, 2006). According to the two main classic texts on Ayurveda, *Charak Samhita* and *Sushruta Samhita*, Amalaki is regarded as "the best among rejuvenative herbs", "useful in relieving cough and skin disease", and "the best among the sour fruits". The fruits have been reported to contain constituents with variable biological activity. In Unani medicine, it is described as a tonic for heart and brain (Kapoor, 1990; Kirtikar and Basu, 2001).

The Indian gooseberry fruits are sour, astringent, bitter, acrid, sweet, cooling, anodyne, ophthalmic, carminative, digestive, stomachic, laxative, alterant, aphrodisiac, rejuvenative, diuretic, antipyretic and tonic. They are useful in vitiated conditions of tridosha, diabetes, cough, asthma, bronchitis, cephalalgia, ophthalmopathy, dyspepsia, colic, flatulence, hyperacidity, peptic ulcer, erysipelas, skin diseases, leprosy, haematogenesis, inflammations, anemia, emaciation, hepatopathy, jaundice, strangury, diarrhoea, dysentery, hemorrhages, leucorrhoea, menorrhagia, cardiac disorders, intermittent fevers and greyness of hair. Emblica fruit is well accepted by consumers for its special taste. It has abundant amounts of vitamin C and superoxide dismutase (Verma and Gupta, 2004; Scartezzini *et al.*, 2006), and is used in many traditional medicinal systems, such as Chinese herbal medicine, Tibetan medicine and Ayurvedic medicine (Zhang *et al.*, 2001, 2004). Experiments conducted with the fruit of amla have been shown to possess antioxidant (Bhattacharya *et al.*, 1999), adaptogenic (Rege *et al.*, 1999), and hepato-protective (Jeena *et al.*, 1999; Scartezzini and Speroni, 2000; Sultana *et al.*, 2008), antibacterial and anti HIV (Eldeen *et al.*, 2010) and anti-tumour activities (Jose *et al.*, 2001; Jeena *et al.*, 2001). Leaf extracts have been shown to possess anti-inflammatory activity (Asmawi *et al.*, 1993; Ihantola-Vormisto *et al.*, 1997). Mishra *et al.* (1981) reported that amla has hypocholesterolemic activity. Emblica fruit is reported to have hypolipidemic (Thakur *et al.*, 1988; Jacob *et al.*, 1988; Mathur *et al.*, 1996; Anila and Vijayalakshmi, 2002, 2003) and hypoglycemic activities (Anila and Vijayalakshmi, 2000; Abesundara *et al.*, 2004), and acts as a important constituent of many hepatoprotective formulations available (Antarkar *et al.*, 1980; De *et al.*, 1993; Panda and Kar, 2003). It is also used as antimicrobial agent (Godbole and Pendse, 1960; Dutta *et al.*, 1998; Rani and Khullar, 2004), anticancer (Jeena *et al.*, 2001; Zhang *et al.*, 2004), and anti-inflammatory agent (Asmawi *et al.*, 1993; Lampronti *et al.*, 2004; Perianayagam *et al.*, 2004), and can improve the metal induced clastogenic effects (Dhir *et al.*, 1990; Biswas *et al.*, 1999). It was reported that emblica has a strong antioxidant activity (Jose and Kuttan, 1995; Anila and Vijayalakshmi, 2003; Bafna and Balaraman, 2004), which may be partially due to the existence of flavonoids and several gallic acid derivatives including epigallocatachin gallate (Anila and Vijayalakshmi, 2002; Sabu and Kuttan, 2002).

Phytochemistry

In recent decades, natural antioxidants have attracted great attention from consumers all over the world due to their lower toxicity compared to synthetic antioxidants (Zhang *et al.*, 2000a,b; Peschel *et al.*, 2006). Many medicinal herbs exhibiting good antioxidant activities have been employed as the source of natural antioxidants. Amla is one of the most celebrated herbs in the Ayurveda and is known for its high levels of vitamin C, which is resistant to storage and heat damage due to cooking. It is found natively in India. Indian gooseberry has been used as valuable ingredient of various medicines in India and abroad.

Chemical Composition/Key Active Constituents

Amla is highly nutritious and is an important dietary source of vitamin C, minerals and amino acids. The edible fruit tissue contains protein concentration 3-fold and ascorbic acid concentration 160-fold high compared to that of the apple and also contains considerably higher concentration of most minerals and amino acids than apples. Glutamic acid, proline, aspartic acid, alanine, and lysine are 29.6 per cent, 14.6 per cent, 8.1 per cent, 5.4 per cent and 5.3 per cent respectively of the total amino acids. The pulpy portion of fruit, dried and freed from the nuts contains: gallic acid 1.32 per cent, tannin, sugar 36.10 per cent; gum 13.75 per cent; albumin 13.08 per cent; crude cellulose 17.08 per cent; mineral matter 4.12 per cent and moisture 3.83 per cent. Amla fruit ash contains chromium 2.5 ppm; zinc 4 ppm; and copper 3 ppm (Ghosal, 1996; Mathur *et al.*, 1996; Kumar *et al.*, 2006).

The fruits of *Emblica officinalis* are rich in tannins. The fruits have 28 per cent of the total tannins distributed in the whole plant. The fruit contains two hydrolysable tannins emblicanin A and B, which has antioxidant properties, one on hydrolysis gives gallic acid, ellagic acid and glucose. The fruit also contains phyllemblin1-3, vitamin C derivatives like puniglucanin, pedunculagin, 2-keto-gluconolactone (vitamin-C equivalents), Hexahydroxy-diphenic acid and conjugates. The main active principles are the tannins and gallic acid (Ghosal *et al.*, 1996; Bhattacharya *et al.*, 2002; Khatoon *et al.*, 2006; Kumar *et al.*, 2006).

Amla's mineral and vitamin contents include calcium, phosphorous, iron, carotene, thiamine, riboflavin, and niacin. The seeds of the Indian gooseberry contain a fixed oil, phosphatides, and an essential oil. The fruits, leaves and bark are rich in tannins. The root contains ellagic acid and lupeol and bark contains leucodelphinidin. The seeds yield a fixed oil (16 per cent) which is brownish-yellow in colour. It has the following fatty acids: linolenic (8.8 per cent), linoleic (44.0 per cent), oleic (28.4 per cent), stearic (2.15 per cent), palmitic (3.0 per cent) and myristic (1.0 per cent) (Thakur *et al.*, 1989). The ethanol soluble fraction contains free sugars like D-glucose, D-fructose, D-myo-inositol. The acidic water soluble fraction contains pectin with D-galacturonic acid, D-arabinosyl, D-rhamnosyl, D-xylosyl, D-glucosyl, D-mannosyl and D-galactosyl residues (Thakur *et al.*, 1989). The low molecular weight hydrolyzable tannins (<1,000), namely Emblicanin A and Emblicanin B, along with pedunculagin and punigluconin are the key ingredients in Emblica (Chaudhuri, 2004).

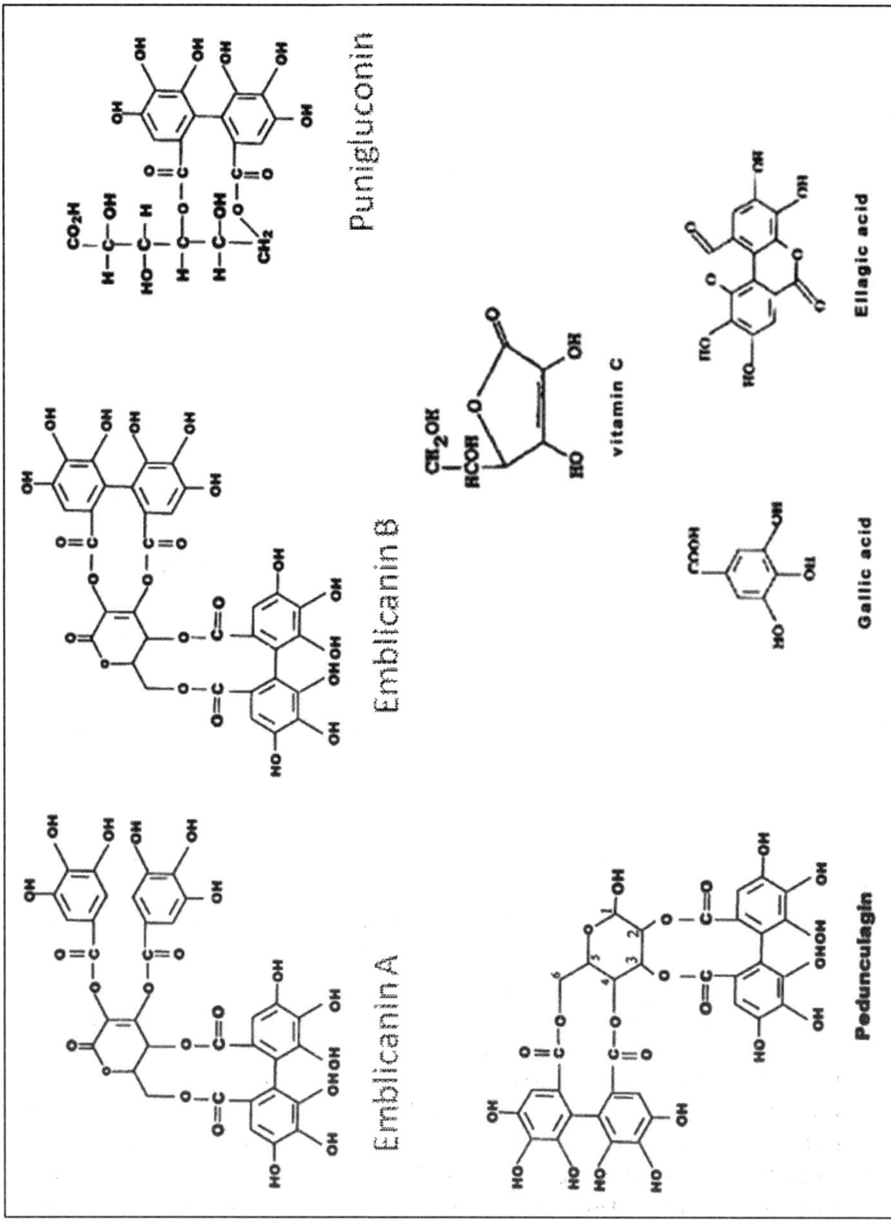

Figure 2.1: Key Constituents of *Emblica officinalis*

It is also known that emblica is a good source of polyphenols, flavones, tannins and other bioactive substances (Zhang *et al.*, 2001; Anila and Vijayalakshmi, 2003); which are strong antioxidants and might be responsible for the protective effects of emblica. It is therefore of interest to investigate the bioactive compounds in the fruit. Air-dried hulls of emblica fruit were extracted with 95 per cent ethanol, and then the extract was partitioned by diethyl ether and ethyl acetate (EA) (Luo *et al.*, 2009) and the EA fraction was purified by silica gel column and thin layer chromatography (TLC) to obtain six compounds. They were identified as cinnamic acid (C1), quercetin (C2), 5-hydroxymethylfurfural (C3), gallic acid (C4), β-daucosterol (C5) and ellagic acid (C6) using mass spectrometry and nuclear magnetic resonance (NMR) spectroscopy. Cinnamic acid and 5-hydroxymethylfurfural were identified as components of emblica fruit for the first time (Luo *et al.*, 2009). The DPPH and ABTS+ radical scavenging activities of components were evaluated. All the compounds showed significant DPPH and ABTS+ radical scavenging activity except for cinnamic acid. Gallic acid showed the highest DPPH radical scavenging activity while ellagic acid showed the highest ABTS+ scavenging activity amongst all the compounds tested.

Ghosal *et al.* (1996) found that *emblica* fruits do not contain ascorbic acid, either in the free or in the conjugated form, but contain two new hydrolysable tannins of low molecular weight, namely emblicanin A (2,3-di-*O*-galloyl-4,6-(*S*)-hexahydroxydiphenoyl-2-keto-glucono-β-lactone) and emblicanin B (2,3,4,6-bis-(*S*)-hexahydroxydiphenoyl-2-keto-glucono-β-lactone), and other tannins, such as punigluconin (2,3-di-*O*-galloyl-4,6-(*S*)-hexahydroxy diphenoyl gluconic acid) and pedunclagin (2,3,4,6-bis-(*S*)-hexahydroxydiphenoyl-d-glucose). The two emblicanins exhibited a very strong antioxidant action; moreover, they improved the efficacy of vitamin C in reducing dehydroascorbic acid to ascorbic acid (Ghosal *et al.*, 1996; Bhattacharya *et al.*, 2000a,b; Raghu *et al.*, 2007). The later studies examined the pharmacological activities of these tannins and reported that they exhibit antioxidant activity *in vitro* and *in vivo*. In particular, they preserve erythrocytes against oxidative stress induced by asbestos (Ghosal *et al.*, 1996), show antioxidant effects in rat brain (Bhattacharya *et al.*, 2000a), exert a prophylactive effect against neuroleptic-induced tardive dyskinesia (Bhattacharya *et al.*, 2000b,c), show antioxidant activity against ischemia reperfusion (Bhattacharya *et al.*, 2002), antiulcerogenic effects (Sairam *et al.*, 2002b), and anticataractogenic effects *in vitro* (Suryanarayana *et al.*, 2004). Pozharitskaya *et al.* (2007) demonstrated that *E. officinalis* extract contains several antioxidants such as emblicanin A and B, gallic acid, ellagic acid, ascorbic acid that possesses strong antioxidative activity. A recent study also shows that emblica extract has potent antioxidant activity in term of free radical scavenging properties (Jain *et al.*, 2008). Amla is an important dietary source of minerals, amino acids, tannin and sugar. Although fruits are reputed to contain high amounts of ascorbic acid (vitamin C), 45 mg/100g (Tarwadi and Agte, 2007), the specific contents are disputed and the overall antioxidant strength of amla may derive instead from its high density of tannins and other polyphenols. The fruit also contains flavanoids, kaempferol, ellagic acid and gallic acid (Habib-ur-Rehman *et al.*, 2007). In the studies of Liu *et al.* (2008a,b) the phenolic contents of methanolic extracts of emblica (*Phyllanthus emblica* L.) fruit from six regions in China were measured in their work. Total phenolic content was ranged from 81.5 to 120.9 mg gallic acid equivalents (GAE)/g and the flavonoids content was varied from 20.3 to 38.7mg quecetin equivalent (QE)/g, while proanthocyanidin content was ranged from 3.7 to 18.7mg catechin equivalents (CE)/g. Among all the methanolic extracts analyzed, the Huizhou sample exhibited a significantly higher phenolic content than other samples. The results of Kumar *et al.* (2006) clearly suggested the presence of potent antioxidants such as gallic acid in *E. officinalis* and protocatechuic acid and ferulic acid in *C. longa*, in addition to the known ascorbic acid and curcumin in *E. officinalis* and *C. longa*, respectively.

For many years, the activity of the fruits was attributed to the high content of ascorbic acid; however, this has recently been questioned. However, the studies of Scartezzini *et al.* (2006) clarified through a reliable and feasible HPLC method with diode array detection has been developed for the determination of ascorbic acid in emblica fruit and particularly in emblica fruit processed according to the Ayurvedic method. The antioxidant effects have also been evaluated in comparison to the real levels of vitamin C by different antioxidant tests. The data obtained show that the emblica fruit contains ascorbic acid (0.40 per cent w/w), and that the Ayurvedic method of processing increases the healthy characteristics of the fruit thanks to a higher antioxidant activity and a higher content of ascorbic acid (1.28 per cent w/w). It has also been found that vitamin C accounts for approximately 45–70 per cent of the antioxidant activity.

Pharmacology

Ayurvedic pharmacology classifies medicinal plants into different groups according to their actions. One of these is the 'Rasayana' group. The word 'Rasayana' literally means the path that 'Rasa' takes. 'Rasayana' drugs act inside the human body by modulating the neuro-endocrino-immune systems and have been found to be a rich source of antioxidants (Brahma and Debnath, 2003). These Rasayana plants are said to possess the following properties: they prevent ageing, re-establish youth, strengthen life, brain power and prevent diseases (Sharma, 1983; Ghanekar, 1981; Vasudevan and Parle, 2007), all of which imply that they increase the resistance of the body against any onslaught. Plenty of study has been undertaken to provide scientific evidence to the 'Rasayana' drugs as immunomodulators and adaptogens (Jayaram *et al.*, 1993; Wagner, 1994; Kumar *et al.*, 1994).

According to the two main classic texts on Ayurved, Charaka Samhita and Sushruta Samhita, Amalaki (Indian gooseberry) is regarded as "the best among rejuvenative herbs", "useful in relieving cough and skin disease" and "the best among the sour fruits". All parts of the plant are used for medicinal purpose. Amla is a major ingredient in several important medicinal preparations including Triphala ("three fruits") and the famous Chyawanprash, a general tonic for people of all ages, which improves mental and physical well being (Manjunatha *et al.*, 2001; Vasudevan and Parle, 2007). Triphala has been reported to possess anti-aging properties and improves the mental abilities (Jagetia *et al.*, 2002). Chyavanprash, a drug preparation in which *E.O* is a major component and is widely used as a health tonic. Low molecular weight hydrolysable gallotannins (EOT) comprising emblicanin A, emblicanin B, punigluconin and pedunculagin, isolated from the fresh juice or solvent extracts of *Emblica* fruits, were shown to have significant antioxidant effects *in vitro* (Ghosal *et al.*, 1996) and *in vivo* (Bhattacharya *et al.*,1999). EOT was shown to exert antioxidant effects against iron-overload hepatotoxicity (Bhattacharya *et al.*,2000a) and to elevate rat frontal cortical and striatal concentrations of superoxide dismutase (SOD), catalase (CAT) and glutathione peroxidase (GPx), and reduce lipid peroxidation in these brain areas (Bhattacharya *et al.*, 1999). In recent decades, natural antioxidants have attracted great attention from consumers over the world due to their lower toxicity than synthetic antioxidants (Peschel *et al.*,2006). As an important dietary fruit source, emblica commonly grows in the subtropical and tropical area of southeast Asia, particularly in south China and India (Zhang *et al.*, 2000).

It has been used for thousands of years in traditional Chinese and Indian medicine for the treatment of jaundice (Scartezzini and Speroni, 2000; Pramyothin *et al.*, 2006), diarrhoea (Rani and Khullar, 2004) or as an antifungal agent (Dutta *et al.*, 1998). Furthermore, extract of emblica has been reported to have antioxidant (Scartezzini and Speroni, 2000; Anila and Vijayalakshmi, 2003), hypolipidemic (Anila and Vijayalakshmi, 2000), anti-diabetic (Sabu and Kuttan, 2002), anti- diarrheal (Perianayagam *et al.*, 2005), anti-tumor (Jeena *et al.*, 2001) and anti-inflammatory activities (Perianayagam *et al.*, 2004). It has been well documented that most of these diseases or disorders are due to oxidative stress, which leads to oxidative damage to biomolecules and cells (Doll, 1990; Temple, 2000; Willett, 2002). It is known that emblica is a good source of polyphenols, flavones, tannins and other bioactive substances (Zhang *et al.*,2001; Anila and Vijayalakshmi, 2003); while these substances are strong antioxidants and might contribute to the healthy effects of emblica.

Indian gooseberry has undergone preliminary research, demonstrating *in vitro* antiviral and antimicrobial properties (Saeed and Tariq, 2007). There is preliminary evidence *in vitro* that its extracts induce apoptosis and modify gene expression in osteoclasts involved in rheumatoid arthritis and osteoporosis (Penolazzi *et al.*,2008). The leaves, bark and fruit have been shown to possess efficacy against laboratory models of disease, such as inflammation, cancer, age-related renal disease, and diabetes (Ganju *et al.*, 2003; Rao *et al.*, 2005; Yokozawa *et al.*, 2007). A human pilot study demonstrated reduction of blood cholesterol levels in both normal and hypercholesterolemic men (Jacob *et al.*,1988). Another very recent study with alloxan-induced diabetic rats that were administered an aqueous extract of amla fruit has shown significant decrease of the blood glucose as well as triglyceridemic levels and an improvement in the liver function (Qureshi *et al.*,2009). Phyllembin, isolated from the ethanolic extract of the fruit pulp has been found to potentiate the action of adrenaline *in vitro* and *in vivo*. It showed a mild depressant action on central nervous system (CNS) and also had a spasmolytic activity. The drug also revealed mild stimulant action on isolated frog heart, short and insignificant rise in cat's blood pressure, contraction of the nictitating membrane, the reduction of outflow of the perfusate in the hind limb of the rat and ear of rabbit, mild cerebral depressant action and anti-spasmodic activity.

Clinical studies were conducted to investigate the effect of crude amla in gastritis syndrome. The crude amla was given in 20 cases in a dose of 3 g, 3 times a day for 7 days. The drug was found effective in 85 per cent of the cases. It was observed that the drug did not have any significant beneficial effect in cases of hypochlorhydria. Only cases of hyperchloridia with burning sensation in abdominal and cardiac regions and epigastric pain were benefited (Singh and Sharma, 1971). Alcoholic extract of a plant (1g/kg) has shown an increase in the cardiac glycogen and a decrease in serum GOT, GPT and LDH in isoprotenol pretreated rats, suggesting a cardioprotective action. It showed a reduction in serum cholesterol levels and a significant antiatherogenic effect. This study suggests that vitamin C content alone may not responsible for the antiatherogenic effect of the plant in animals (Thakur, 1985). The lipid lowering and antiatherosclerotic effects of amla fresh juice were evaluated in cholesterol fed rabbits. Amla fresh juice was administered at a dose of 5ml/kg body weight per rabbit per day for sixty days. Serum cholesterol, triglycerides, phospholipid and low-density lipoprotein levels were lowered by 82 per cent, 66 per cent, 77 per cent and 90 per cent respectively. Similarly, the tissue lipid level showed a significant reduction following amla juice administration. Aortic plaques were regressed. Amla juice treated rabbits excreted more cholesterol and phospholipids, suggesting that the mode of absorption was affected. Amla juice is an effective hypolipidemic agent and can be used as a pharmaceutical tool in hyperlipidemic subjects (Mathur *et al.,* 1996). The crude extract of *Emblica officinalis* was reported to counteract hepatotoxic effects of metals due to anti-oxidant activity (Roy *et al.,* 1991).

The ether extract and alcoholic extract of fruits acidified with hydrochloric acid were found to have antibacterial activity. The other extract of acidified alcoholic extract showed the highest activity, inhibiting the growth of *M. pyogenes* var. *S. typhosa* and *S. paratyphi* at a concentration of 0.21mg/ml and that of *M. pyogenes* var. *albus; S. schottmmellari* and *S. dysenteriae* at a concentration of 0.42mg/ml. The effect of crude amla on total serum protein and its fractions was studied in rabbits. The drug had no significant effect on the levels of serum protein fractions, but it raised the total protein level and increased the body weight. The studies indicated that the increase in the body weight was due to positive nitrogen balance. The drug was found to have only anabolic effect without affording resistance against diseases (Tewari *et al.,* 1968).

The fruit extract has many pharmacological activities for the treatment of a number of diseases and is a constituent of many hepatoprotective formulations (De *et al.,* 1993). Increase in scientific investigations into indigenous wealth of herbal medicines gives ample evidence of medicinal plants as sources of drugs (Bannerman, 1980). The evaluation of various components of traditional drugs or medicinal plants in the light of modern science have revealed their efficacy in certain diseases thus forming a valuable source of therapeutic agents in armory of modern medicine (Hikino, 1991; Lamartimere *et al.,* 1998). Screening of crude extracts of several edible plants revealed the mechanism of several compounds acting together in additive, synergistic or antagonistic manner to suppress tumor promotion (Koshimizu *et al.,* 1988). Several medicinal plants that are prescribed as constituents of liver protective herbal drugs have been shown to inhibit DEN-induced hepatocarcinogenicity in experimental animals (Bhattracharya and Chatterjee, 1998; Jeena *et al.,* 1999; Sultana *et al.,* 2008). *Emblica officinalis* of Euphorbiaceae family is also one such plant that has been used as major constituent of various valuable Indian polyherbal formulations for liver protecting activity. Its fruits are rich sources of vitamin C and are found to be effective as hypolipidemic and antiatherosclerotic agents (Mathur *et al.*, 1996) and reported to reduce serum aortic and hepatic cholesterol in rabbits (Thakur, 1985). *Emblica officinalis* fruits also possess antimutagenic and anticarcinogenic properties owing to the combined presence of β-carotene (Jeena *et al.*, 1997), ascorbic acid (Counsell and Hornig, 1981) and chlorophylin (Ong *et al.*, 1986) and have also been shown to modulate several biochemical events associated with tumor promotion such as alteration of protein kinase C activity (Gschwendt *et al.*, 1983). Phytochemical analysis of the plant revealed the presence of tannins (Brahmachari and Gupta, 1958), flavonoids like quercetin (Khanna *et al.*, 1982) and ellagic acid (Brahmachari and Gupta, 1958). Flavonoids have been described as health-promoting, disease-preventing dietary supplements, and have activity as cancer preventive agents. Dietary administration of *Emblica officinalis* fruit extract to mice significantly reduces clastogenic effect of benz(a)pyrene (Nandi *et al.*, 1997).

The active tannoids of *Emblica officinalis* consisting of emblicanin A (37 per cent), emblicanin B (33 per cent), punigluconin (12 per cent) and pedunculagin (14 per cent), administered in the doses of 5 and 10 mg/kg, i.p., and deprenyl (2 mg/kg, i.p.), induced an increase in both frontal cortical and striatal SOD, CAT and GSH-px activity, with concomitant decrease in LPO in brain areas when administered once daily for 7 days (Bhattacharya *et al.*, 1999). Fresh juice of Emblica fruits (50 and 100 mg/kg body weight) given orally twice daily for 14 days increased the activities of cardiac SOD, CAT and GSH-px, with a concomitant decrease of LPO in Ischemia-reperfusion-induced rats (Bhattacharya *et al.*, 2002). *Emblica officinalis* inhibited LPO induced with Fe(2+)/ascorbate along with inhibition of hydoxyl and superoxide radical (Sabu and Kuttan, 2002). A standardized extract of *Emblica officinalis* was found to havea long-lasting and broad-spectrum antioxidant activity, thus showing that *Emblica* is suitable for use in anti-aging, sunscreen and general purpose skin care products (Chaudhuri *et al.*, 2003). Administration of *Emblica* tannoids (10 and 20 mg, po) for 21 days, concomitant with the stress procedure, induced a dose-related alteration in the stress effects. Thus, antistress 'Rasayana' activity of *Emblica officinalis* may be, at least partly due to its tendency to normalize stress-induced perturbations in oxidative free radical scavenging activity (Bhattacharya *et al.*, 2000b). The presence of 'Amlaki' resulted in an enhanced cell survival, decreased free radical production and higher antioxidant levels (Sairam *et al.*, 2003). *Emblica officinalis* causes myocardial adaptation and protects against oxidative stress in ischemic-reperfusion injury in rats (Rajak *et al.*, 2004).

The fruit extract has many pharmacological activities: it inhibits micronuclei formation, sister chromatid exchanges, clastogenicity and mutagenicity induced by metals such as lead, aluminum, cadmium, nickel, arsenic and caesium; it preserves against radiations (Dhir *et al.*, 1991, 1993; Scartezzini and Speroni, 2000; Sharma *et al.*, 2009; Adil *et al.*, 2010), possesses antidiabetic activity (Sabu and Kuttan, 2002), inhibits clastogenicity of benzopyrene and cyclophosphamide (Sharma *et al.*, 2000; Haque *et al.*, 2001), is gastroprotective (Al-Rehaily *et al.*, 2002), cytoprotective, and immunomodulating (Sai Ram *et al.*, 2002a,b). In recent years, new pharmacological activities have been found for *Emblica*: it has cytoprotective activity against chromium

(Sai Ram *et al.*, 2003), protects against oxidative stress in ischemic-reperfusion injury (Rajak *et al.*, 2004), shows antivenom capacity (Alam and Gomes, 2003), ameliorates hyperthyroidism and hepatic lipid peroxidation (Panda and Kar, 2003), displays antiproliferative activity on MCF7 and MDA-MB-231 breast cancer cell lines (Lamartimere *et al.*, 1998), shows antitussive activity (Nosal'ova *et al.*, 2003), and induces apoptosis in Dalton's Lymphoma Ascites and CeHa cell lines (Rajeshkumar *et al.*, 2003).

Therapeutics

It is a plant that is used in its entirety and so presents the herbalist with excellent value for money. The dried fruit, the nut or seed, leaves, root, bark and flowers are frequently employed. The ripe fruits are generally used fresh, but dried fruit are also used.

The health promotive, disease preventive and rejuvenation approach available in the Indian systems of medicine like 'Ayurveda' is gaining greater attention and popularity in many regions of the world. A majority of the present day diseases are reported to be due to the shift in the balance of the pro-oxidant and the antioxidant homeostatic phenomenon in the body. Pro-oxidant conditions dominate either due to the increased generation of the free radicals caused by excessive oxidative stress of the present day life, or due to the poor scavenging/quenching in the body caused by depletion of the dietary antioxidants (Schulz *et al.*, 2000; Govindarajan *et al.*, 2005). Ancient Ayurvedic physicians had developed certain dietary and therapeutic measures to arrest/delay ageing and rejuvenating whole functional dynamics of the body system. This revitalization and rejuvenation is known as the 'Rasayan chikitsa' (rejuvenation therapy). Traditionally, Rasayana drugs are used against a plethora of seemingly diverse disorders with no pathophysiological connections according to modern medicine. Though, this group of plants generally possesses strong antioxidant activity, only a few have been investigated in detail.

For many years, the therapeutic potential of the amla fruits was attributed to their high ascorbic acid content, contains about 1 g vitamin C per 100 mL of fresh juice (Kapoor, 1990). Because of the presence of tannins, the ascorbic acid is not oxidized even in dried fruit, thus maintaining its antiscurvy property unchanged. The fresh or the dry fruit is used in traditional medicines for the treatment of diarrhea, jaundice and inflammations (Deokar, 1998; Sultana *et al.*, 2008). The pulp of the fruit is smeared on the head to dispel headache and dizziness (Perry, 1980). *Emblica officinalis* leaves and fruit have been used for fever and inflammatory treatments by rural populations in its growing areas. The earlier study have demonstrated potent anti-microbial (Ahmad *et al.*, 1998; Eldeen *et al.*, 2008), anti-oxidant (Bhattacharya *et al.*, 1999), adaptogenic (Rege *et al.*, 1999), hepatoprotective (Jeena and Kuttan, 2000; Jeena *et al.*, 1999), anti-tumour (Jose *et al.*, 2001) and anti-ulcerogenic activities (Sairam *et al.*, 2002) in the fruits of *Emblica officinalis*. Leaf extracts have been shown to posses anti-inflammatory activity (Asmawi *et al.*, 1993; Ihantola-Vormisto *et al.*, 1997). The ethanol and aqueous extract of *Emblica officinalis* has shown significant anti-inflammatory activity (Sharma *et al.*, 2003).

A large series of human drugs derive from botanical therapeutics, since medicinal plants have been used for centuries as remedies for human diseases. Indian gooseberry has been used as a valuable ingredient of various medicines in India and Middle East from time immemorial. The fruits are sour, astringent, bitter, acrid, sweet, cooling, anodyne, ophthalmic, carminative, digestive, stomachic, laxative, alterant, aphrodisiac, rejuvenative, diuretic, antipyretic and tonic. They are useful in vitiated conditions of tridosha, diabetes, cough, asthma, bronchitis, cephalalgia, ophthalmopathy, dyspepsia, colic, flatulence, hyperacidity, peptic ulcer, erysipelas, skin diseases, leprosy, haematogenesis, inflammations, anemia, emaciation, hepatopathy, jaundice, strangury, diarrhoea, dysentery, hemorrhages, leucorrhoea, menorrhagia, cardiac disorders, intermittent fevers and greyness of hair (Udupa, 1985; Thakur, 1989; Treadway, 1994; Nadkarni and Nadkarni, 1999; Bhattacharya *et al.*, 1999; Chaudhuri *et al.*, 2003).

The fruit extract has been reported to have hypolipidemic, antidiabetic and anti-inflammatory activity, and to inhibit retroviruses such as HIV-1, tumour development and gastric ulcer (Sabu and Kuttan, 2002). Emblica fruit extract exhibits antioxidant properties, its aqueous extract being a potent inhibitor of lipid peroxidation and a scavenger of hydroxyl and superoxide radicals *in vitro* (Scartezzini and Speroni, 2000). Contrary to the long-standing belief that Emblica fruits owe their potential pharmacological activity to their vitamin C content, Ghosal *et al.* (1996) employing liquid chromatography, asserted that emblica fruits do not contain ascorbic acid, either in the free or in the conjugated form, but contain two hydrolysable tannins of low molecular weight, namely, Emblicanin A and Emblicanin B, and other tannins such as punigluconin and pedunclagin. The two Emblicanins are shown to exhibit a very strong antioxidant action (Ghosal *et al.*, 1996). The therapeutic effect has been suggested to be ascribed to its high vitamin 'C' content and possibly to tannin like structures.

Different plant parts of Amla are ethnobotanically reported to have various therapeutic activities *e.g.* leaves as expectorant, diaphoretic and useful in strangury and sweats; the seeds as carminative, laxative, astringent to the bowels, tonic to the liver, diuretic, diaphoretic, useful in bronchitis, earache, griping, opthalmia and ascites (Kirtikar and Basu, 2001; Khatoon *et al.*, 2006). The fresh roots and leaves species have been reported to be potent remedy for jaundice (Satyavati *et al.*, 1987; Kirtikar and Basu, 2001). Phyllanthin and hypophyllanthin present in *Phyllanthus amarus* are also reported as hepatoprotective agents and protect hepatocytes against carbon tetrachloride (CCl_4) and galactosamine induced cytotoxicity in rats (Syamsundar *et al.*, 1985). Amla is one of the strongest rejuvenatives in Indian pharmacopoeia. It contains 30 times the amount of vitamin C found in oranges and also contains tannins, phyllembelic acid, phyllemblin, rutin, curcuminoides and emblicol and phenolic compounds (Jeena and Kuttan, 1995, 2000; Zhang *et al.*, 2000). The pharmacological studies showed the ability of the fruits to lower the lipid levels in the liver of rabbits. The therapeutic efficacy of Amla in cases of dyspepsia was evaluated (Chawla *et al.*, 1982) with promising results in human subjects. It was therefore, thought worthwhile to undertake antisecretory, antiulcer and cytoprotective studies in rats, using various experimental models to substantiate the claims of its use in traditional medicine of many countries including Saudi Arabia.

Khare (2007) described the key actions that the amla fruits an important source of vitamin C, minerals and amino acids. The fruit gave cytokinine-like substances identified as zeatin, zeatin riboside and zeatin nucleotide; suspension culture gave phyllembin. Phyllembin exhibits CNS depressant and spasmolytic activity, potentiates action of adrenaline and hypnotic action of Nembutal. The leaves contain gallic acid, besides ascorbic and mucic acid. The methanol extract of the leaves is found to be effective in rat paw inflammation. The bark contains tannin identified as mixed type of proanthocyanidin. The fruit contains superoxide dismutase and exhibits antisenescent (anti-aging) activity. Fruit, juice, its sediment and residue are antioxidant due to gallic acid. EtOH extract–antiviral. Aqueous extract of the fruit increases cardiac glycogen level and decreases serum GOT, GPT and LDH in rats having induced myocardial necrosis. Preliminary evidence suggests that the fruit and its juice may lower serum cholesterol, LDL, triglycerides and phospholipids without affecting HDL levels and may have positive effect on atherosclerosis.

Conclusions and Future Perspectives

In recent decades, natural antioxidants have attracted great attention from consumers over the world due to their lower toxicity than synthetic antioxidants. Many medicinal herbs exhibiting good antioxidant activities have been employed as the source of natural antioxidants. Emblica plant as medical and dietary use, commonly grows in the subtropical and tropical area of southeast Asia, particularly in south China and India. It has been used for thousands of years in traditional Chinese and Indian medicine for the treatment of broad spectrum of disorders. It is also well documented that most of these disorders or disorders are due to oxidative stress, which leads to oxidative damage to biomolecules and cells. It is known that emblica is a good source of polyphenols, flavones, tannins and other bioactive substances while these substances are strong antioxidants and might contribute to the healthy effects of emblica. In this area, the scientists can investigate the lead bioactive compounds in this fruit and develop drugs for treatment of diseases.

Several studies are going on throughout the world to identify antioxidant compounds that are pharmacologically potent with low profile of side effects. Ayurveda, the oldest medical system in the world, provides lots of lead to find active and therapeutically useful compounds from plants. 'Rasayana' formulations in Indian traditional medicine may have antioxidant activity arising from individual plants including Indian gooseberry, and may act synergistically to prevent aging and related degenerative diseases. Further studies to isolate active principles from these plants and their pharmacological validation in terms of modern medicine will be of great medicinal importance in future.

References

Abesundara, K. J. M., Matsui, T., and Matsumoto, K. (2004). α-Glucosidase inhibitory activity of some Sri Lanka plant extracts, one of which, *Cassia auriculata*, exerts a strong anti hyperglycemic effect in rats comparable to the therapeutic drug acarbose. *Journal of Agricultural and Food Chemistry*, **52:** 2541–2545.

Rani, P., and Khullar, N. (2004). Antimicrobial evaluation of some medicinal plants for their anti-enteric potential against multi-drug resistant *Salmonella typhi*. *Phytotherapy Research*, **18:** 670–673.

Rao, T.P., Sakaguchi, N., Juneja, L.R., Wada, E., and Yokozawa T (2005). Amla (*Emblica officinalis* Gaertn.) extracts reduce oxidative stress in streptozotocin-induced diabetic rats. *J Med Food*, **8** (3): 362–8.

Rege, N.N., Thatte, U.M., and Dahanukar, S.A. (1999). Adaptogenic properties of six rasayana herbs used in Ayurvedic medicine. *Phytotherapy Research*, **13:** 275–291.

Roy A. K., Dhir, H., Sharma, A., and Talukder, G. (1991). *Phyllanthus emblica* Fruit extract and Ascorbic acid modify Hepatotoxic and Renotoxic effects of metals in mice" *Ind. J. Pharmacog.*, **29:** 117-126.

Sabu, M. C., and Kuttan, R. (2002). Anti-diabetic activity of medicinal plants and its relationship with their antioxidant property. *Journal of Ethnopharmacology*, **81:** 155–160.

Saeed, S., and Tariq, P. (2007). Antibacterial activities of *Emblica officinalis* and *Coriandrum sativum* against Gram negative urinary pathogens. *Pak J Pharm Sci.*, **20** (1): 32–5.

Sai Ram, M., Neetu, D., Deepti, P., Vandana, M., Ilavazhagan, G., Kumar, D., and Selvamurthy, W. (2003). Cytoprotective activity of amla (*Emblica officinalis*) against chromium (VI) induced oxidative injury in marine macrophages. *Phytotherapy Research*, **17:** 430–433.

Sai Ram, M., Neetu, D., Yogesh, B., Anju, B., Dipti, P., Pauline, T., Sharma, S.K., Sarada, S.K.S., Ilavazhagan, G., Kumar, D., Selvamurthy, W. (2002a). Cyto-protective and immunomodulating properties of amla (*Emblica officinalis*) on lymphocytes: an *in-vitro* study. *Journal of Ethnopharmacology*, **81:** 5–10.

Sairam, K., Rao, Ch.V., Dora Babu, M., Vijay Kumar, K., Agrawal, V.K., and Goel, R.K. (2002b). Antiulcerogenic effect of methanolic extract of *Emblica officinalis*: an experimental study. *Journal of Ethnopharmacology*, **82:** 1–9.

Satyavati, G.V., Gupta, A.K., and Tandon, N. (1987). Medicinal plants of India. Indian Council of Medical Research New Delhi 2, 405–411.

Scartezzini, P., and Speroni, E. (2000). Review on some plants of Indian traditional medicine with antioxidant activity. *Journal of Ethnopharmacology*, **71:** 23–43.

Scartezzini, P., Antognoni, F., Raggi, M.A., Poli, F., and Sabbioni, C. (2006). Vitamin C content and antioxidant activity of the fruit and of the Ayurvedic preparation of *Emblica officinalis* Gaertn. *Journal of Ethnopharmacology*, **104:** 113–118.

Schulz, J.B., Lindnau, J., Seyfriend, J., and Dichgans, J. (2000). Glutathione oxidative stress and neuro-degeneration. *European Journal of Biochemistry*, **267:** 4904–4911.

Sharma, S.K., Perianayagam, J.B., Joseph, A., and Christina, A.J.M. (2003). Antiinflammatory activity of ethanol and aqueous extracts of *Emblica officinalis* Gaertn fruits. *Hamdard Med.*, **46:** 71–3.

Sharma, A., Sharma, M.K., and Kumar, M. (2009). Modulatory role of *Emblica officinalis* fruit extract against arsenic induced oxidative stress in Swiss albino mice. *Chemico-Biological Interactions,* **180**: 20–30.

Sharma, N., Trikha, M., and Raisuddin, S. (2000). Inhibitory effect of *Emblica officinalis* on the *in vivo* clastogenicity of benzo(*a*)pyrene and cyclophosphamide in mice. *Human and Experimental Toxicology,* **19:** 377–384.

Sharma, P. (1983). Chikithsasthana. In: Charaka Samhita. Chaukhamba Orientalia, Varanasi.

Singh, B.N., and Sharma, P.V. (1971). Effect of Amalaki on amalapitta. *J. Res. Ind. Med.,* **5:** 223.

Sultana, S., Ahmed, S., and Jahangir, T. (2008). *Emblica officinalis* and hepatocarcinogenesis: A chemopreventive study in Wistar rats. *Journal of Ethnopharmacology,* **118:** 1–6.

Suryanarayana, P., Kumar, P.A., Saraswat, M., Petrash, J.M., and Reddy, G.B. (2004). Inhibition of aldose reductase by tannoid principles of *Emblica officinalis*: implications for the prevention of sugar cataract. *Molecular Vision,* **10:** 148–154.

Syamsundar, K.V., Singh, B., Thakur, R.S., Hussain, A., Kiso, Y., and Hikino, H. (1985). Antihepatotoxic principles of *Phyllanthus niruri* herb. *J. Ethnopharmacology,* **14:** 41–44.

Tarwadi, K., and Agte, V. (2007). Antioxidant and micronutrient potential of common fruits available in the Indian subcontinent. *Int J Food Sci Nut.r,* **58 (5):** 341–9.

Temple, N.J. (2000). Antioxdants and disease. *Nutrition Research,* **20:** 449–459.

Tewari, A. Sen, S.P., and Guru, L.V. (1968). The effect of Amalaki (*Phyllanthus emblica*) rasayana on biologic system. *J. Res. Ind. Med.,* **2:** 189.

Thakur, C.P. (1985). *Emblica officinalis* reduces serum, aortic and hepatic cholesterol in rabbits. *Experientia,* **41:** 423.

Thakur, C.P., Thakur, B., Singh, B., Singh, S., Sinha, P.K., and Sinha, S.K. (1988). The Ayurvedic medicines, Haritaki, Amla and Bahira reduce cholesterol induced atherosclerosis in rabbits. *Indian J Cardiol.,* **21:** 167–75.

Thakur, R.S., Puri, H.S., and Akhtar, H. (1989). Major Medicinal Plants of India. Central Institute of Medicinal and Aromatic Plants, Lucknow, India.

Treadway, L. (1994). Amla Traditional food and medicine. *HerbalGram.,* **31:** 26.

Udupa, K. N. (1985). Ayurveda for Promotion of Health. *Journal of Ayurveda,* **3.**

Vasudevan, M., and Milind, P. (2007). Memory enhancing activity of Anwala churna (*Emblica officinalis* Gaertn.): An Ayurvedic preparation. *Physiology and Behavior,* **91:** 46–54.

Verma, R.C., and Gupta, A. (2004). Effect of pre-treatments on quality of solar-dried amla. *Journal of Food Engineering,* **65:** 397–402.

Wagner, H. (1994). Therapy and Prevention with Immunomodulatory and Adaptogenic Plant Drugs. Update – Ayurveda, Bombay.

Willett, W.C. (2002). Balancing life-style and genomics research for disease prevention. *Science*, **296:** 695–698.

Yang, Y. (2010). Chinese Herbal formulas. Treatment principles and composition strategies. Churchil livingstone. USA.

Yokozawa, T., Kim, H.Y., Kim, H.J. *et al.* (2007). Amla (*Emblica officinalis* Gaertn.) attenuates age-related renal dysfunction by oxidative stress. *J Agric Food Chem.*, **55**: 7744–52.

Zhang, Y.J., Tanaka, T., Iwamoto, Y., Yang, C.R., and Kouno, I. (2000a). Phyllaemblic acid, a novel highly oxygenated norbisabolane from the roots of *Phyllanthus emblica*. *Tetrahedron Letters*, **41:** 1781–1784.

Zhang, Y.J., Tanaka, T., Iwamoto, Y., Yang, C.R., and Kouno, I. (2000b). Novel norsesquiterpe-noids from the roots of *phyllanthus emblica*. *J Nat Prod.,* **63(11):** 1507–1510.

Zhang, Y.J., Tanaka, T., Iwamoto, Y., Yang, C.R., and Kouno, I. (2001). Novel sesquiterpenoids from the roots of *Phyllanthus emblica*. *Journal of Natural Products,* **64:** 870-873.

Zhang, Y.J., Nagao, T., Tanaka, T., Yang, C.R., Okabe, H., and Kouno, I. (2004). Antiproliferative activity of the main constituents from *Phyllanthus emblica*. *Biological and Pharmaceutical Bulletin,* **27:** 251–255.

Medicinal Plants: Phytochemistry, Pharmacology and Therapeutics Vol. 2 (2012) *Pages* **41–51**
Editor-in-Chief: **V.K. Gupta**
Published by: **DAYA PUBLISHING HOUSE, NEW DELHI**

3

Chemical Constituents from *Phyllanthus amarus* Schum & Thonn and its Pharmacological Effectiveness

M.A.M. Maciel[1*], A.F. Cunha[1], C.R. Kaiser[2], E.A. Costa[3], F.F. Rocha[4] and F.A. Vanderlinde[4*]

ABSTRACT

Phyllanthus niruri L. and Phyllanthus amarus Schum and Thonn are targets of current phytopharmacological researches around the world, in which they have been cited as synonymous. However, a recent botanic study indicated significant differences between these specie, the main of them were found to be in base, seed and stigma type. In this work Phyllanthus amarus Schum and Thonn was unambiguously identified and a phytochemical investigation of its methanolic extract obtained from the whole plant, revealed the presence of six bioactive lignans such as isolintetralin (2,3-demethoxy-seco-isolintetralin diacetate), demethylenedioxy-niranthin, 5-demethoxy-niranthin, niranthin, phyllanthin and hypophyllanthin] and one triterpene (2Z, 6Z, 10Z, 14E, 18E, 22E-farnesil farnesol). The main pharmacological activities were correlated to those lignans and carried out to evaluate in vivo gastrointestinal transit

1 Departamento de Química, Universidade Federal do Rio Grande do Norte, Campus Universitário, 59078-970, Natal, RN, Brazil

2 Instituto de Química, Universidade Federal do Rio de Janeiro, 21941-972, Rio de Janeiro, RJ, Brazil

3 Instituto de Ciências Biológicas, Departamento de Ciências Fisiológicas, Universidade Federal de Goiás, Goiânia, GO, Brazil

4 Instituto de Biologia, Departamento de Ciências Fisiológicas, Universidade Federal Rural do Rio de Janeiro, Seropédica, RJ, Brazil

* *Corresponding author*: E-mail: M.A.M. Maciel: mammaciel@hotmail.com; F.A. Vanderlinde: favanderlinde@gmail.com.

influence of Phyllanthus amarus methanolic extract (MeOH). The oral administration of mice (0.1, 0.3 or 1 g/kg) of MeOH caused a significant dose-related reduction of charcoal intestinal transit (6.8±0.4 per cent, 35.6±2.9 per cent and 58.5±6.2 per cent), respectively, compared to the control vehicle group (IC_{50} = 631 mg/kg). Atropine used as positive control reduced this parameter by 80 per cent. The found pharmacological results justify the traditional uses of Phyllanthus amarus Schum & Thonn against gastrointestinal disorders.

Keywords: *Phyllanthus amarus* Schum & Thonn, Euphorbiaceae, Bioactive lignans, Gastrointestinal transit.

Introduction

Phyllanthus (Euphorbiaceae) a native genus of the American continent is a representative medicinal plant with a higher concentration (about 750 species) in tropical and subtropical countries (Castro-Chaves *et al.*, 2002; Guerra *et al.*, 2003). This genus is widely distributed in Brazilian territory and has long been used in folk medicine (Matos *et al.*, 2004). *Phyllanthus niruri* L. and *Phyllanthus amarus* Schum & Thonn have been frequent targets of ethnopharmacological work all over the world, mainly in U.S.A, Malaysia, Cuba, Peru, Caribbean, China, Nigeria, Africa, India and Brazil. Despite the large number of literature register these species are cited as being synonymous. However, a recent botanic study performed in Brazil, proved to exist significant differences between *Phyllanthus niruri* L. and *Phyllanthus amarus* Schum & Thonn. According to this study, the main differences were evidenced to its base, seed and stigma type. Specifically, *Phyllanthus niruri* L. presents asymmetric base of lamina, capitated stigma and seeds with many *verrucula* in longitudinal lines. Meanwhile, *Phyllanthus amarus* Schum & Thonn has asymmetric base of lamina, but the stigma is not capitated and the seeds are striated (Silva, 2006; Silva *et al.*, 2004). Additionally, it is important to highlight that Webster, in 1957, notified that *Phyllanthus niruri* L. species had never been confirmed out of the American continent (Webster, 1957). Considering these reports it becoming important an extensive evaluation of the whole published chemistry, pharmacology and therapeutic potential of *Phyllanthus niruri* L. and *Phyllanthus amarus* Schum & Thonn, as well as *Phyllanthus sellowianus* Mull. Arg. Taking into account that *P. amarus* and *P. sellowianus* are considered a variation of *P. niruri*, and/or synonymous, an over general revision aiming to identify in literature reports which properties really pretence to *Phyllanthus niruri* L., represents a very difficult task, and could result in unsatisfactory results.

Concerning to the pharmacological potential reports of *Phyllanthus niruri* L., *Phyllanthus amarus* Schum & Thonn and *Phyllanthus sellowianus* Mull. Arg., many of their traditional therapeutic properties were scientifically validated, being *Phyllanthus niruri* L. an effective agent in uric acid elimination and liver diseases which cause jaundice (icterus), as well as diuretic, antioxidant, antitumoral, anticarcinogenic, antigenotoxic, antimicrobial, antiplasmodial, antiinflammatory, antinociceptive, analgesic, antimalarial, antiviral (including action against HIV), hepatoprotector, hypoglycemic and hypolipidemic (Calixto *et al.*, 1998; Cimanga *et al.*, 2004; Gilbert *et al.*, 2005; Harish and Shivanandappa, 2006; Khanna *et al.*, 2002; Ogata *et al.*, 1992;

Qian-Cutrone *et al.*, 1996; Santos *et al.*, 2000; Subeki *et al.*, 2005; Tona *et al.*, 1999; Venkateswaran *et al.*, 1987).

The species *Phyllanthus amarus* Schum & Thonn proved to be diuretic, antiinflammatory, antioxidant, antiviral, antitumoral, antimutagenic, antispasmodic, antiulcerogenic, hepatoprotector, hypoglycemic and hypotensive (Blumberg *et al.*, 1990; Calixto *et al.*, 1998; Gilbert *et al.*, 2005; Gowrishanker and Vivekanandan *et al.*, 1994; Jayram *et al.*, 1997; Kassuya *et al.*, 2003; Kiemer *et al.*, 2003; Lee *et al.*, 1996; Odetola and Akojenu, 2000; Ott *et al.*, 1997; Rajeshkumar and Kuttan, 2000; Rajeshkumar *et al.*, 2002; Raphael *et al.*, 2002; Raphael and Kuttan *et al.*, 2003; Santos *et al.*, 2000; Srividya and Periwal, 1995; Thyagarajan and Jayaram, 1992).

The previously mistakable identification of *Phyllanthus amarus* Schum & Thonn, and its medicinal importance motivated the present work, in which this plant was submitted to classical phytochemical evaluation using a specimen collected in the northern region of Brazil, as well as its investigation on gastrointestinal transit.

Material and Methods

Plant Material

Phyllanthus amarus Schum & Thonn was collected in Natal, the capital city of Rio Grande do Norte, Brazil. The plant identification was unambiguously performed by Dr. Maria Iracema Bezerra Loiola and a voucher specimen (no. 1645) has been deposited in Herbarium of the Departamento de Botânica, Ecologia and Zoologia da UFRN.

The dried vegetal material (124.5 g of the whole plant) was submitted to extraction (by percolation method) with MeOH. The obtained filtrate was reduced under vacuum leading 13.6 per cent of the *Phyllanthus amarus* alcoholic extract (16.9g). The chromatographic procedure was performed with silica gel (230-80 Mesh) column, giving a total of 43 fraction. The triterpene 2Z, 6Z, 10Z, 14E, 18E, 22E-farnesil farnesol was identified in the F_{11-16} fraction group, eluted with a mixture of hexane:$CHCl_3$ (90:10). The obtained lignans were identified in the fraction F_{36} to F_{43}, in that F_{36-40} fraction group was eluted with a mixture of hexane:EtOAc in polarity gradient (50:50 – 0:100); whilst F_{41-43} fraction group was eluted using EtOAc.

Spectra Data

The infrared spectra were registered on Fourier transform BioRad Excalibur Series FTS 3000MX spectrophotometer and KBr was used for solid substances with approximately 1 per cent of sample. The absorption frequencies were measured in units of wave number (cm^{-1}). The ^{1}H-NMR and ^{13}C-NMR spectra were recorded in Varian Gemini Spectrometer, at 300 and 75 MHz, respectively. The signal of the solvent, which was employed to solubilize the samples, was used as a reference pattern. Sigma and Merck deuterated solvents were used in NMR spectroscopy. Merck silica gel (230-80 Mesh) and, Queel and Vetec, Brazil, solvents (MeOH, hexane and ethyl acetate) were utilized for the chromatographic column separations. The TLC was realized with Vetec, Brazil, silica gel 60H, chloroform, hexane and ethyl acetate. TCL revelation procedure was performed with sulphuric acid and methanol (1:1).

Pharmacological Procedures

Animals

Adult male Swiss mice (25–35 g) were housed in plastic cages, with food and tap water available *ad libitum* in the colony room. Mice were acclimatized in the laboratory for at least 60 min prior to the test procedure and left without food for 12 h before the gavages. All experiments were carried out in accordance with current guidelines for the care of laboratory animals and the ethical guidelines on the use of animals in pain research (CIOMS, 1985; Zimmermann, 1986). Experimental protocols were approved by the local Animal Care and Use Committee (012/2007/CEPEB/UFRuralRJ) and the minimum number of animals and duration of observation required to obtain consistent data was employed.

Drugs

The used drugs were atropine sulfate and charcoal from Merck AG (Darmstadt, Germany). Test solutions of *Phyllanthus amarus* methanolic extract (MeOH), charcoal and atropine were diluted in water in such a concentration as to allow the administration of constant volumes of 10 mL/kg for each dose employed. Control animals received similar volume of vehicle (water). The oral pre-treatment (p.o.) was always done 1 h before charcoal administration.

Gastrointestinal Transit Charcoal Method

Groups of 10 mice were orally treated with water, *Phyllanthus amarus* methanolic extract (MeOH - 0.1, 0.3 or 1 g/kg) or atropine (5 mg/kg), 60 min prior to administration of the charcoal suspension (10 per cent). Thirty minutes after receiving the charcoal meal, mice were euthanized and the small intestine was removed. The length of the small intestine was measured by laying out the small intestine on a measuring tape and measuring the distance from the pyloric sphincter to the ileo-cecal valve. The distance traveled by the charcoal was measured from the pyloric sphincter to the most caudal edge of the charcoal. Values for gastrointestinal transit were expressed as a percent total intestinal length and calculated according to the following methodology: the distance traveled by the charcoal in centimeters was subtracted by the total length of the intestines in centimeters (pylorus to cecum) and then evaluated for each mice (STICKNEY; NORTHUP, 1959). Mean values were calculated for each group and statistical comparisons were made between treatment groups using parametric statistics (one-way analysis of variance, Dunnett's t test). Statistical significance was considered to be $p < 0.05$.

Results and Discussion

The phytochemical study performed with the methanolic extract obtained from the whole plant of *Phyllanthus amarus* Schum & Thonn lead to the identification of the triterpene 2Z, 6Z, 10Z, 14E, 18E, 22E-farnesil farnesol and six bioactive lignans: isolintetralin (2,3-demethoxy-*seco*-isolintetralin diacetate), niranthin, 5-demethoxy-niranthin, demethylenedioxy-niranthin, phyllanthin and hypophyllanthin (Figure 3.1), which presented antioxidant, antiinflammatory and hepatoprotector effects (Huang and Chen, 1992; Satyanarayana and Venkateswarlu, 1991; Sharma *et al.*,

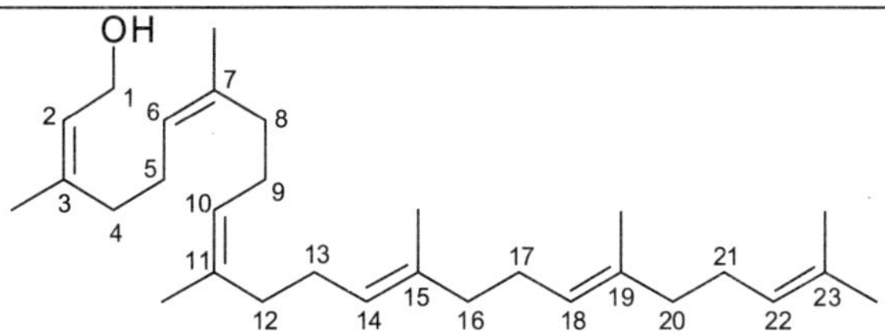

Farnesil farnesol

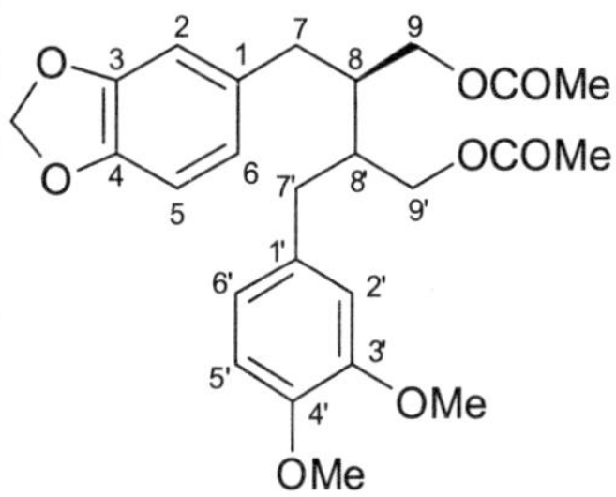

Isolintetralin

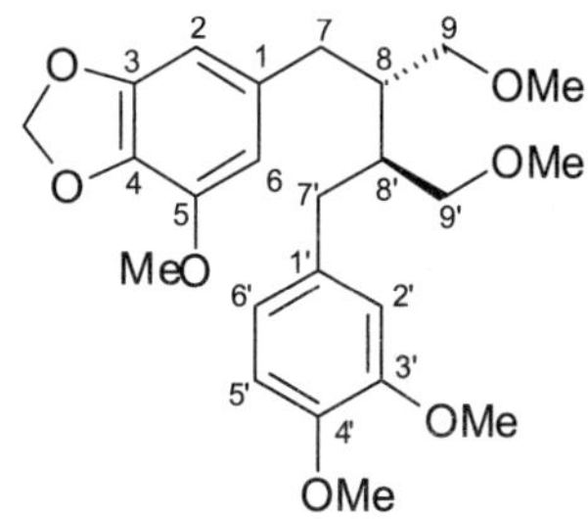

Niranthin

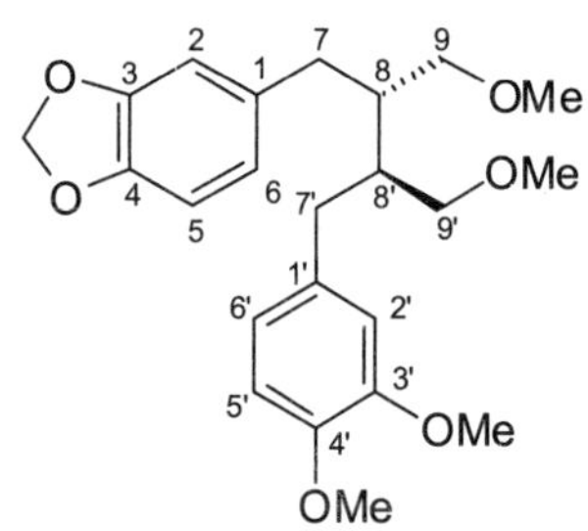

5-Demethoxy-niranthin

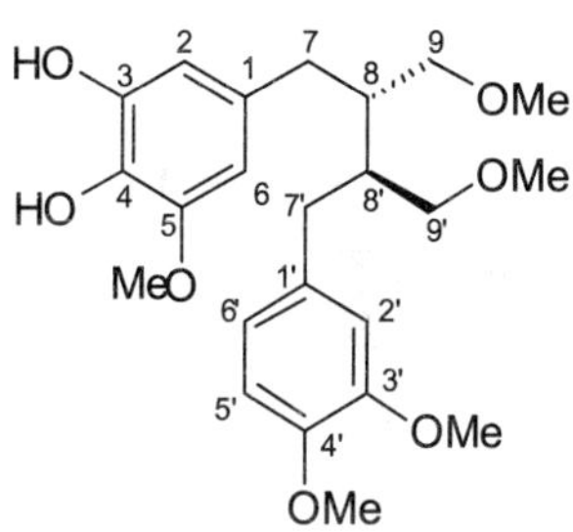

Dimethylenodioxy-niranthin

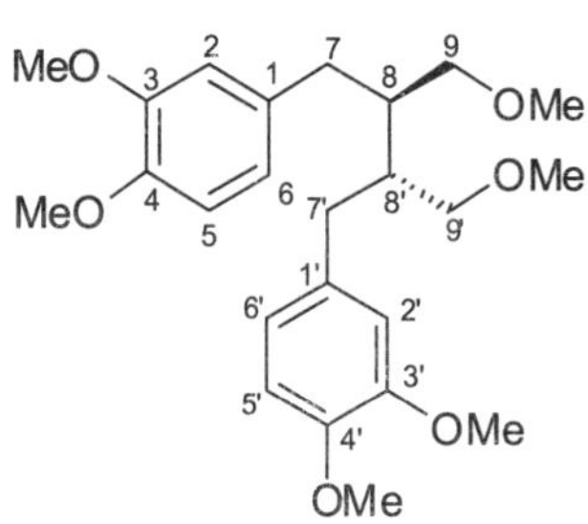

Phyllanthin

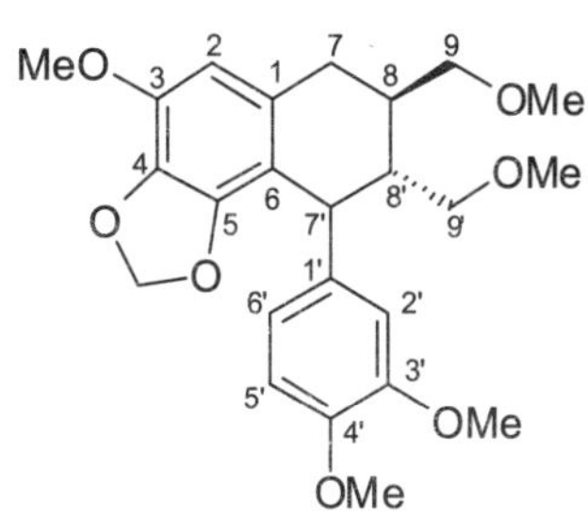

Hypophyllanthin

Figure 3.1. *Phyllanthus amarus* chemical constituents.

1993; Somanbadhu *et al.*, 1993). The triterpene was identified in the F_{11-16} fraction group [its infrared (IR) and NMR data showed to be coherent to those literature reports (Singh *et al.*, 1991)].

The cited above lignans were identified in the both F_{36-40} and F_{41-43} fraction groups. The IR spectrum of the isolintetralin, demethylenedioxy-niranthin, 5-demethoxy-niranthin, niranthin, phyllanthin and hypophyllanthin lignans mixture showed distinctive bands of CH_2 and CH-alkyl groups, through a large and intense band in 2926 cm^{-1} that suggested the presence of more than one substance, C=C aromatic ring groups (1591, 1508 and 1454 cm^{-1}) and C-O groups (1250, 1112 and 1030 cm^{-1}). Hydroxyl groups of demethylenedioxy-niranthin absorbed in 3502 and 3306 cm^{-1}, and the ester carbonyl moiety equivalent for the 5-demethoxy-niranthin lignan, in 1726 cm^{-1}. The ^1H-NMR data of isolintetralin, demethylenedioxy-niranthin, 5-demethoxy-niranthin and niranthin presented distinctive aromatic hydrogen region [H-Ar: δ 6.72 – 6.53 (m)]; methylenedioxy moieties [O-CH_2-O: δ 5.85 (s)]; methoxyl groups bonded to the aromatic ring (OMe-Ar: δ 3.81 – 3.73, 3.51); methoxyl groups bonded to the alkyl moieties (OMe-alkyl: δ 3.31 – 3.19); methynic groups [CH: δ 2.00 – 1.94 (m)]; methylenic groups [CH_2: δ 3.00 – 2.54, 2.26 (m)]; and hydroxylic groups [particularly the demethylenedioxy-niranthin OH: δ 5.66 (s) and 5.58 (s)]. Isolintetralin, and 5-demethoxy-niranthin (detected in the F_{36-40} fraction group) only differ in C-9 and C-9′ (CH_2-alkyl) substituted groups, which contain ester and methoxyl moieties, respectively. The observed ^1H-NMR differences data of these lignans are coherent with the literature data, as well as their ^{13}C-NMR data (Satyanarayana and Venkateswarlu, 1991; Chang *et al.*, 2003). Niranthin and demethylenedioxy-niranthin only differ in C-3 and C-4 substituted groups, which contain cyclic dioxymethylene and hydroxyl moieties, respectively. Significant differences were observed among the C-2, C-4, C-6 and C-7 carbon absorbances, as a result of mesomeric effects (electron delocalization) caused by the oxygen of the cyclic or hydroxyl groups, which might have encountered in a hydrogen binding. The observed differences were in accordance with previously reported data (Satyanarayana and Venkateswarlu, 1991).

Concerning to the ^1H-NMR spectrum of the F_{41-43} fraction group confirmed the presence of aromatic hydrogen; deoxymethylene moieties; methoxyl groups bonded to the aromatic ring; methoxyl groups bonded to alkyl moieties; methynic and methylenic groups; and hydroxylic groups, suggesting the presence of isolintetralin, demethylenedioxy-niranthin, 5-demethoxy-niranthin and niranthin mixed with two other lignans phyllanthin and hypophyllanthin. These last lignans were specially detected through the ^{13}C-NMR data analysis; the attributed data was in accordance with previously reports data (Somanbadhu *et al.*, 1993). The assignments of the ^1H and ^{13}C NMR spectra of the triterpene farnesil farnesol were performed by one- and two-dimentional NMR analysis. The other absorbance evidences that support the presence of this triterpene in *Phyllanthus amarus* Schum & Thonn, as well as those cited above lignans were previously reported (Maciel *et al.*, 2007).

The evaluation of the *Phyllanthus amarus* Schum & Thonn methanolic extract influence in charcoal gastrointestinal transit demonstrated that oral administration of mice (0.1, 0.3 or 1 g/kg) of this MeOH extract, caused a significant dose-related reduction (6.8±0.4 per cent, 35.6±2.9 per cent and 58.5±6.2 per cent, respectively), when compared to the control vehicle group. Atropine used as positive control reduced this parameter by 80 per cent (Figure 3.2) and the calculated IC_{50} (50 per cent inhibitory concentration) was 631 mg/kg (Figure 3.3).

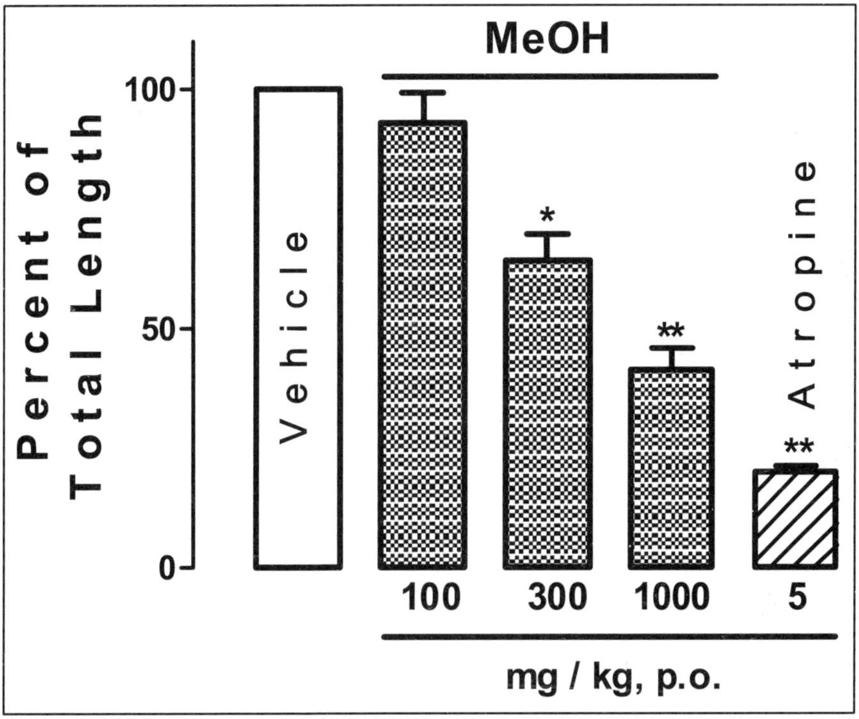

Figure 3.2. Effect of *Phyllanthus amarus* methanolic extract (MeOH) or atropine (5 mg/kg) on gastrointestinal transit. Plots of mean and S.E.M. (n = 10) per cent of total intestinal length. Measurements were made 30 min after oral administration of charcoal. *Significantly different (* $p < 0.01$; ** $p < 0.001$) than vehicle.

Conclusions

The present phytochemical study performed with *Phyllanthus amarus* Schum & Thonn (a specimen collected in the northern region of Brazil) indicated a strong chemical compatibility with other *Phyllanthus* specimen. Six special metabolites from the lignan class, and one acyclic triterpene were identified and characterized by NMR spectra data. The lignans phyllanthin and hypophyllanthin were previously isolated from *Phyllanthus amarus* Schum & Thonn (a specimen from different origin); isolintetralin (2,3-demethoxy-seco-isolintetralin diacetate), niranthin, 5-demethoxy-niranthin, and demethylenedioxy-niranthin were isolated from *Phyllanthus niruri* L. and other specimens from *Phyllanthus* genera and the triterpene (2Z, 6Z, 10Z, 14E, 18E, 22E-farnesil farnesol) from *Phyllanthus niruri*. The pharmacological results determined by charcoal meal method demonstrate a dose related inhibition of gastrointestinal transit and may account for the wide popular use of this plant as

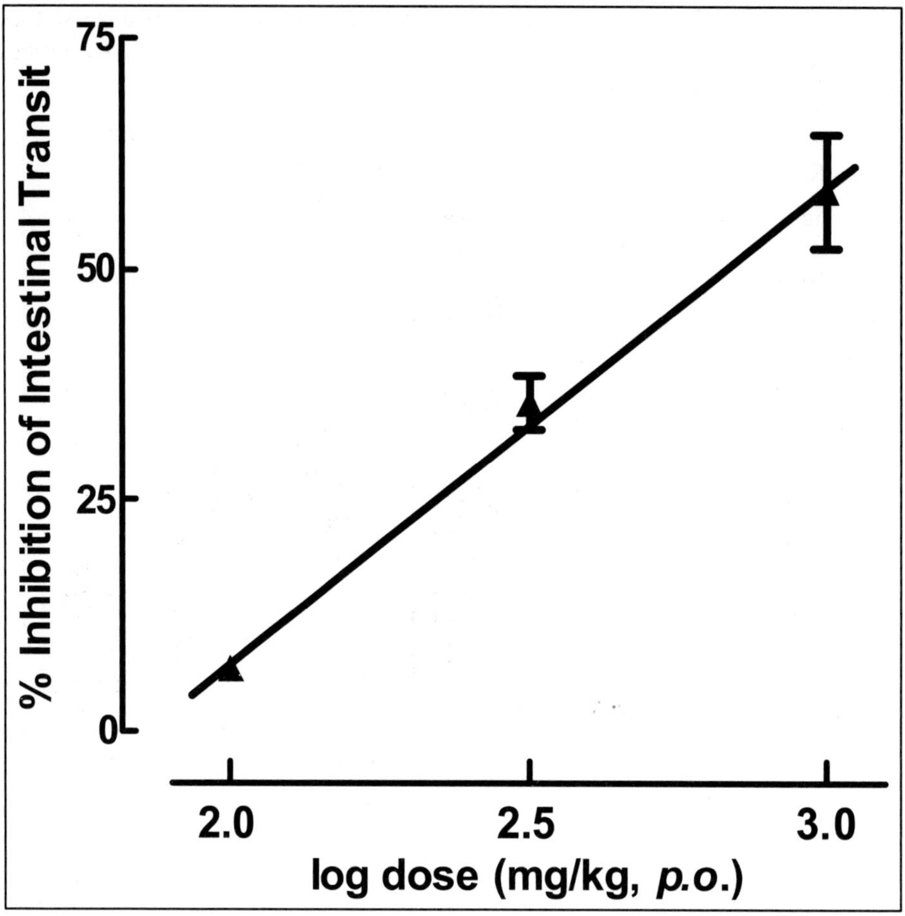

Figure 3.3. Dose-effect inhibitory produced by *Phyllanthus amarus* methanolic extract (MeOH) administration on gastrointestinal transit after oral administration of charcoal. The symbol and vertical bars are means ± *S.E.M.* of 10 animals.

antidiarrheal agent. Since, *Phyllanthus niruri* L. and *Phyllanthus amarus* Schum & Thonn are not any more considered synonymous, this present work bring satisfactory phytochemical and pharmacological results, contributing to the scientific advancement of this broadly used medicinal species *P. amarus* Schum & Thonn.

Acknowledgments

The authors thank Professor Dr. Maria Iracema Bezerra Loiola (UFRN) for the botanic identification and CNPq for scholarship and financial support.

References

Blumberg, B.S., Millman, I., Venkateswaran, P.S., and Thyagarajan, S.P. (1990). Hepatitis B virus and hepatocellular carcinoma-treatment of HBV carriers with *Phyllanthus amarus*. *Cancer Detection and Prevention*,**14(2):** 195–201.

Calixto, J.B., Santos, A.R., Cechinel Filho, V., and Yunes, R.A. (1998). A review of the plants of the genus *Phyllanthus*: their chemistry, pharmacology, and therapeutic potential. *Medicinal Research Reviews*, **8(4):** 225-258.

Castro-Chaves, C., Cunha, A.M.F., Cruz, G.M.C., and Oliveira, D.V.O. (2002). *Phyllanthus niruri* L. Induz Caliurese Dissociada da Diurese e da Natriurese em Ratos Acordados. *Revista* Brasileira de *Farmacognosia*, **12**: 2-4.

Cimanga, R.K., Tona, L., Luyindula, N., Mesia, K., Lusakibanza, M., Musuamba, C.T., Apers, S., De Bruyne, T., Van Miert, S., Hermans, N., Totté, J., Pieters, L., and Vlietinck, A.J. (2004). *In vitro* antiplasmodial activity of callus culture extracts and fractions from fresh apical stems of *Phyllanthus niruri* L. (Euphorbiaceae) (Part 2). *Journal of Ethnopharmacology*, **95**: 399-404.

CIOMS- Council for International Organization of Medical Sciences. International Guiding Principles for Biomedical Research Involving Animals, 1985. <http: / /http: / /www.cioms.ch/ frame_1985_texts_of_guidelines.htm>, accessed 26 July 2010.

Chang, Chia-Chuan., Lien, Yu-Chin., Karin, C.S., Liu, C., and Lee, Shoei-Sheng (2003). Lignans from *Phyllanthus urinaria*. *Phytochemistry*, **63(7):** 825-833.

Gilbert, B., Ferreira, J.L.P., and Alves, L. F. (2005). *Monografias de plantas medicinais brasileiras e aclimatadas*. Curitiba: *Abifito*, 115-142.

Gowrishanker, B., and Vivekanandan, O.H. (1994). *In vivo* studies of a crude extract of *Phyllanthus amarus* L. by tannery effluents. *Mutation Research,* **322**: 185-192.

Guerra, M.P., and Nodari, R.O. (2003). Biodiversidade: aspectos biológicos, geográficos, legais e éticos (Cap. 1) 2003. In: Simões, C.M.O.; Schenkel, E.P.; Gosmann, G.; Melo, J.C.P.; Mentz, L.A.; Petrovick, P.R. (Org.) Farmacognosia da Planta ao Medicamento, 5ª. ed., Editora UFRGS, Editora UFSC, Porto Alegre, Florianópolis, p.15.

Harish, R., and Shivanandappa, T. (2006).Antioxidant activity and hepatoprotective potential of *Phyllanthus niruri. Food Chemistry,* **95**: 180-185.

Huang, Y.L., Chen, C.C., and Ou J.C. (1992). Isolintetralin: a new lignan from *Phyllanthus niruri. Planta Medica,* **58**: 473-474.

Jayram, S., Thyagarajan, S.P., Sumathi, S., Manjula, S., Malathi, S., and Madanagopalan, N. (1997). Efficiency of *Phyllanthus amarus* treatment in acute viral Hepatitis A, B and non A and non B: an open clinical trial. *Indian Journal of Viorology,* **13**: 59-64.

Kassuya, C.A.L., Silvestre, A.A., Rehder, V.L.G., and Calixto, J.C. (2003). Anti-allodynic and anti-oedematogenic properties of the extract and lignans from *Phyllanthus amarus* in models of persistent inflammatory and neuropathic pain. *European Journal of Pharmacology,* **478**: 145-153.

Khanna, A.K., Rizvi, F., and Chander, R. (2002). Lipid lowering activity of *Phyllanthus niruri* in hyperlipemic rats. *Journal of Ethnopharmacology,* **82**: 19-22.

Kiemer, A. K., Hartung, T., Huber, C., and Vollmar, A. M. (2003). *Phyllanthus amarus* has anti-inflammatory potential by inhibition of Inos, COX-2, and cytokines via the NF-Kappab pathway. *Journal of Hepatology*, **38(3):** 289-297.

Lee, C.D., Ott, M., Thyagarajan, S.P., Shafritz, D.A., Burk, R.D., and Gupta, S. (1996). *Phyllanthus amarus* down regulates hepatitis B virus RNAm transcription and translation. *European Journal of Clinical Investigations*, **26(12):** 1069–1076.

Maciel, M.A.M., Cunha, A.F., Dantas, T. N.C., and Kaiser, C.R. (2007). NMR Characterization of Bioactive Lignans from *Phyllanthus amarus* Schum & Thonn. *Annals Magnetic Resonnance*, **6(3):** 76-82.

Matos, F.J.A., Sousa, M.P., Matos, M.E.O., Machado, M.I.L., and Craveiro, A.A. (2004). *Constituintes químicos qtivos e propriedades biológicas de plantas medicinais brasileiras*, 2ª ed., Editora UFC.

Odetola, A.A., and Akojenu, S.M. (2000). Anti-diarrhoeal and gastro-intestinal potentials of the aqueous extract of *Phyllanthus amarus* (Euphorbiaceae). *Afr. J. Med. Med Sci.*, **29(2):** 119-122.

Ogata, T., Higuchi, H., Mochida, S., Matsumoto, H.,Kato, A., Endo, T., Kaji, A., and Kaji, H. (1992). HIV-1 reverse transcriptase inhibitor from *Phyllanthus niruri*. *AIDS Research and Human Retroviruses*, **8(11):** 1937-1944.

Ott, M., Thyagarajan, S.P., and Gupta, S. (1997). *Phyllanthus amarus* supress hepatitis B virus by interrupting interactions between HBV enhancer I and cellular transcription factors. *European Journal of Clinical Investigation*, **27(11):** 908-915.

Qian-Cutrone, J., Huang, S., Trimble, J., Li, H.; Lin, P., Masud, A., Klohr, S.E., and Kadow, K.F. (1996). Niruside, a new HIV REV/RRE binding inhibitor from *Phyllanthus niruri*. *Journal of Natatural Product*, **59(2):** 196-199.

Rajeshkumar, N.V., Joy, K.L., Kuttan, G., Ramsewak, R.S., Nair, M.G., and Kuttan, R. (2002). Antitumour and Anticarnogenic Activity of *Phyllanthus amarus* Extract. *Journal of Ethnopharmacology*, **81**: 17-22.

Rajeshkumar, N.V., and Kuttan, R. (2000). *Phyllanthus amarus* extract administration increases the life span of rats with hepatocellular carcinoma. *Journal of Ethnopharmacology*, **73**: 215-219.

Raphael, K.R., and Kuttan, R. (2003). Inhibition of experimental gastric lesion and inflammation by *Phyllanthus amarus* extract. *Journal of Ethnopharmacology*, **87**: 193-197.

Raphael, R.K., Ajith, T.A., Joseph, S., and Kuttan, R. (2002). Anti-mutagenic activity of *Phyllanthus amarus* Schum and Thonn in vitro as well as *in vivo*. *Teratogenesis, Carcinogeneses, and Mutagenesis*, **22(4):** 285-291.

Santos, A.R.S., De Campos, R.O.P., Miguel, O.G., Filho, V.C., Siani, A.C., Yunes, R.A., and Calixto, J.B. (2000). Antinociceptive properties of extracts of new species of plants of the genus *Phyllanthus* (Euphorbiaceae). *Journal of Ethnopharmacology*, **72**: 229-238.

Satyanarayana, P., and Venkateswarlu, S. (1991). Isolation, structure and synthesis of new diarylbutane lignans from *Phyllanthus niruri*: synthesis of 5′-desmethoxy niranthin and an antitumor extractive. *Tetrahedron*, **47(42):** 8931-8940.

Sharma, A., Singh, R.T., and Handa, S.S. (1993). Determination of phyllantin and hypophyllanthin by performance liquid chromatography in *Phyllanthus amarus*. *Phytochemical Analysis*, **4(5):** 226-229.

Silva, M.J. (2006).O gênero *Phyllanthus* L. (Phyllanthaceae Martynov) no Nordeste do Brasil, com ênfase nas espécies de Pernambuco, Dissertação de Mestrado, Recife, PE, UFPE.

Silva, M.J., and Sales, M.F. (2004). O. gênero *Phyllanthus* L. (Phyllantheae – Euphorbiaceae Juss.) no bioma caatinga do estado de PE -Brasil. *Rodriguésia*, **55(84):** 101-126.

Singh, B., Agrawal, P.K., and Thakur, R.S. (1991). Isolation of *trans*-phytol from *Phyllanthus niruri*. *Planta Medica*, **57(1):** 98.

Somanabandhu, A., Nityangkuru, S., and Mahidol, C. (1993). ^{1}H and ^{13}C NMR assignments of phyllanthin and hypophyllanthin lignans that enhance cytotoxic responses with cultured multidrug-resistant cells. *Journal of Natural Product*, **56**: 233-239.

Srividya, N., and Periwal, S. (1995). Diuretic, hypotensive and hypoglycemic effect of *Phyllanthus amarus*. *Indian Journal of Experimental Biology*, **33(11):** 861-864.

Stickney, F.O., and Northup, D.W. (1959). Effect of gastric emptying upon propulsive motility of small intestine in rat. *Proc. Soc. Exp. Biol. Med.*, **101**: 582.

Subeki; H.M., Takahashi, K., Yamasaki, M.; Yamato, O., Maede, Y., Katakura, K., Kobayashi, S., Trimurningsih; Chairul, and Yoshihara, T. (2005). Anti-Babesial and anti-plasmodial compounds from *Phyllanthus niruri*. *Journal of Natural Product*, **68**: 537-539.

Thyagarajan, S.P., and Jayaram, S. (1992). Natural history of *Phyllanthus amarus* in the treatment of hepatitis B. *Indian Journal of Medical Microbiology*, **10**: 64–84.

Tona, L.; Ngimbi, N.P., Tsakala, M.; Mesia, K., Cimanga, K., Apers, S., De Bruyne, T., Pieters, L., Tollé, J., and Vlietinck, A.J. (1999). Antimalarial activity of 20 crude extracts from nine african medicinal plants used in Kinshasa, Congo. *Journal of Ethnopharmacology*, **68**: 193-203.

Venkateswaran, P.S., Millman, I., and Blumberg, B.S. (1987). Effects of an extract from *Phyllanthus niruri* on Hepatitis B and Woodchuck Hepatitis viruses: in vitro and *in vivo* studies, *Proceedings of the National Academy of Sciences USA*, **84(1):** 274-278.

Webster, G.L. (1957). A monographic study of the West Indian species of *Phyllanthus* (continued). *Journal of the Arnold Arboretum*, **38**: 51-80.

Zimmermann M. (1986). Ethical considerations in relation to pain in animal experimentation. *Acta Physiol Scand Suppl.*, **554**: 221-233.

Medicinal Plants: Phytochemistry, Pharmacology and Therapeutics Vol. 2 (2012) *Pages* **53–67**
Editor-in-Chief: **V.K. Gupta**
Published by: **DAYA PUBLISHING HOUSE, NEW DELHI**

4

Antiulcerogenic Activity of *Citrus lemon* Essential Oil on Acetic Acid-Induced Gastric Ulcer in Rats

Ariane Leite Rozza[1], Marcia Ortiz Mayo Marques[2], Clélia Akiko Hiruma-Lima[3] and Cláudia Helena Pellizzon*[1]

ABSTRACT

Citrus lemon belongs to Rutaceae family and is popularly known in Brazil as limão siciliano. The present study aimed to evaluate healing effects of Citrus lemon essential oil (CL) on acetic acid-induced gastric ulcer in Wistar male rats. After gastric ulcer induction, animals (n=7) were orally treated with vehicle (8 per cent Tween 80, negative control), cimetidine (100 mg/kg, positive control) or CL (250 mg/kg) for 14 days. The rats were sacrificed, the ulcer was measured and the stomachs were destined to histology. The CL components were identified by gas chromatography/mass spectrometry. ANOVA, Dunnett, $p<0.01$. CL reduced the internal ulcer area in 42 per cent and the external ulcer area in 59 per cent compared to the vehicle group. In CL group, immunohistochemical analyses displayed marked area for PCNA statistically higher (17543.0 ± 2275.4 μm^2) than Cimetidine (6810.4 ± 1684.0 μm^2) or vehicle group (6710.1 ± 2337.6 μm^2), indicating cell proliferation activity. CL stimulated cellular but not neutrophils infiltration in submucosa of the ulcer region. There was COX-2 expression and the PGE_2 production in CL group (18.25 ± 2.58 ng/mL) was

1 Morphology Department, Biosciences Institute, UNESP – Univ Estadual Paulista, Botucatu/SP, Brazil.
P.O. Box 510, Zip Code 18618-970, Botucatu/SP, Brazil

2 Campinas Agronomic Institute, Campinas/SP, Brazil.
P.O. Box 28, Zip Code 13020-902, Campinas/SP, Brazil

3 Physiology Department, Biosciences Institute, UNESP – Univ Estadual Paulista, Botucatu/SP, Brazil.
P.O. Box 510, Zip Code 18618-970, Botucatu/SP, Brazil

* *Corresponding author*: E-mail: claudia@ibb.unesp.br

Histological Analysis

After removing the stomachs, each one of them was sectioned and fixed in ALFAC solution (80 per cent alcohol, acetic acid and formaldehyde) for 24h at 4°C. Then the samples were routinely processed for embedding in paraplast, cut into 5 mm-thick sections and put into histological slides. These sections were stained with Haematoxylin-Eosin (HE), Periodic Acid-Schiff (PAS) or destined for immunohistochemistry. After staining, slides were analyzed with a Leica microscope, associated with Leica Qwin Software (Leica-England), in which regeneration epithelium height was measured to evaluate cicatrization.

Cell and Neutrophils Counts

After capturing images using a Leica microscope associated with Leica Qwin Software, the total number of cells in ulcer submucosa was counted automatically by the software AVSoft BioView through 15 fields. Neutrophils were counted manually in the same 15 fields.

Immunohistochemistry

Representative sections were deparaffinized, rehydrated and immunostained with ABC method. Nonspecific reaction was blocked with H_2O_2 and goat serum prior to incubation with the specific antiserum. After rinsing in phosphatase buffer saline (PBS 0.01mol/L, pH 7.4), the section was incubated in secondary antiserum (ABC kit). They were washed in PBS buffer and finally the ABC complex was prepared, and the reaction was carried out in a DAB solution (3,3′-diaminobenzidine-tetrahydrochloride) containing 0.01 per cent H_2O_2 in PBS buffer. After immunostaining, the sections were lightly counterstained with haematoxylin and the immunoreactive cells were observed under a Leica microscope associated with Leica Qwin Software (Leica-England). For the control reaction, some slides were processed omitting the primary antibody and other slides omitting the primary and secondary antibodies. These procedures were done for PCNA (Proliferating Cell Nuclear Antigen - Novo Castra) and COX-2 (Cyclooxygenase-2 - Cayman Chemical). Twenty slides were used for each antibody. Marked area were measured with the aid of AVSoft BioView software.

Electron Microscopy

Samples of stomachs were fixed in 3 per cent glutaraldehyde in PBS solution, post-fixed in osmium solution and ultrathin sections obtained by the ultramicrotome Ultra Cut UCT-Leica, stained with uranyl acetate and lead citrate and observed in Philips electron microscope model CM 10 from the Laboratory of Electron Microscopy–Institute of Biosciences, UNESP, Botucatu.

Toxicological Analysis

During the treatment period (14 days), body weight progression and possible alterations in hair and mucosa were observed daily. After animal death, the heart, kidneys, liver, lungs and spleen were weighed to detect any effect from the treatment. Biochemical analyses were performed on the animals' serum, to quantify AST (aspartate aminotransferase), ALT (alanine aminotransferase) and g-GT (gamma glutamyltransferase) to evaluate liver damage, and creatinine and urea to evaluate kidney damage, using the automated biochemical analyzer SBA-200, CELM, Brazil. These analyses were done according to Calvo *et al.* (2007).

Assessment of Prostaglandin E_2 Synthesis

Wistar male rats (n=7), fasted for 24 h prior to the experiment, were randomly distributed into five groups: sham, VEH, VEH + indomethacin, CL, CL + indomethacin. The rats received subcutaneous indomethacin (30 mg/kg) or VEH injections and, after 30 minutes, orally received CL or VEH. Sham group did not receive any drug or treatment. Thirty minutes after the treatment, the rats were killed, the abdomen was opened and a sample of the corpus (full thickness) was excised, weighed and then placed in 1ml 10mM-sodium phosphate buffer, pH 7.4. Finally, the tissue was minced and then incubated at 37°C for 20 min. PGE_2 in the buffer solution was measured by enzyme immunoassay (R&D Systems), with the absorbance being read at 420 nm (Curtis *et al.*, 1995). Results were expressed in µg/mL.

Statistical Analysis

Results were expressed as mean ± s.e.m. Statistical significance was determined by ANOVA one-way analysis of variance followed by Dunnett's test, with minimum significance level of $P<0.01$. All analyses were accomplished via GraphPad Instat software, 3.02 version, San Diego, California, USA.

Results

Components Identification

Thirteen substances were identified in CL by gas chromatography. The majority consists of limonene (70,75 per cent) and β-pinene (13,19 per cent). They are listed in Table 4.1.

Table 4.1. Identification of *Citrus lemon* essential oil components by gas chromatography/mass spectrometry and their relative abundance (per cent).

Peak	*Substance*	*(per cent)*
1	α-tujene	0.26
2	α-pinene	1.72
3	Sabinene	1.71
4	β-pinene	13.19
5	β-mircene	1.35
6	α-terpinolene	0.11
7	p-cimene	0.10
8	Limonene	70.75
9	n.i.	0.11
10	γ-terpinene	9.19
11	Terpinolene	0.22
12	n.i.	0.14
13	n.i.	0.32
14	Neral	0.30
15	α-trans-bergamotene	0.20
16	β-bisabolene	0.16
17	n.i.	0.17

n.i. = Not identified.

Gastric Ulcer Measures

Macroscopic measures showed significant reduction in internal and external ulcer area of CL in comparison with CIM and VEH group. Gastric pH measures in CL group were not different from CIM or VEH groups (Table 4.2).

Histological Analysis and Electron Microscopy

Morphometric analysis of linear distance from the ulcer base to the stomach lumen showed that in CL group mucosa was significantly smaller than the VEH group (Table 4.2). HE staining displayed that in CIM and VEH groups the lesions were still observed, but in the CL group the gastric ulcer was recovered by a regeneration epithelium (Figures 4.1 A, B, C).

Table 4.2. Macroscopic and microscopic analyses in rats' stomach treated for 14 days with vehicle, cimetidine (100 mg/kg) or *Citrus lemon* essential oil (250 mg/kg) (n=7) after acetic-acid induced gastric ulcer.

Treatments	*Vehicle*	*Cimetidine*	*Citrus Lemon*
Internal area (mm^2)	4.18 ± 0.29	3.27 ± 0.27	2.41 ± 0.39 **
External area (mm^2)	9.29 ± 0.80	6.64 ± 0.62 *	3.82 ± 0.58 **
pH	2.75 ± 0.48	3.25 ± 0.48	2.90 ± 0.58
Mucosal height (μm)	1102.40 ± 44.61	1247.40 ± 57.91	825.04 ± 32.40 **
Cells count	925.8 ± 85.6	1137.7 ± 85.9	1243.0 ± 46.3 **
Neutrophils count	12.00 ± 0.44	9.83 ± 0.43 **	9.42 ± 0.58 **
Immunoreactive area for PCNA (μm^2)	6710.1 ± 2337.6	6810.4 ± 1684.0	17543.0 ± 2275.4 **
Immunoreactive area for COX-2 (μm^2)	11433 ± 0.28	11625 ± 0.72	12413 ± 0.74

Mean±sem, ANOVA followed by Dunnett, **$p<0.01$.

PAS staining showed more intense and homogeneous secretion in mucus production in the CL group than control groups (Figures 4.1 D, E, F). Electron microscopy confirmed high mucus production in the CL group, which showed several empty mucous vesicles in the mucous neck cells and intense alteration of cell apical surface, indicating exocytosis. The CIM group displayed a large number of intracellular vesicles, but no vesicle eliminated in the gastric lumen. VEH group showed little mucous granule production on the apical surface but no effective exocytosis (Figures 4.1 G, H, I).

Cell and Neutrophils Counts

The CL group had a significant increase in cells counted in the submucosa of the ulcer in comparison VEH group. However, there was a significant decrease of neutrophils registered in regions under the regenerative stomach mucosa of animals treated with CL (Table 4.2).

Immunohistochemistry

PCNA expression showed increased cell proliferation (Figures 4.2 A, B, C) in the CL group, as confirmed by measuring the immunoreactive area (Figure 4.7), which was significantly augmented in the CL group.

The COX-2 expression (Figures 4.2 D, E, F) was observed in all groups. The marked area was not different between the CL, CIM or VEH group (Table 4.2).

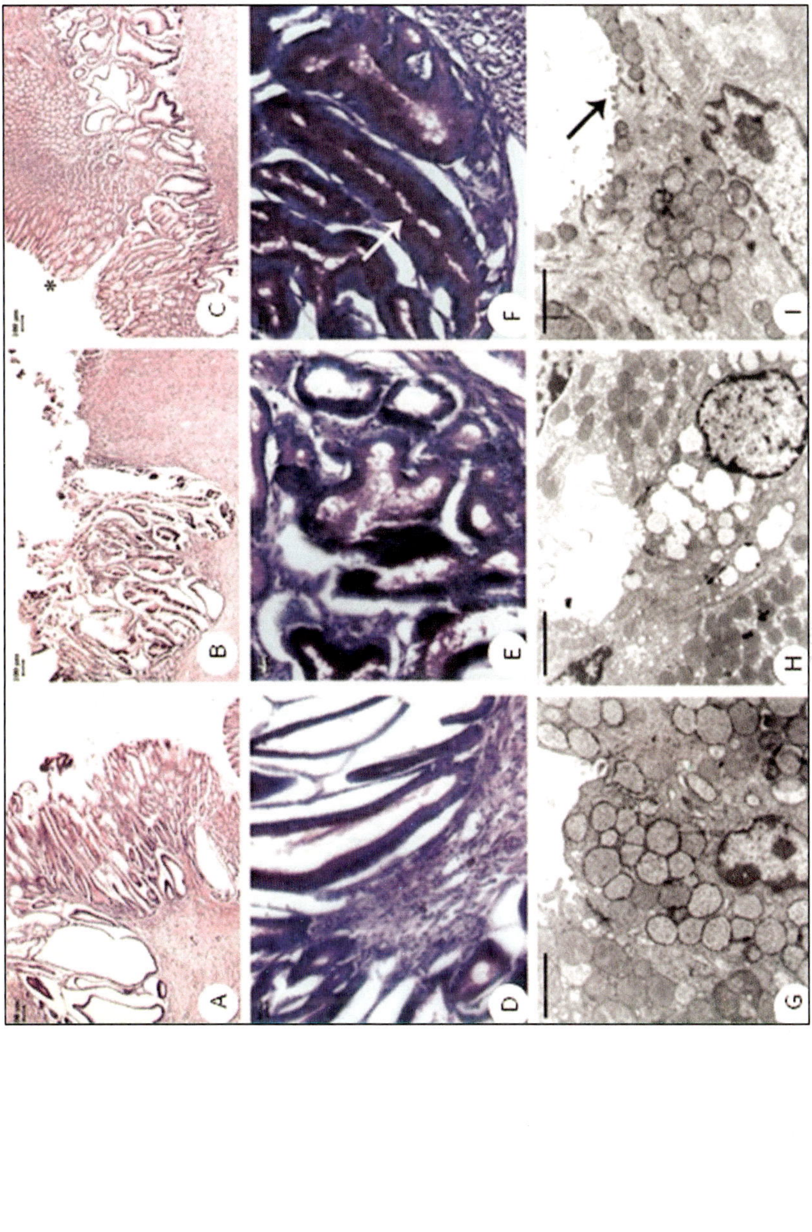

Figure 4.1. Histological analysis of rats' stomachs treated with vehicle (A, D, G), Cimetidine (B, E, H) and *Citrus lemon* (C, F, I) for 14 days. In HE staining (A, B, C) notice different stages for gastric ulcer healing in each treatment and in C the ulcer is recovered by a regeneration epithelium (*). Bar = 100 µm. In PAS staining (D, E, F) notice mucus secretion (arrow) to the lumen almost inexistent in D and higher in E and F. Bar = 20 µm. In electron microscopy (G, H, I) note exocitosis of mucus vesicles (arrow) in F. Bar = 1 µm.

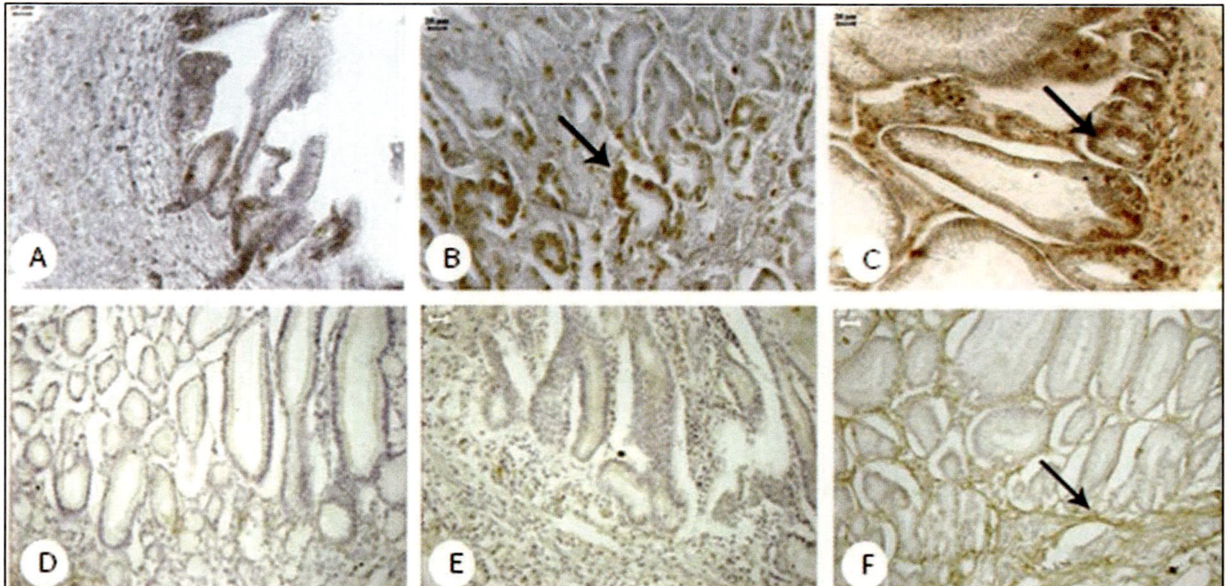

Figure 4.2. Immunohistochemistry for Proliferating Cell Nuclear Antigen (PCNA) in vehicle (A), Cimetidine (B) and *Citrus lemon* (C) groups. Note great number of cells undergoing mitosis (arrow) in B and C. Bar = 20 µm. Immunohistochemistry for COX-2 in vehicle (D), Cimetidine (E) and *Citrus lemon* (F) groups. Arrow indicates immunoreaction. Bar = 20 µm.

Toxicological Analysis

There were no alterations in body weight progression of the rats neither in their appearance. Biochemical analysis to AST, ALT, γ-GT, creatinine and urea of the animals' serum showed no significant difference among all groups, evidencing no toxicological alterations. The heart, liver, lungs and spleen weight were not different between the three groups. However, the kidneys of the rats from CL group were statistically heavier than the kidneys of the rats from the control groups (Table 4.3).

Table 4.3. Evaluation of the toxicity in rats orally treated for 14 days with vehicle, cimetidine (100 mg/kg) or *Citrus lemon* essential oil (250 mg/kg) (n=7) after acetic-acid induced gastric ulcer.

Treatments		*Vehicle*	*Cimetidine*	*Citrus lemon*
Biochemical	AST	243.12 ± 41.13	258.74 ± 34.28	179.23 ± 21.30
parameters	ALT	37.73 ± 5.37	35.23 ± 0.63	35.30 ± 1.76
	γ-GT	11.50 ± 5.11	4.56 ± 1.03	9.36 ± 2.31
	Creatinine	0.43 ± 0.03	0.46 ± 0.06	0.37 ± 0.02
	Urea	62.00 ± 6.92	60.67 ± 14.34	49.60 ± 9.75
Organ	Heart	3.56 ± 0,15	3.60 ± 0.08	3.73 ± 0.10
	Kidneys	4.86 ± 0.07	4.92 ± 0.06	5.20 ± 0.12**
	Liver	9.15 ± 1.04	9.49 ± 1.24	9.80 ± 0.44
	Lungs	4.64 ± 0.56	4.40 ± 0.24	4.48 ± 0.30
	Spleen	2.99 ± 0.40	3.05 ± 0.25	3.19 ± 0.19

AST, ALT, g-GT expressed in U/L, creatinine and urea and expressed in mg/dL. Organs weight were expressed in Arcsine. All parameters were measured through animals' serum. ANOVA followed by Dunnett, $^{**}p<0.01$.

Assessment of Prostaglandin E_2 Synthesis

Validating the result obtained for COX-2 immunohistochemistry, CL was able to maintain PGE_2 level near to sham group, even with indomethacin administration. Indomethacin was able to statistically reduce PGE_2 level when administered with VEH in comparison with the level in the VEH alone (Figure 4.3).

Discussion

The acetic acid-induced gastric ulcer model is the one most similar to human gastric ulcers, since it is difficult to treat and it requires a long time for healing (Okabe and Amagase, 2005). Histologically, an ulcer consists of two major structures: a distinct ulcer margin formed by the adjacent non-necrotic mucosa (the epithelial component) and the granulation tissue at the ulcer base (the connective tissue component) (Cotran, 1999; Tarnawski, 2000). Ulcer healing is a complex process that involves cell migration, proliferation, reepithelization, angiogenesis, and matrix deposition (Tarnawski, 2005).

Woollard *et al.* (2007) reviewed evidence in the literature on the influence of essential oils on wound healing and their potential application in clinical practice.

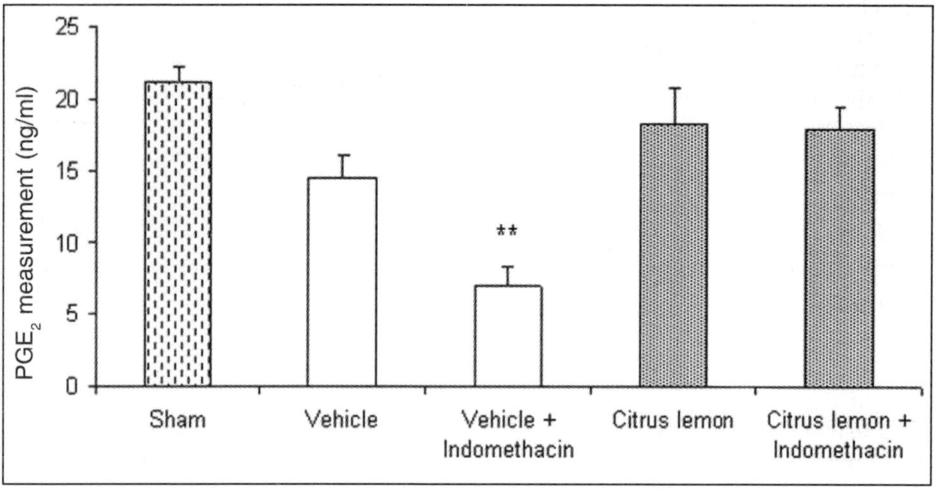

Figure 4.3. PGE_2 measurement (ng/ml) in gastric mucosa of rats treated with *Citrus lemon* essential oil (250 mg/kg) or vehicle, alone or in association with nonselective COX inhibitor (indomethacin) (n=7). ANOVA followed by Dunnett, **p<0.01.

Essential oils has been very effective in treatment of hyperacidity, gastric and duodenal ulcer and our group has demonstrated effective healing and gastroprotective effects of essential oils of some medicinal plants (Hiruma-Lima *et al.,* 2002; Paula *et al.,* 2006). As essential oils from Citrus genus are composed mainly of terpenes that have shown antiulcerogenic effects in several species, we decided to evaluate the gastric ulcer healing effect of CL essential oil considering macroscopic and microscopic alterations and mechanism of action.

The treatment with CL was able to reduce the external ulcer area in 59 per cent and the internal ulcer area in 42 per cent, while the positive control CIM reduced the external ulcer area in 28 per cent and the internal in 22 per cent. The significant reduction in these macroscopic measures means reduction in exposed submucosa in CL group, and it was confirmed by the microscopic analyses. The ulcers were less profound in CL group, as shown by the reduced mucosal height. As could be seen in the Figure 4.1, in the CL group the gastric mucosa was recovered by a regeneration epithelium and the gastric glands showed more efficient organization.

The significant increase in cells counted in the submucosa of the ulcer in CL group denotes cell proliferation at that site, contributing to the formation of a new epithelium. Increased cellularization is an important indication of healing process efficacy because, besides denoting increased vascularization at that site (Tarnawski, 2005), some cells are especially important to secretion of specific proteins that respond to local injuries, such as COX (Tsukimi and Okabe, 2001; Sánchez-Fidalgo *et al.,* 2004). Both the immunohistochemistry and the measured immunoreactive area for PCNA confirmed the accelerated epithelial regeneration shown by HE staining and cell counts, which allows us to conclude that CL stimulates mitosis for the formation of a new epithelium that will scar the ulcer. PCNA is nuclear peptide expressed in proliferating cells (Celis and Celis, 1985).

The significant decrease of neutrophils was also a beneficial effect from the treatment with CL. Neutrophil accumulation can result in impaired tissue regeneration (Pizza *et al.*, 2001), because it produces excessive oxygen-derived free radicals, which cause lipid peroxidation, tissue damage (Butterfield *et al.*, 2006) and inflammation. The inflammatory process cells and also the mitogenic agents can induce the expression of the COX-2 enzyme in lesions (Motilva *et al.*, 2005). COX-2 promotes epithelial cell proliferation and granulation tissue formation by increasing blood flow and stimulating growth factor expression that together accelerate ulcer healing and protects the mucosa (Sánchez-Fidalgo *et al.*, 2004).

Furthermore, COX-2 stimulates PGE_2 production (Shen *et al.*, 2005). Prostaglandins are produced in response to several extrinsic stimuli and regulate cellular growing and differentiation and homeostasis (Fukushima, 1990). CL was able to maintain PGE_2 level near to sham group, even with indomethacin administration. Indomethacin is a non-steroidal anti-inflammatory drug that injuries the gastric mucosa through inhibition of PGE_2 production through COX enzyme. This result evidenced that CL healing effect includes PGE_2 production. Moraes *et al.* (2009) also found the involvement of PGE_2 in the gastroprotective effect of the essential oil of another specie of Citrus. The protective effects of PGE_2 on gastric mucosa are a consequence of various mechanisms that include enhancement in the mucosal sulfhydryl compounds (Brzozowski *et al.*, 2005), amelioration of mucosal blood flow and increased epithelial mucus secretion (Motilva *et al.*, 2005), that is specially favorable to ulcer healing, since the mucus layer protects the newly formed cells against damage caused by acid pH and proteolytic potential of gastric secretions (Valcheva-Kuzmanova *et al.*, 2005). PAS staining and electron microscopy (Figure 4.1) showed intense and homogenous mucus secretion in the CL group, with several empty mucous vesicles in the mucous neck cells and intense alteration of cell apical surface, indicating exocytosis. Release of preformed mucus plays a role in promoting epithelial recovery by forming a mucoid cap beneath which re-epithelization occurs (Banerjee *et al.*, 2008).

Limonene and β-pinene were the majoritary substances identified in CL by gas chromatography. Limonene is a monocyclic monoterpene and is a major constituent of several Citrus oils. It has been used for relief of heartburn and gastroesophageal reflux disorder (GERD) because of its gastric acid neutralizing effect and improvement of peristalsis (Sun, 2007). It has also demonstrated chemopreventive activity against many types of cancer including gastric (Yano *et al.*, 1999) and colorectal (Vigushim *et al.*, 1998) cancer. Recent reports (Riyazi *et al.*, 2007; Liapi *et al.*, 2007) have shown that the monoterpene β-pinene exerts an antispasmodic effect at the rat ileum and provokes antinociceptive actions in rats.

The balance between the therapeutic versus the toxicological effects of a drug is an important parameter in assessing its applicability as an antiulcer or a pharmacological agent. Although acetic acid-induced gastric ulcer model was not a specific method to analyze toxicological effects from drugs, this method simulates the treatment condition for 14 days and aids in the acquisition of these important toxicological parameters. None of the treatments showed toxicity in rats given that body weight normally progressed during the treatment in all groups. Although biochemical analysis of the animals' serum showed no significant difference among all groups, organ weights showed that, in the CL group, kidneys were heavier relative to body weight in comparison with control groups. It occurred probably because limonene, the major constituent of this essential oil, could produce tumors only in the kidneys of male rats in association with hyaline-droplet nephropathy, which is due to the accumulation of the rat-specific, low molecular weight protein alpha(2μ)-globulin in the P_2 segment cells of renal proximal tubules. Mice of both genders and female rats showed no evidence of any tumor (Sun, 2007). Human urine contains no alpha(2μ)-globulin and, compared with the male rat, much less protein and almost no low-molecular-weight protein. Thus, there is no risk of kidney cancer for humans from limonene, since the binding of limonene to alpha(2μ)-globulin would not occur (Whysner and Williams, 1996). Besides relatively heavier kidneys, CL was not harmful to rats because biochemical analyses did not show alteration in creatinine or urea values that would indicate kidney lesion.

Finally, we can conclude that essential oil from CL could be a good option for the treatment of gastric ulcer and exerts its action by stimulating COX-2 production and PGE_2 secretion, which are important factors to epithelial cell proliferation, granulation tissue formation and mucus production and secretion, thus protecting the mucosa against the lesive effects of gastric secretions. This essential oil also stimulates cell recruitment to submucosa, which renews the epithelium, accelerating ulcer healing. This is the first study elucidating the effect of a Citrus essential oil in gastric ulcer healing.

Acknowledgements

This work was supported by Fundação de Amparo à Pesquisa do Estado de São Paulo (FAPESP).

References

Adams, R.P. (1995). Identification of essential oil Components by Gas Cromatography/ Mass Spectroscopy. Allured Publ Corp, Carol Stream, Illinois.

Aloisi, A.M., Ceccarelli, I., Masi, F., and Scaramuzzino, A. (2002). Effects of the essential oil from *Citrus lemon* in male and female rats exposed to a persistent painful stimulation. *Behavioral Brain Research*, **136(1):** 127-135.

Arun, M., and Asha, V.V. (2008). Gastroprotective effect of *Dodonaea viscosa* on various experimental ulcer models. *Journal of Ethnopharmacology*, **118:** 460–465.

Banerjee, D., Maity, B., Nag, S.K., Bandyopadhyay, S.K., and Chattopadhyay, S. (2008). Healing potential of *Picrorhiza kurroa* (Scrofulariaceae) rhizomes against indomethacin-induced gastric ulceration: a mechanistic exploration. *BMC Complementary and Alternative Medicine*, **8:** 3.

Brzozowski, T., Konturek, P.C., Konturek, S.J., Brzozowska, I., and Pawlik, T. (2005). Role of prostaglandins in gastroprotection and gastric adaptation. *Journal of Physiology and Pharmacology*, **56(5):** 33-55.

Butterfield, T.A., Best, T.M., and Merrick, M.A. (2006). The dual roles of neutrophils and macrophages in inflammation: a critical balance between tissue damage and repair. *Journal of Athletic Training*, **41(4):** 457–465.

Calvo, T.R., Lima, Z.P., Silva, J.S., Ballesteros, K.V., Pellizzon, C.H., Hiruma-Lima, C.A., Tamashiro, J., Brito, A.R., Takahira, R.K., and Vilegas, W. (2007). Constituents and antiulcer effect of *Alchornea glandulosa*: activation of cell proliferation in gastric mucosa during the healing process. *Biological and Pharmaceutical Bulletin*, **30(3):** 451-459.

Ceccarelli, I., Lariviere, W.R., Fiorenzani, P., Sacerdote, P., and Aloisi, A.M. (2004). Effects of long-term exposure of lemon essential oil odor on behavioral, hormonal and neuronal parameters in male and female rats. *Brain Research*, **1001(1-2):** 78-86.

Celis, J.E., and Celis, A. (1985). Individual nuclei in polykaryons can control cyclin distribution and DNA synthesis. *EMBO Journal*, **4(5):** 1187-1192.

Cotran, R.S. (1999). Gastric ulceration. *In:* Robbins Pathologic Basis of Disease, Ed by Cotran, R.S., Kumar, V., Robbins, S.L., Saunders, USA, pp. 298–299.

Curtis, G.H., Macnaughton, W.K., Gall, D.G., and Wallace, J.L. (1995). Intraluminal pH modulates gastric prostaglandin synthesis. *Canadian Journal of Physiology and Pharmacology*, **73:** 130-134.

Fukushima, M. (1990). Prostaglandin J2-anti-tumour and anti-viral activities and the mechanisms involved. *Eicosanoids*, **3:** 189-199.

Hiruma-Lima, C.A., Gracioso, J.S., Bighetti, E.J.B., Kassisse, D.M.G., Nunes, D.S., and Souza-Brito, A.R.M. (2002). Effect of essential oil obtained from *Croton cajucara* Benth. on gastric ulcer healing and protective factors of the gastric mucosa. *Phytomedicine*, **9:** 523-529.

Liapi, C., Anifantis, G., Chinou, I., Kourounakis, A.P., Theodosopoulos, S., and Galanopoulou, P. (2007). Antinociceptive properties of 1,8-Cineole and β-pinene, from the essential oil of *Eucalyptus camaldulensis* leaves, in rodents. *Planta Medica*, **73(12):** 1247-1254.

Lu, H., and Graham, D.Y. (2006). New development in the mechanistic understanding of peptic ulcer diseases. *Drug Discovery Today*, **3(4):** 431-437.

Martelli, A., Mattlioli, F., Mereto, E., Brambilla, C.G., Sini, D., Bergamaschi, R., and Brambilla, G. (1998). Evaluation of omeprazole genotoxicity in a battery of *in vitro* and *in vivo* assays. *Toxicology*, **30:** 29–41.

Moraes, T.M., Kushima, H., Moleiro, F.C., Santos, R.C., Rocha, L.R.M., Marques, M.O., Vilegas, W., Hiruma-Lima, C.A. (2009). Effects of limonene and essential oil from *Citrus aurantium* on gastric mucosa: Role of prostaglandins and gastric mucus secretion. *Chemico-Biological Interactions*, **180:** 499–505.

Motilva, V., La Lastra, C.A., Bruseghini, L., Herrerias, J.M., and Sánchez-Fidalgo, S. (2005). COX expression and PGE(2) and PGD(2) production in experimental acute and chronic gastric lesions. *International Immunopharmacology*, **5(2):** 369-379.

Medicinal Plants: Phytochemistry, Pharmacology and Therapeutics Vol. 2 (2012) *Pages* **69–79**
Editor-in-Chief: **V.K. Gupta**
Published by: **DAYA PUBLISHING HOUSE, NEW DELHI**

5

The Importance of Dietary Plant Lectins: The Blood Type Diet Revisited

Sunniva B.L. Helleland[1] and Ian F. Pryme[1*]

ABSTRACT

Plant lectins resist proteolysis and survive passage through the alimentary tract in a biologically and immunologically active form due to their inherent structural and functional features as complex glycoproteins. Since the gut surface is glycosylated, orally ingested lectins have the potential to interact with different parts of the gastrointestinal tract and exert powerful effects on its structure, function, digestive capacity, immune state and bacterial flora. Dietary lectins can therefore influence the nutritional state and health of humans and animals. These molecules are generally poorly recognised as important dietary constituents but an understanding of their biological properties is gradually making an impact on scientists and physicians. Since lectins are proteins they are denatured by heat and thereby lose their biological activity. Processing of plant-based material using high temperature (cooking, frying, grilling etc.) will thus drastically reduce the lectin content. Many national campaigns (for example "Eat 5 a day") have been aimed at mounting the public awareness of the importance of increasing the dietary content of fruit, nuts and vegetables. Such campaigns, however, have largely failed. Unfortunately "fast food" has become more and more popular resulting in a further decrease in our intake of fresh fruit and vegetables. Concerning the scientific basis regarding the importance of dietary lectins many people have undoubtedly been confused by the writings of D´Adamo who has coupled the 4 blood types up against specific diets where certain lectin-containing food commodities are recommended in the diet, or should be lacking. Using in vitro tests lectins have been shown to agglutinate red blood cells. If this were to occur in the body then D´Adamo warns that emboli produced could well be life-threatening. There

1 Department of Biomedicine, University of Bergen,Jonas Liesvei 91, N-5009 Bergen, Norway.

* *Corresponding author*: E-mail: ian.pryme@biomed.uib.no

is no clinical indication that this is the case. In this review our current knowledge of the importance of dietary lectins is considered in light of the blood type diet hypothesis lanced by D´Adamo.

Keywords : Agglutination, Blood groups, Fruit, Glycoproteins, Health, Immunomodulation, NK-cells, Vegetables.

Introduction

Stillmark (1888) reported that components in castor bean extracts were able to agglutinate red blood cells from different animal species. The seed extracts were found to contain haemagglutinating proteins, defined as haemaglutinins or agglutinins. During the early part of the last century it was demonstrated that some haemaglutinins had the property of selectively agglutinating *in vitro* red blood cells from particular blood groups in the ABO-system (see Sharon, 1998). This led to the introduction of the term lectin since this means to select or choose. The group of proteins termed lectins has become a very heterogeneous group of proteins of non-immune origin and have gone through several definition steps resulting in lesser strictness over the years. Some years ago Van Damme *et al.* (1997) defined lectins as "carbohydrate-binding proteins possessing at least one non-catalytic domain, which bind reversibly to a specific mono- or oligosaccharide". The continuous discovery of new and diverse lectins with similarities found in several different classes of proteins seems to call for even less strict definitions in the future. Maybe the most accurate lectin definition would simply be: "proteins that specifically bind or cross-bind carbohydrates". Van Damme *et al.* (1997) have introduced a new and unambigous classification system of lectins.

A large number of plant, animal and microbe lectins have now been isolated (Prokop *et al.*, 1968; Ashwell and Morell, 1974; Barondes, 1981; Liener *et al.*, 1986; Mirelman and Ofek, 1986; Van Damme *et al.*, 1997). Lectins are widespread in the plant kingdom (fruits, nuts, vegetables), occurring in seeds and all kinds of vegetative tissues, and often take part in the plants defence system against predators such as insects, worms etc. (Chrispeels and Raikhel, 1991; Debenham, 2005). In many cases lectins severely interfere with digestive processes in such predators. Lectins and many other low molecular weight components in foodstuffs are thus called antinutrients because they often have a negative impact on the nutritional value of diets containing them. However, most of the antinutritional effects can be eliminated or substantially reduced with proper storage, heat treatment, soaking, germinating and cooking. As biologically active proteins some are able to modify and sometimes improve gut function and body metabolism, and thus can also improve health status as well. Animal lectins are usually secreted from the cells where they may participate in cell-cell-interactions, recognition of immune defence system, immunoregulation and prohibition of autoimmunity (Petersen *et al.*, 2001; Holmskov *et al.*, 2002; Wallis, 2002). Due to the homology between plant and animal lectins, it is likely that the dietary plant lectins to some extent can mimic and amplify the effects normally exerted by their lectin counterparts produced by the animals themselves.

Oral Intake of Lectins

Lectins are found in almost all fruits, nuts and vegetables that are present in our every day diets (Table 5.1). The dietary intake of lectins can therefore be quite considerable (Gonzalez de Mejía and Prisecaru, 2005). Lectins are often heavily glycosylated such that many lectins taken orally are resistant to the low pH in the stomach and to attack by the proteolytic enzymes present in the digestive juices in the small intestine. They thus remain fully biologically and immunogenically active during their passage through the entire alimentary canal (Table 5.2; Pusztai *et al.*, 1990).

Table 5.1. Examples of some important dietary lectins.

Lectins	*Lectin–Abbreviation*	*Plant of Derivation*	*Latin Name*
Banana lectin	BanLek	Banana	*Musa acuminata* L.
Phytohemagglutinin, leukoagglutinin	PHA, PHA-L	Kidney bean	*Phaseolus vulgaris* L.
Pea agglutinin	PSA	Pea	*Pisum sativum* L.
Peanut	PNA	Peanut	*Arachis hypogaea*
Potato	STL	Potato	*Solanum tuberosum*
Rice bran agglutinin	RBA	Rice bran	*Oryza sativa* L.
Soya bean agglutinin	SBA	Soya bean	*Glycine max*
Lycopersicon esculentum agglutinin	LEA	Tomato	*Lycopersicon esculentum*

Table 5.2. Survival of some dietary lectins in the gastrointestinal tract.

Lectins	*Plant of Derivation*	*Latin Name*	*% Recovery**
Concanavalin (Con A)	Castor bean	*Canavalia ensiformis*	>90
Phytohemagglutinin, leukoagglutinin (PHA/PHA-L)	Kidney bean	*Phaseolus vulgaris* L	>90
SNA-II	Elderberry	*Sambucus nigra*	>60
SNA-I	Elderberry	*Sambucus nigra*	50-60
Wheat germ agglutinin (WGA)	Wheat	*Triticum vulgare*	50-60
SBA	Soya bean	*Glycine max*	40-50
Lycopersicon esculentum (LEA) agglutinin	Tomato	*Lycopersicon esculentum*	40-50
Pea agglutinin (PSL)	Pea	*Pisum sativum* L	30-40

* The per cent recovery of the individual lectins is based on the percentage lectin remaining 1h after intragastric intubation of a solution of pure lectin (10mg in PBS) to rats fasted for 16h prior to the experiment. Adapted from Pusztai *et al.* (1996).

The surface of the mammalian gut is highly glycosylated and the epithelium is covered by glycolipids and glycoproteins. Through their saccharide binding, lectins bind to epithelial membrane glycoproteins, including receptors of hormones, growth factors and cytokines, transport proteins and brush-border membrane enzymes, glycolipids, gangliosides and secreted mucins (Pusztai *et al.*, 1990, 1995). Although lectins binding is most extensive in the small intestine, similar binding does occur throughout the entire digestive system from the oral cavity to the distal colon. The lectins, following binding to the cell, can send information into the cell´s interior via second messengers, often modulating gene expression (Bardocz *et al.*, 1995), or by the lectins itself entering the cell through endocytosis.

Among the major effects mediated by lectin binding in the digestive tract are hyperplasia and an increase in crypt cell production rate (Bardocz *et al.*, 1994a,b; Pryme *et al.*, 1998a), and immunostimulation (Lavelle *et al.*, 2000). Both hyperplasia and immunostimulation are indeed interesting aspects in cancer research.

Oral Immunogenicity

The function of the gut associated lymphoid tissue is to absorb minute samples of oral antigens via M-cells of Peyers patches and activate the gut immune system. As lectins are able to bind to M-cells (Sharma *et al.*, 1996), their endocytosis is more extensive, which makes them more powerful immunogens than other antigens. Lectins influence the immune system by evoking local and systemic immune responses (Bardocz *et al.*, 1999). In a series of publications Lavelle *et al.* (Lavelle, 1999; Lavelle *et al.*, 2000, 2001, 2002) have clearly shown that lectins when administered either orally or intranasally can result in the production of specific serum IgG and IgA antibodies to the lectins. Mitogenic lectins are inducers of lymphocyte proliferation. Several components of the immune system, such as mast cells, basophils, eosinophils and others produce or release cytokines and chemokines (Ebisawa *et al.*, 1997) when exposed to appropriate lectins.

Functions of Dietary Lectins

Sharma *et al.* (1996) demonstrated that a series of plant lectins can bind to receptors on the surfaces of human intestinal cells (biopsy material). Following binding to appropriate receptors lectins can then propagate release of intracellular second messenger molecules that ultimately instigate a series of different biological responses (Bardocz *et al.*, 1995; Pryme *et al.*, 2007; Winge *et al.*, 2010). This unique group of proteins thus possesses potent biological activity following their ingestion. Several lectins, for example, have been found to possess anticancer properties both *in vitro, in vivo*, and in human case studies (Gonzalez de Mejía and Prisecaru, 2005; Pryme *et al.*, 1998b, 2004, 2007). Some lectins can preferentially bind to cancer cell membranes or their receptors, causing cytotoxicity upon internalization and activation, resulting in apoptosis and cessation of tumour growth (González De Mejía, and Dia, 2010). Lectins are able to modify the cell cycle by inducing non-apoptotic G1-phase accumulation mechanisms, G2/M phase cell cycle arrest and apoptosis, and can activate the caspase cascade. Lectins can also down-regulate telomerase activity and result in an inhibition of angiogenesis (González De Mejía, and Dia, 2010). Ingestion of specific lectins can lead to a sequestration of the available body pool of polyamines, resulting in reduced cancer cell growth (Pryme *et al.*, 1999; Pryme, 2007). Many lectins have been shown to stimulate the immune system by altering the production of various interleukins. This may indeed be an extremely important property of the dietary lectins since they are able to prime the immune system, thus keeping it activated.

Winge *et al.* (2010) performed a small pilot study to evaluate whether or not a lectin-containing preparation taken orally was able to modulate the immune system in healthy adults. Eight healthy individuals took the preparation daily for a period of three months. Blood samples were taken both before and during the study. All individuals demonstrated the presence of anti-lectin antibodies in the blood at day 84, showing the occurrence of an immune response. No antibodies were identified at the onset of the study. During the period of observation four cell types showed a marked response: activated IL-2 helper cells, memory cells, activated T-cells and activated natural killer (NK) cells. In general the levels of activated IL-2 helper cells and memory cells were elevated on day 28 with a return to normal levels on day 84. The levels of activated T-cells and the activated NK cells, however, were still elevated on day 84. At the start of the investigation four of the individuals had levels of NK cells that were well below normal values. At 84 days, however, three of these had values that were now within the normal range. It is likely that keeping the NK cell level within normal levels is of major importance in order to maintain a potent first line of attack against virus and bacterial infections. Furthermore, it has been known for many years that in animals with low levels of NK cell activity there is an increased number of both spontaneous and experimental tumours (Talmadge *et al.*, 1980; Gorelik *et al.*1982; Okumura *et al.*, 1982). It would seem likely that NK cells have a similar role in the immunologic surveillance against cancer in humans and that plant lectins here play a vital role (Takeda and Okumura, 2004). There is, therefore, a strong indication of the importance of keeping the number of activated NK cells in the blood within normal limits. It is thus evident that to ensure long-term good health the diet needs to have an adequate content of plant lectins. Pusztai *et al.* (2008) have expressed the opinion that lectins will almost certainly have a major impact in biomedicine in forthcoming years. Pryme *et al.* (2007) have advocated the use of oral mistletoe lectins in cancer therapy.

According to current nutritional guidelines one is recommended to consume a diet consisting of a high intake of fruit, nuts and vegetables. National campaigns encouraging people to eat "Five a day", equivalent to about 400g of fruit and vegetables, have not been particularly successful. In Scotland, for example, daily consumption between 1993 and 2000 only increased from 190g to 200g. Since there is considerable evidence that consumption of sufficient amounts of fruit and vegetables has an impact on preventing many chronic diseases (heart disease, stroke, several form of cancers – for example see Johnsen *et al.*, 2003 and Rissanen *et al.*, 2003) such results are extremely disheartening. It is also important to remember that plant lectins, being proteins, will be subject to denaturation when heated. Thus cooking, frying, grilling, heating in a microwave oven etc. will drastically reduce the active lectin content of the food.

Conclusions

It is evident that there are major differences of opinion between the claims of D´Adamo and the scientific community, both with respect to the scientific content and the manner by which D´Adamo has founded his approach in formulating the blood type diet. There is also a difficulty in coming to terms with the positive results that have been reported.

Industrially processed food forms an increasing part of every day life. The means by which such food is prepared will often result in a loss (degradation, denaturation etc.) of biologically active molecules *e.g.*, lectins. As mentioned above lectins can have extremely important functions and their "removal" from the diet would therefore not be desirable. A person closely following the blood type diet would probably eat lower amounts of processed food than non-followers, meaning that their diet would have a higher active lectin content. This may then afford an explanation for some of the positive effects that D´Adamo has described. The positive results that people have reported may well be explained by a general improvement in life style and health attitudes such as less fat, salt, sugar, more fruit and vegetables, reduced smoking, a lower alcohol consumption, and a higher level of physical activities. It is thus quite possible that the overall effect of D´Adamo´s dietary recommendations have in fact been positive by increasing public awareness of what they eat. On the other hand his warning of the potential hazards of dietary lectins would seem to be unfounded. Accumulating scientific evidence in fact clearly indicates that dietary lectins are important constituents of our diet, along with vitamins, minerals, trace elements, antioxidants and the 3 and 6-omega fatty acids.

References

Ashwell, G. and Morell, A.G. (1974). The role of surface carbohydrates in the hepatic recognition and transport of circulating glycoproteins. *Advances in Enzymology and Related Areas in Molecular Biology,* **41** : 99-128.

Bardocz, S., Grant, G., Duguid, T. J., Brown, D. S., Pusztai, A. and Pryme, I.F. (1994a). Effect of phytohaemagglutinin on the growth of Krebs II tumour cells, body metabolism and internal organs of mice. *International Journal of Oncology,* **5** : 1369-74. I. F. (1994a) *Int. J. Oncol. 5,* 1369-1374.

Bardocz, S., Grant, G., Duguid, T. J., Brown, D. S., Sakhri, M., Pusztai, A., Pryme, I. F., Mayer, D. and Wayβ, K. (1994b). Phytohaemagglutinin in the diet induces growth of the gut and modifies some organ weights in mice. *Medical Science Research,* **22**: 101-3.

Bardocz, S., Ewen, S.W.B., Grant, G. and Pusztai, A. (1995). Lectins as growth for the small intestine and the gut. *In;* Lectins : Biomedical Perspectives. *Ed.* by Pusztai, A. and Bardocz, S., Taylor and Francis, London, UK, pp. 103-16.

Bardocz, S., Grant, G., Pusztai, A. and Ewen, S.W.B. (1999). Lectins as gut growth factors – a summary. *In;* Effects of antinutrients on the nutritional value of legume diets. *Ed.* by Bardocz, S., Hajós, G., and Pusztai, A., *COST 98,* Vol. **6**, Luxembourg. pp. 61-4.

Barondes, S. H. (1981). Lectins: their multiple endogenous cellular functions. *Annual Reviews Biochemistry*, **50** : 207-31.

Chrispeels, M.J. and Raikhel, N.V. (1991). Lectins, lectin genes and their role in plant defence. *The Plant Cell*, **3** : 1-9.

D´Adamo, P.J. and Whitney, P.C. (1996). *Eat Right 4 Your Type*. G.P. Putnam´s Sons

Debenham, M. (2005). Waiting to fight? Lectins´ passive defence role in plants. *Biologist*, **52** : 74-9.

Ebisawa, M., Tachimoto, H., Iikura, Y., Akiyami, K. and Saito, H. (1997), *Progress in Allergy and Clinical Immunology*, Vol. **4**, Hogrefe and Huber Publishers, Seattle, Toronto, Bern, Göttingen.

González De Mejía, E. and Prisecaru, V.L. (2005). Lectins as bioactive plant proteins: A potential in cancer treatment. *Critical Reviews in Food Science and Nutrition*, **45**: 425–45.

González De Mejía, E. and Dia, V.P. (2010). The role of neutraceutical proteins and peptides in apoptosis, angiogenesis, and metastasis of cancer cells. *Cancer Metastasis Reviews*, **29** : 511-28.

Gorelik, E., Wiltrout, R.H., Okumura, K., Habu, S. and Herberman, R.B. (1982). Role of NK cells in the control of metastatic spread and growth of tumor cells in mice. *International Journal of Cancer*, **30**: 107–12.

Holmskov, U., Thiel, S. and Jensenius, J.C. (2003). Collectins and ficolins: humoral lectins of the innate immune defense. *Annual Reviews Immunology*, **21** : 547-78.

Johnsen, S.P., Overvad, K., Stripp, C., Tjønneland, A., Husted, S.E. and Sørensen, H.T. (2003). Intake of fruit and vegetables and the risk of ischemic stroke in a cohort of Danish men and women. *American Journal of Clinical Nutrition*, **78** : 57-64.

Lavelle, E. C. (1999). Lectins in oral vaccination. *In;* Effects of antinutrients on the nutritional value of legume diets. *Ed.* by Bardocz, S., Hajós, G., and Pusztai, A., *COST 98*, Vol. **6**, Luxembourg. pp. 148-59.

Lavelle, E. C., Grant, G., Pusztai, A., Pfuller, U. and O'Hagan, D.T. (2000). Mucosal immunogenicity of plant lectins in mice. *Immunology*, **99** : 30-7.

Lavelle, E.C., Grant, G., Pusztai, A., Pfüller, U. and O'Hagan, D.T. (2001). The identification of plant lectins with mucosal adjuvant activity. *Immunology*, **102**: 77–86.

Lavelle, E.C., Grant, G., Pusztai, A., Pfüller, U., Leavy, O., McNeela, E., Mills, K.H. and O'Hagan, D.T. (2002). Mistletoe lectins enhance immune responses to intranasally co-administered herpes simplex virus glycoprotein D_2. *Immunology*, **107**: 268–74.

Liener, I. E., Sharon, N., and Goldstein, I. J. (1986). *The lectins, properties, functions and application in biology and medicine*, Academic Press, New York.

Mirelman, D. and Ofek, I. (1986). *Microbial Lectins and Agglutinins*, Willey Sons, New York.

Okumura, K., Habu, S. and Kasai, M. (1982). The role of NK cells in resistance of *in vivo* tumors. *Advances in Experimental Medicine and Biology*, **155**: 773–84.

Petersen, S. V., Thiel, S., Jensen, L., Steffensen, R. and Jensenius, J. C. (2001). An assay for the mannan-binding lectin pathway of complement activation. *Journal of Immunological Methods*, **257** : 107-16.

Prokop, O., Uhlenbruck, G. and Kohler, W. (1968). A new source of antibody-like substances having anti-blood group specificity. A discussion on the specificity of Helix agglutinins. *Vox Sanguinis*, **14** : 321-33.

Pryme, I. F., Pusztai, A., Bardocz, S. and Ewen, S.W.B. (1998a). The induction of gut hyperplasia by phytohaemagglutinin in the diet and limitation of tumour growth. *Histology and Histopathology*, **13** : 575-83.

Pryme, I.F., Bardócz, S., Grant, G., Duguid, T.J., Brown, D.S. and Pusztai, A. (1998b). The effect of PHA on the growth and polyamine content of Krebs II non- Hodgkin lymphoma tumour in mice. *In* : Biogenically Active Amines in Food, *Ed.* by Bardócz, S., White, A. and Hajós, G., *COST 917, Vol.* 2. Luxembourg, pp. 123-9.

Pryme, I. F., Grant, G., Pusztai, A. and Bardocz, S. (1999). Limiting the availability of polyamines for a developing tumour : An alternative approach to reducing tumour growth. In : Polyamines in Health and Nutrition, *Ed.* by Bardocz, S. and White, A., Kluwer Academic Publishers, Nirwell, Mass. USA, pp 283 -91.

Pryme, I. F., Bardocz, S., Pusztai, A., Ewen, S.W.B. and Pfüller, U. (2004). A mistletoe lectin (ML-1)-containing diet reduces the viability of a murine non-Hodgkin lymphoma tumor. *Cancer Detection and Prevention*, **28** : 52-6.

Pryme, I. F. (2007). Reducing the availability of polyamines for a developing tumour. *Biochemical Society Transactions*, **35** : 340-2.

Pryme, I.F., Dale, T.M. and Tilrem, P. (2007). Oral mistletoe lectins : A case for their use in cancer therapy. *Cancer Therapy*, **5**: 287–300.

Pusztai, A., Ewen, S. W., Grant, G., Peumans, W. J., van Damme, E. J., Rubio, L. and Bardocz, S. (1990). Relationship between survival and binding of plant lectins during small intestinal passage and their effectiveness as growth factors. *Digestion*, **46** : 308-16.

Pusztai, A., Ewen, S. W., Grant, G., Peumans, W. J., Van Damme, E. J., Coates, M. E. and Bardocz, S. (1995). *Glycoconjugate Journal*, **12** : 22-35.

Pusztai, A., Ewen, S. W., Grant, G. and Bardocz, S. (1996). Effects of lectins on digestion of food and body metabolism. *In;* Effects of antinutrients on the nutritional value of legume diets. *Ed.* by Bardocz, S., Gelencsér, É. and Pusztai, A., *COST 98*, Vol. **1**, Luxembourg. pp. 22-8.

Pusztai, A., Bardocz, S. and Ewen, S.W.B. (2008). Uses of plant lectins in bioscience and biomedicine. *Frontiers in Bioscience*, **13**: 1130–40.

Rissanen, T.H., Voutilainen, S., Virtanen, J.K., Venho, B., Vanharanta, M., Mursu, J. and Salonen, J.T. (2003). Low intake of fruits, berries and vegetables is associated with excess mortality in men: the Kuopio Ischaemic Heart Disease Risk Factor (KIHD) Study. *Journal of Nutrition*, **133** : 199-204

Sharma, R., van Damme, E. J., Peumans, W. J., Sarsfield, P., and Schumacher, U. (1996). Lectin binding reveals divergent carbohydrate expression in human and mouse Peyer's patches. *Histochemistry and Cell Biology*, **105** : 459-65.

Sharon, N. (1998). Glycoproteins now and then : A personal account. *Acta Anatomica Basel*, **161** : 1-4, 7-17.

Stillmark, H. (1888). Über Ricin, ein giftiges Ferment aus dem Samen von *Ricinus comm.* und einigen anderen Euphorbiaceen, *Inaug Diss Dorpat University.*

Takeda, K. and Okumura, K. (2004). CAM and NK cells. *Evidence based Complimentary and Alternative Medicine*, **1** : 17-27

Talmadge, J.E., Meyers, K.M., Prieur, D.J. and Starkey, J.R. (1980). Role of NK cells in tumour growth and metastasis in beige mice. *Nature*, **284**: 622–4.

Wallis, R. (2002). Structural and functional aspects of complement activation by mannose-binding protein. *Immunobiology*, **205** : 433-45.

Winge, I., Dale, T.M., Tilrem, J.P.P. and Pryme, I.F. (2010). A mistletoe lectin-containing preparation for oral use provokes an immune response and induces an increase in the population of activated natural killer cells. *In* : Comprehensive Bioactive Natural Products. *Ed.* by Gupta, V.K. Vol. **5**, Immune-modulation and vaccine adjuvants. Studium Press LLC, USA, pp. 283-99.

Van Damme, E. J. M., Peumans, W. J., Pusztai, A., and Bardocz, S. (1997). Handbook of Plant Lectins: Properties and Biomedical Applications, Wiley and Sons Ltd, Chichester, UK.

Yamamoto, F., Clausen, H., White, T., Marken, J. and Hakomori, S. (1990). Molecular genetic basis of the histo-blood group ABO system, *Nature*, **345** : 229-33.

Medicinal Plants: Phytochemistry, Pharmacology and Therapeutics Vol. 2 (2012) *Pages* **81–95**
Editor-in-Chief: **V.K. Gupta**
Published by: **DAYA PUBLISHING HOUSE, NEW DELHI**

6

Labisia pumila (Kacip Fatimah), a Malaysian Medicinal Herb: An Update

G.D. Singh[1]*, S. Singh[1], A. Koul[1], P. Kaul[1] and V.K. Gupta[1]

ABSTRACT

Labisia pumila (Myrsinaceae), known as "Kacip Fatimah", is popular medicinal herb amongst the local womenfolk in Malaysia. For over 400 years, a decoction of the whole plant is used in folk medicine by Malay women one to two months prior to childbirth as well as a post-partum medicine. The plant was found to exert uterotrophic action and significantly decreased stress hormones. Furthermore, immunomodulatory, antioxidative and skin protection activities have been reported of this plant. Recently many commercial products are available in the form of capsules and canned drinks containing the powdered plant and its extracts in the Malaysian market for human use. This review highlights the importance and significance of Labisia pumila as potential source of traditional medicine in Malaysia.

Keywords: *Labisia pumila,* Antioxidant, Antistress, Immunomodulatory, Skin protection, Postpartum medication.

Introduction

Labisia pumila (Myrsinaceae), popularly known as "Kacip Fatimah", has been used by many generation of the Malay women to induce and facilitate childbirth as well as a post-partum medicine (Burkill, 1935). *Labisia pumila* is a member of the small genus of slightly woody plants of the family Myrsinaceae. Although the common name of the plant is Kacip Fatimah but is also known by the other names such as

1 Division of Pharmacology and Natural Product Chemistry, Indian Institute of Integrative Medicine (CSIR), Canal Road, Jammu-Tawi – 180 001, J&K State, India.

* *Corresponding author*: E-mail: singh_gd@iiim.ac.in

Selusoh Fatimah, Rumpur Siti Fatimah, Kacit Fatimah, Pokok Pinggang, Rumput Palis, Tadah Matahari, Mata Pelanduk Rimba (Malay); Sangkoh (Iban). There are at least four known varieties of *Labisia pumila* found in Malaysia. Though, only three of them are popularly used by the Malays and are recognized as *Labisia pumila* var. *pumila* (LPP), *Labisia pumila* var. *alata* (LPA) and *Labisia pumila* var. *lanceolata* (LPL) (Stone, 1988). It is imperative to differentiate the three varieties in terms of their physical and chemical characteristics as well as biological activity, in order to determine the proper plant material for use, hence producing quality herbal medicines with proven safety and efficacy. Mainly the plant is wild, cultivation just started and research is being conducted to improve the planting stock and propagation techniques.

The current high rate of demand and methods of harvesting medicinal plants, particularly from the wild, for the herbal market has lowered natural population sizes for many species. Even for wild American ginseng (*Panax quinquefolius*), regardless of its historical abundance, in some locations it has been reduced to populations of a few dozen individuals (Van der Voort, 1998). This has made research on the propagation of medicinal plants more urgent than ever. There is, presently a great local market demand for Kacip Fatimah especially as afterbirth tonic. However, paucity exists in technical information on plant identification, propagation techniques, agronomy and silvicultural aspects (Jaganath and Ng, 2000). Each variety commands a different use and thus, it is important to ensure that the right variety is used in each case.

Species identification is made difficult by the lack of difference in the leaves and petioles between var. *alata* and var. *pumila*. Thus, an efficient method of authentification needs to be developed. Preliminary studies had been conducted previously on *Labisia pumila* using the agroforestry approach involving intercropping of *Labisia pumila* under rubber and rattan (pers. Comm. Khozirah Shaari). However, the planting of *Labisia pumila* as a monoculture crop has yet to be studied but nonetheless, these studies showed that *Labisia pumila* was best propagated by seeds or root cuttings. The plants thrive best in shady areas and non-waterlogged, humus rich soil. *Labisia pumila* has also been used by the indigenous people of the Malay Archipelago for menstrual irregularities and post partum. The plants are usually boiled and water soluble extract taken as a drink. Interest has recently been shown in the herbal preparation to determine its mode of action and potential pharmacological application.

Labisia pumila, or Kacip Fatimah, is part of a genus of approximately seven species and is found in Southeast Asia in the lowlands and hill forests of Malaysia at an altitude of 300 to 700 m. It is a small sub-herbaceous perennial shrub with creeping stems growing from 30 to 40 cm in height (Figure 6.1). The leaves are elliptical-lanceolate in shape. The upper side of the leaf is dark green and the underside is light green to reddish-purple. The whole leaf can be more than 30 cm long and 13 cm wide. The clustered whitish to pink flowers are 6 to 30 cm long with sepals, petals, and stamens. The flowers produce a round, bright red to purple fruit 0.5 cm in diameter when ripe (Foster *et al.*, 2009; Mannerås *et al.*, 2010). Although this plant has not been subjected to a detailed pharmacological investigation, some biological activities have recently been documented which have attracted enormous attention of researchers worldwide to experimentally validate the therapeutic uses of this medicinal herb.

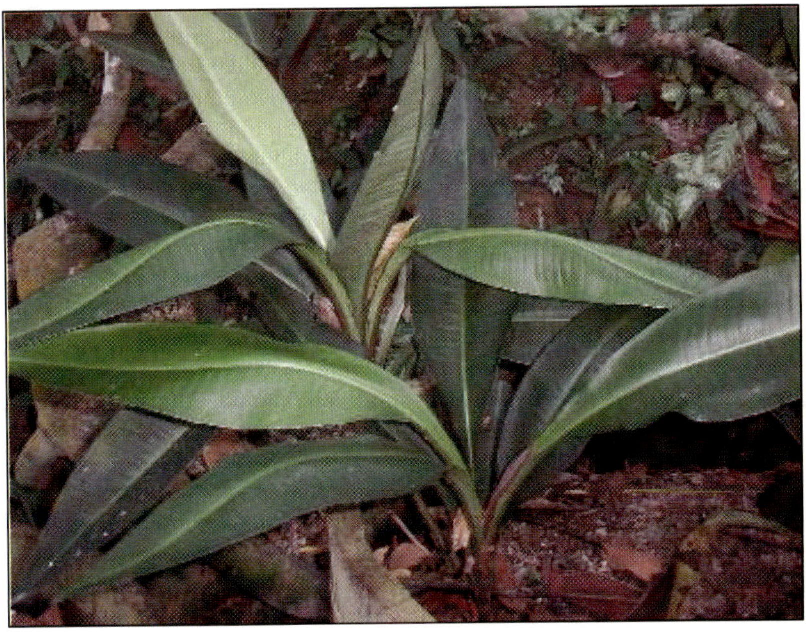

Figure 6.1. *Labisia pumila* (Kacip Fatimah).

Labisia pumila has been utilized by many generations of Malay women for the purpose of inducing and in the facilitation of labour. Water decoctions of the root or whole plant were and are still given to pregnant woman one to two months prior to childbirth (Burkill, 1935; Stone, 1988). It is also used as a postpartum medication (Stone, 1988) in the form of mixed preparation to help in the contraction of uterus. Further, *Labisia pumila* is reported to delay fertility and to help regain body strength of mothers (Zakaria and Mohd, 1994). It is very popular amongst the local womenfolk in Malaysia and is frequently consumed by women of reproductive age. As a result of this popularity, recently several commercial products in the form of capsules (Houghton *et al.*, 1999) and canned drinks containing this herb have emerged in the Malaysian market (Nazaimoon, 2002). This herb has been widely used in the herbal and pharmaceutical industries as a health tonic especially for women (Latiff, 1997; Houghton *et al.*, 1999). These products are claimed to contain the grinded or extracted parts of the plant (Houghton *et al.*, 1999; Nazaimoon, 2002). Although *Labisia pumila* is normally used by women, it has been reported that men from several ethnic group in Sarawak consume it to maintain and increase stamina (Runi, 2001).

Characteristics Features of the Plant

Labisia pumila (Figure 6.1) is a small herbaceous shrub with a rooting system starting from the stem. The plants thrive best in shady areas and non- waterlogged humus rich soil. The planting of Kacip Fatimah best propagate by seeds or root cuttings. The leaves are few in number which point upwards. The tip of the leaf is pointed with a base that is tapered or rather broad and rounded. The leaf has a slight odor and taste. The whole leaf is about 5-35cm long and 2-8cm wide finely toothed with numerous veins. It is of a dark green color on adaxial and lighter green on the abaxial. The root is tough and woody with long primary roots and few secondary roots. Flowers of the shrub are very small, generally white or pink in colour, in spike like panicle of small clusters. They range from 6-30 cm long with sepals, petals and stamens. The petals wrap around and enclose the stamens. The fruit are about 0.5cm in diameter and are either bright red or purple. In Malaysia three varieties of Kacip Fatimah exist and each variety commands a different use, thus, it becomes important to ensure that the right variety of the plant be used in each case. There are very few charactristic features for the identification of different species on the basis of the leaves and petioles between var. *alata* and var. *pumila*.

Microscopic Characteristics of the Root and Leaf

Root

The fairly abundant sclereid, which occur singly are elongated rectangular in outline and have thickened and pitted wall. Lumen may be present or absent. Sometimes starch is present inside the large lumen. The abundant starch granules are simple and spherical to oval or sometimes rectangular in shape. No bilium or striation is present. The abundant sclereids are found in large fragments.

Leaf

The fragments of the upper epidermis are composed of cells with straight or slightly sinuous walls; stomata are absent. The cells of the lower epidermis are rather more sinuous in outline, stomata are numerous, paracytic types. Both the upper and lower epidermis show numerous cicatrices where the peltate trichomes were attached.They appear as circular scars around which the epidermal cells occur in a radiating arrangement. The cicatric has an evenly thickened wall. The fairly abundant trichomes from the leaf epidermis are two types; the peltate and covering trichomes, which are found scattered in the powder. The covering trichomes are large with numerous thin walled cells radiating form the tip of the central axis. They show considerable variation in size and characteristic feature. The starch granules are not very abundant, they are found scattered but more usually are seen in masses in some of the parenchymatous cells. The granules are simple and spherical. No bilum is present. The very occasional fibre is thick walled with irregular lumen and few pits. Very few sclerid are found singly, individual cells are elongated and irregular in outline with moderately thickened walls and numerous pits. The prisms and cluster crystals of calcium oxalate are found scattered as well as associated with the fibre. They vary in size and are sometimes quite large.

Ethno-botanical Information/Folklore Usage

Ayurveda is the most ancient health care system and is practiced widely in India, Srilanka and other countries (Chopra and Doiphode, 2002). Atharveda (around 1200 BC), Charak Samhita and Sushruta Samhita (100 – 500 BC) (Bhagvan and Sharma, 2001) are the main classics which have given the detailed descriptions of over 700 herbs. Researchers on pharmacognosy, chemistry, pharmacology and clinical therapeutics have been carried out on ayurvedic medicinal plants and many of the major pharmacological corporations have renewed their strategies in favour of natural products drug discovery (Sapna and Ravi, 2007). Numerous drugs have entered the international pharmacopoeia through the study of ethnopharmacology and traditional medicine (Waxler, 1988).

In traditional medicine of Malaysia, *Labisia pumila* (Roots, leaves or whole plant) has been traditionally used by the Malay women for many generations in childbirth in inducing and eases delivery, as a post partum medication to help contract the birth channel, to regain body strength, regulate menstrual cycle and avoid painful or difficult menstration, and to alleviate menopausal symptoms. The plant is traditionally boiled and the water extraction is taken as a drink. Other traditional uses include treating dysentery, rheumatism, and gennoehoea. It is also used as antiflatulence by helping to drive away and prevent the formation of gas. The plant also help to firm and tone the abdominal muscles. Scientific studies have established that the medicinal properties and biological activities of *Labisia pumila* are due to the presence of phytoestrogen (plant estrogen) that is naturally found in the plant (Burkill, 1966; Stone, 1988; Zakaria and Mohammad, 1994; Zaizuhana *et al.*, 2006).

Chemistry

A very scarce chemistry has been carried out on *Labisia pumila*. The major components isolated from the roots and leaves of the plant are benzoquinoid alkenyl resorcinols, and triterpenoid (Jamia *et al.*, 2004; Foster *et al.*, 2009; Ezumi *et al.*, 2007). The root also contains high iron content (Foster *et al.*, 2009). The alkenyl resorcinols were previously described compounds, however, never had been isolated before from a member of the Myrsinaceae family. The substitution pattern of all 4 compounds is highly lipophilic and thus, the compounds are practically insoluble in water (Figure 6.2). For this reason, those compounds cannot be used as marker compounds for the standardization of aqueous extracts of *Labisia pumila*.

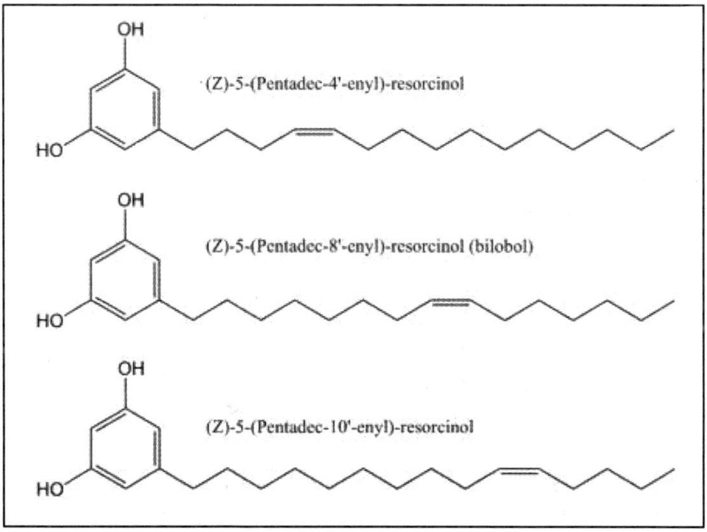

Figure 6.2. Highly lipophilic alkenyl resorcinols isolated from *Labisia pumila* var. *alata*.

The ultra-performance liquid chromatography coupled with electrospray ionisation tandem mass spectrometry (UPLC–ESI-MS/MS) study was used for the determination of flavonoids and phenolic acids from *Labsia pumila* extracts. Nine flavonols (quercetin, myricetin and kaempferol), two flavanols (catechin and epigallocatechin) (Table 6.1, Figure 6.2) and nine phenolic acids (Table 6.2, Figure 6.3) were identified from this active fraction by UPLC–ESI-MS/MS, and confirmed by comparison with the mass spectra of standard aglycones, theoretical fragments generated from MS Fragmenter software, and literature values (Lee *et al.*, 2011).

Table 6.1. Flavonoids of *Labisia pumila* as determined by negative ion mode EPI scan.

Flavonoid, (CF, MW)	*Retention Time (min)*	*Collision Energy (V)*	*Molecular Ion [M]⁻ (m/z)*	*Product Ion (m/z)*
Flavonols				
Quercetin	7.62	30	600	447(–pentose)/**301**(–deoxyhexose)/179/151
($C_{15}H_{10}O_7$, 302)	10.32	40	609	463(–deoxyhexose)/**301**(–hexose)/271/255/179/151
	9.53	40	615	463(–pentose)/**301**(–hexose)/271/255/179/151
	10.11	45	761	615(–deoxyhexose)/609/**301**/271/255/179/151
Myricetin,	9.89	40	463	**317**(–deoxyhexose)/271/179/151
($C_{15}H_{10}O_8$, 318)	10.90	40	479	461/**317**(–hexose)/271/179/151
	4.72	40	625	463(–hexose)/**317**(–deoxyhexose)/271/179/151
	3.71	55	778	632(–deoxyhexose)/463/**317**(–deoxy-hexose)/271/179/151
Kaempferol,	5.53	50	593	549/**285**/267/255/223/149/117
($C_{15}H_{10}O_6$, 286)	8.00	50	583	493/383/300/**285**/271/179/151/117
Flavanols				
Catechin,	3.65	30	289	**289**/151/137/123
($C_{15}H_{14}O_6$, 290)				
Epigallocatechin	6.25	20	305	**305**/287/261/233/169/169/151
($C_{15}H_{14}O_7$, 306)				

In addition to the polyphenols discussed above, nine phenolic acids and two organic acids were also identified (Figure 6.4). The phenolic acids included benzoic acids and cinnamic acids. The fragmentation patterns of the acids were predicted using MS Fragmenter 12.0. The theoretical fragment ions corresponded to the experimental mass spectral data and confirmed the structures. It is worth noting that all the acids were detected in the negative ion mode, except chlorogenic acid. Chlorogenic acid belongs to a family of esters of quinic acid and caffeic acid or ferulic acid. Besides chlorogenic acid, a chlorogenic acid derivative was also detected in the negative ion mode with a molecular ion *m/z* 593. The product ions *m/z* 353 (chlorogenic

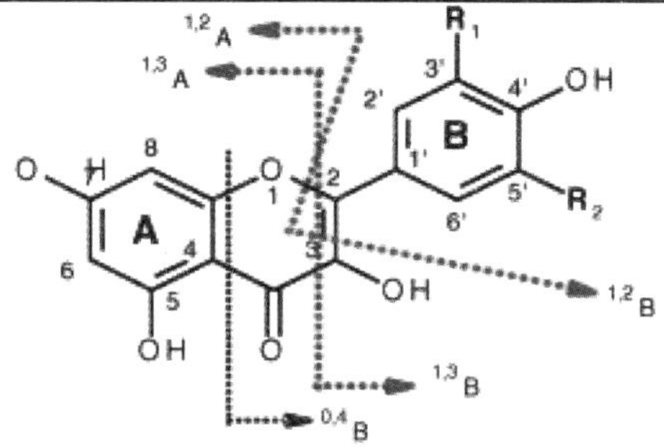

Flavonols	R_1	R_2
Quercetin	OH	H
Myricetin	OH	OH
Kaempferol	H	H

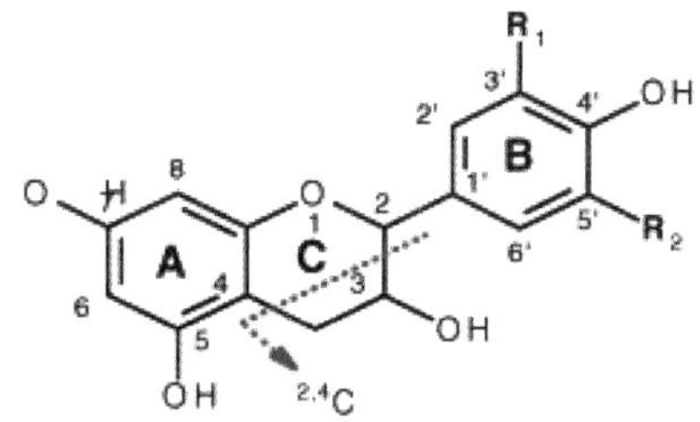

Flavanols	R_1	R_2
Catechin	OH	H
Epigallocatechin	OH	OH

Figure 6.3. Flavonols (quercetin, myricetin and kaempferol), and flavanols (catechin and epigallocatechin) from *Labisia pumila.*

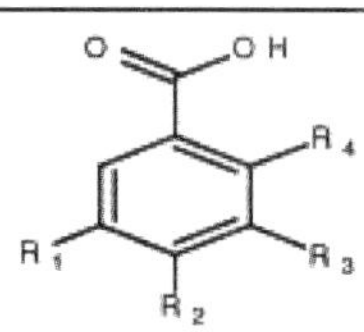

Benzoic acid	R_1	R_2	R_3	R_4
Gallic acid	OH	OH	OH	H
Protoc ate c hin a cid	H	OH	OH	H
Vanil lic a cid	OCH3	OH	H	H
Syringic a cid	OCH3	OH	OCH3	H
Salicylic a cid	H	H	H	OH

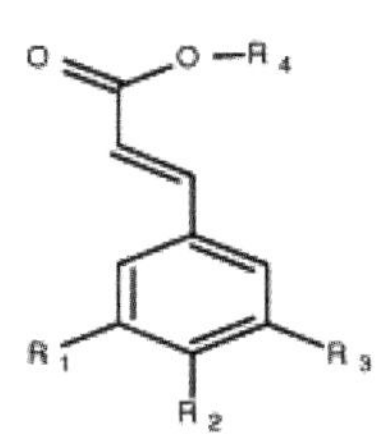

Cinnam ic acid	R_1	R_2	R_3	R_4
Coumaric a cid	H	OH	H	H
Caffeic a cid	H	OH	OH	H
Chlorogenic acid	H	OH	OH	quinic a cid

Figure 6.4. Phenolic acids included benzoic and cinnamic acids.

acid), *m/z* 191 (quinic acid) and *m/z* 179 (caffeic acid) were detected. The 240 Da difference has not been assigned.

Table 6.2. Phenolic acids from the 40% MeOH fraction of the 60% MeOH extract of *Labisia pumila* as determined by negative ion mode EPI scan.

Phenolic Acid	*[M"H]⁻*	*Fragment Ions*	*Retention Time (min)*
Benzoic acid			
Gallic acid	169	125(–CO_2)	2.20
Protocatechuic acid derivative	315	269(–CO_2H_2), 153(–$C_6H_{12}O_6$), 136(–$C_6H_{12}O_6$, –OH), 108(–$C_6H_{12}O_6$, –CO_2H)	3.23
Vanillic acid	167	152(–CH_3), 123(–CO_2), 108(–CO_2, –CH_3)	4.39
Syringic acid	197	182(–CH_3), 180(–OH), 166(–OCH_3), 152(–CO_2H)	4.50
Salicylic acid	137	119(–H_2O), 93(–CO_2)	3.53
Cinnamic acids			
Coumaric acid	163	146(–OH), 119(–CO_2)	4.33
Caffeic acid	179	162(–OH), 135(–CO_2), 134(–CO_2H), 109(–$C_3O_2H_2$), 91(–$C_3O_2H_2$–H_2O)	17.12
Chlorogenic acid	355 $[M+H]^+$	337(–H_2O), 319(–$2H_2O$), 301(–$3H_2O$), 281(–$2H_2O$–C_3H_2), 263(–$3H_2O$–C_3H_2), 245(–$4H_2O$, –C_3H_2)	8.45
Chlorogenic acid derivative	593	353(–240 Da), 191(quinic acid), 179(caffeic acid)	4.56
Organic acid			
Fumaric acid	115	98(–OH), 71(–CO_2)	2.00
Succinic acid	117		

Biological and Pharmacological activity

Antioxidant

Two varieties of *Labisia pumila*; *Labisia pumila* var. *alata* and *Labisia pumila* var. *pumila* (aqueous extracts of leaves) have shown significant activity in number of test methods like using DPPH, FRAP and β-carotene bleaching methods. In addition, ascorbic acid, β-carotene, anthocyanin, total flavonoid and total phenolic content were also analyzed. In eight methods studied, six of them showed high activities of antioxidant in *Labisia pumila* var. *alata* compared to that of *Labisia pumila* var. *pumila* (Norhaiza *et al.*, 2009).

Antistress

Labisia pumila was found to be potential ant-stress activity using a battery of tests widely employed in different stressful situations. Pretreatment of experimental animals with aqueous extract caused an increase in the swimming endurance and hypoxia time and also showed the recovery of physical stress-induced depletion of neuromuscular coordination and scopolamine induced memory deficit. The extract at graded doses reversed the chronic restraint stress (RST), induced depletion of CD4 (+) and CD_8 (+) T lymphocytes, NK cell population, and corresponding cytokines expression besides downregulating the stress-induced increase in plasma corticosterone, a major stress hormone. In addition, *Labisia pumila* reversed the chronic stress-induced increase in adrenal gland weight, serum alanine aminotransferase (ALT), alkaline phosphatase (ALP), and hepatic lipid peroxidation (LP) levels and augmented the RST induced decrease in hepatic glutathione (GSH), thymus and spleen weight. The *Labisia pumila* has the ability to reverse the alterations produced by various stressful stimuli and therefore restores homeostasis (Kour *et al.*, 2010). In another study in pregnant rats, aqueous extract of *Labisia pumila* significantly decreased stress hormone, cortisol level during the pregnancy without altering the immune status of the pregnant rats (Pandey *et al.*, 2009).

Skin Protection

Labisia pumila extract protected against the effects of ultraviolet radiation by protecting dermal fibroblasts from cell death, reducing expression of inflammatory mediators tumor necrosis factor-α and cyclo-oxygenase-2, increasing expression of type 1 procollagen and reducing expression of inflammatory cytokines (Choi *et al.*, 2010).

Immunomodulatory

In one of the study oral treatment *Labisia pumila* aqueous extract showed significant immunopotentiating activity. It produced a dose related increase in the clearance of carbon particles from the reticuloendothelial system and also the hastening in the rate of phagocytosis *in vitro* by marine macrophages, thereby suggesting an increase in the functioning of macrophages (innate response) by causing stimulation of non-specific immune response.

In T cell specific response reaction (cell mediated immunity) it showed the stimulatory effect on 'T' lymphocytes in SRBC induced DTH response. Evidence that leads to support hypothesis of T-lymphocytes stimulation is by the reduction in the homologous skin graft rejection time in mice treated with extract of *Labisia pumila*. The basic mechanism involved in reduction in graft rejection time is the stimulation of T-lymphocytes *i.e.* CD_4 and CD_8 positive T cells. One of the major effectors functions of CD_4+ T cells is the activation of macrophages and this plays an important role in enhancing the activity at sites of insult. CD_4+ T cell activation by *Labisia pumila* may be one of the factors responsible for the increase in the functioning of the macrophages.

The extract also shows a significant increase in expression of Interleukin-2 (IL-2) a growth factor for the T cells (CD_4+ and CD_8+) in serum of the treated animals. The extract also shows a significant up-regulation of interferon-gamma (IFN-α) where the maximum expression was observed. This cytokine is a signature cytokine of the Th1 response and its up regulation shows specific Th1 response (Qazi *et al.*, 2009). In another study, the ethyl acetate fraction of *Labisia pumila* showed selective Th1 upregulation via evaluation of pro-inflammatory cytokines in murine neutrophils followed by expression of T cell-surface markers and corresponding intracellular expression of cytokines related to T helper 1 (Th1) and T helper 2 (Th2). The graded doses of ethanolic extract of leaves of *Labisia pumila* (*in vitro*) showed increased expression of TNF-α, IL-6 and IL-12 is a strong inducer of Th1 response in activated CD_4+ T cells which cause marked stimulation of CD_4+ T helper cells and related cytokine expression like IL-2 and IFN-gamma (a potent Th1 inducer), thereby, having a predominant Th1 upregulation pathway. The study was further validated by suppression of IL-4 and IL-10 expression which are the Th2 pathway cytokines (Pandey *et al.*, 2010).

Estrogenic

In human endometrial adenocarcinoma cells of the Ishikawa-Var I line (*In vitro* study) showed that ethanolic extract of *Labisia pumila* (roots) exhibited a weak but specific estrogenic effect, resulting in secretion of alkaline phosphatase (Jamal *et al.*, 1992). Many studies have demonstrated that *Labisia pumila* extract acts as estrogen receptor modulators (SERMS) which is active on certain tissues.

One of the study showed that aqueous extract of *Labisia pumila* was able to displace estradiol binding to antibodies raised against estradiol, making it similar to other estrogens such as estrone and estradiol (Hasniza *et al.*, 2000). The extract has also been found to produce a dose-response effect on the reproductive hormones of female rats, notably on the estradiol and free testosterone levels (IMR, 2002). In a recent study by Al-Wahabi *et al.* (2007) indicating that aqueous extract of *Labisia pumila* play a role in modulating postmenopausal adiposity (*i.e.* the weight gain commonly associated with menopause) through the initiation of the lipolysis process in adipose tissue. This data indicate that *Labisia pumila* may indeed also have estrogenic activity.

In human trial study aqueous extracts of *Labisia pumila* increased testosterone levels in healthy females. The data showed that in a study involving 220 premenopausal women with regular menstrual cycles, effects of two months administration of freeze-dried aqueous extract of *Labisia pumila* increased total testosterone concentration significantly whereas androstenedione and SHBG were significantly lower in the females receiving *Labisia pumila* extract (Norlela *et al.* 2004).

This finding is extremely significant since it is scientifically well established that there is a positive correlation between testosterone levels and libido and sexual satisfaction and fulfillment in post-as well as pre-menopausal women. As an alternative to hormone treatments as offered by big pharmaceutical companies, *Labisia pumila* seems to provide a natural way to increase (at least pre-menopausal) female testosterone levels and, thus, may provide a way to avoid the side-effects commonly associated with hormone treatments.

Other Pharmacological Activities

In ovariectomized rats, aqueous extract of *Labisia pumila* maintained the integrity and morphology of the aortic wall. In another study, in rats, aqueous extract of *Labisia pumila* may modulate postmenopausal adiposity similar to esterogen by initiating lipolysis in adipose tissue (Faziliana, 2009). The mechanism of action is associated with an uterotrophic effect and regulating body weight gain by changing the expression and secretion of adipokines, leptin and resistin in adipose tissue. In another study, in a rat model of polycystic ovary syndrome, oral treatment with extract of *Labisia pumila* increased insulin sensitivity, reduced triglyceride and total cholesterol levels, increased circulating resistin levels and decreased leptin mRNA expression. Body weight development was not affected, but uterine weight was increased, indicating potential esterogenic effects of *Labisia pumila* (Mannreas *et al.*, 2010).

Safety Studies

Even though the *Labisia pumila* is documented as traditional medicinal herb within Malaysia since centuries clearly indicates that it is safe to take *Labisia pumila* decoction/aqueous extract, but a few scientific studies were undertaken to address safety issues of medicinal herb.

In a human clinical trials, blood pressure, heart beat rate, biochemical as well haematological parameters were not altered by administration of aqueous extract of *Labisia pumila* over a 2 month period in a study involving 220 pre-menopausal women with regular menstrual cycles This clearly demonstrates that *Labisia pumila* is definitely safe over a short period of time (Norlela, 2004).

A 28-day sub-acute toxicity testing in Wistar rats using repeated doses was undertaken to assess any possible health hazard (Singh *et al.*, 2009). The results have revealed that a low dose of 50 mg/kg (NOAEL) of *Labisia pumila* extract was devoid of toxicity, whereas higher doses were associated with some toxicity concerns. An elevated AST and ALP in *Labisia pumila* treated groups are clinically measurable indications of potential risks to normal liver function. Further there were findings of pathological nature in histological profile of liver, kidney and lungs of *Labisia pumila* treated groups. However, some of these were not in a dose-response related manner. Moreover these organs were not subjected to a major injury, as there were no significant alterations in liver-to-body weight ratio, kidney-to-body weight ratio and lungs-to-body weight ratio in *Labisia pumila* treated groups.

Effect of aqueous extract of *Labisia pumila* after 24, 48 and 72 hrs post administration in rats for genotoxic potential of extract on bone marrow cells to study the micronuclei formation as the toxicological end points was studied. No statically significant increase in micronucleated erythrocytes was observed, after 24, 48, 72 hrs of drug administration. There was significant decrease of erythrocytes from the highest dose used (2000 mg/kg of body weight) as 48 hrs period. Mammalian bone marrow cells were used to determined micro-nuclei formation (Shahrim *et al.*, 2006).

Labisia pumila extracts did not alter the estrous cycle and general health of all rats. All the animals proceed towards successful mating and pregnancies. There was no significant difference in the duration of pregnancy and all pregnant rats delivered normally. There were no changes in maternal body weight, number of implantation, litter size and pup body weight. Other parameters measured include pup sex ratio, live birth index, pup viability index and percentage of implantation death and all were found normal. The water based extract of *Labisia pumila* did not pose any reproductive toxicity or complication in pregnancy and the duration of pregnancy in rats (Wan Ezumi *et al.*, 2006). In another study reproductive toxicity of aqueous extract of *Labisia pumila* in rats was studied to determine potential adverse effect of aqueous extract of *Labisia pumila* on estrous cycle, reproductive performance, post natal growth and offspring survival of rats. The present findings indicate that water based extract of *Labisia pumila* var. *alata* do not pose any significant reproductive toxicity or complication in pregnancy and delivery in rats. The extract did not significant alter the duration of pregnancy in rats (Wan Ezumi *et al.*, 2007). In another study, teratogenic potential of aqueous extract of *Labisia pumila* was studied in rodent's gravid uterine weight, number of corpora lutea, number of implantation sites, percentage of total weight and fetal sex ratio showed no significant differences among all groups of animals. None of the fetuses from all dams showed evidence of external congenital malformation. The findings suggest that aqueous extract of *Labisia pumila* up to 1000mg/kg/day do not show any significant teratogenic effect in rat but do affect the maternal body weight and this is dose dependent (Wan Ezumi *et al.*, 2005). Side effect of petroleum ether extract of *Labisia pumila* on liver and kidney of white rats was studied. Liver impairment was indicated by the development of hydrophic degeneration in sinusoid area as early as day 1 post-treatment. Lesion proposed in day 3 and 7. Renal tubules were inflammated. Glomerulonephritis and nephrosis of the kidney were observed on day 7. This abnormality in the liver and kidney tissues suggested the presence of toxin compound in *Labisia pumila* (Efendy *et al.*, 2006). Due to the significantly different way of extract preparation and administration, however, this study is not at all relevant to oral administration of aqueous extracts of *Labisia pumila* and thus can safely be disregarded.

Conclusion

The data presented in this review chapter would further help in utilizing the traditional medicinal and health benefit attributes of *Labisia pumila*, which is finding increasing use in several nutraceutical products that are currently being marketed for women's health care.

References

Al-Wahaibi, A., Nazaimoon, W.W.M., Farihah, H.S. and Azian, A.L. (2007). Effects of water extract of *Labisia pumila* var. *alata* on beta-hydroxysteroid dehydrogenase activity induced fat deposition in the Sprague Dawley rats. *Trop. Med. Plants,* **8:** 21-26.

Bhagvan Dass and Sharma, B.K. (2001). Charak samhita (Chaukhamba Sankrit series office, Varanasi, India 2001) 7th edition.

Burkill, I.H. (1935). A *dictionary of the economic products of the Malay Peninsula.* London: Crown Agent.

Burkill, I.H. (1966). A Dictionary of the Economic Products of the Malay Peninsula, Vol. II (I–Z). Ministry of Agriculture and Co-operatives, Kuala Lumpur, Malaysia. 2444 pp.

Choi, H.K., Kim, D.H., Kim, J.W., Ngadiran, S., Sarmidi, M.R. and Park, C.S. (2010). *Labisia pumila* extract protects skin cells from photoaging caused by UVB irradiation. *J Biosci Bioeng.,* **109(3)**: 291-296.

Chopra, A. and Doiphode, V. (2002). Ayurvedic medicine: Core concept, therapeutic principle and current relevance. *Med. Chem. North Am.,* **86**: 75-89.

Effendy, A.W.M., Siti-Nurtahirah, J., Hussin, J.M. and Zamri-Saad, M. (2006). The side effects of kacip fatimah extract on liver and kidney of white rats. *Journal of Sustainability Science and Management,* **1**: 40–46.

Ezumi, M., Amrah, S., Suhaimi A. and Mohsin, S. (2007). Evaluation of the female reproductive toxicity of aqueous extract of *Labisia pumila* var. *alata* in rats. *Indian J. Pharmacol.,* **39(1):** 30 -32.

Fazliana, M., Wan Nazaimoon, W.M., Gu, H.F. and Ostenson, C.G. (2009). *Labisia pumila* extract regulates body weight and adipokines in ovariectomized rats. *Maturitas,* **20**: 91–97.

Foster, S. (2009). Balancing Nature and Wellness -Malaysian traditions of "Ramuan" – The history, culture, biodiversity and scientific assimilation of medicinal plants in Malaysia. *American Botanical Council. HerbalGram.,* **84:** 30-43.

Houghton, P.J., Jamal, J.A. and Milligan, S. (1999). Studies on *Labisia pumila* herb and its commercial products. *Journal of Pharmacy and Pharmacology,* **51**: 236.

Husniza, H., Wan Nazaimoon, W.M., Khozirah, S., Jamia, A.J., Balaspramaniam, A., Paridah, J. and Khalid, B.A.K. (2000). Estrogenic properties of Kacip Fatimah (*Labisia pumila*: A preliminary study. Proceedings: 3rd Scientific Conference, National Institute of Health, Malaysia. pp.77.

Jaganath, I.B. and Ng, L.T. (2000). Herbs: The green pharmacy of Malaysia. *Vinpress Sdn. Bhd. and Malaysian Agricultural Research and Development Institute,* 95-99.

Jamal, Z., Martin, A., Gomez-Munoz, A., Hales, P., Chang, P., Russell, J. C. and Brindley, D. N. (1992). Phosphatidate phosphohydrolase in the liver, heart and adipose tissue of the JCR: LA Corpulant rat and the lean genotypes: implications for glycerolipid synthesis and signal transduction. *Int. J. Obesity* **16**: 789-799.

Jamia, A. J., Ibrahim, J., Khairana, H. and Juriyati, J., (2004). Progress of Research and Development of Kachip Fatimah. pp 13-19. In: Chang, Y. S., Mastura, M. and Nurhanan, M. Y. (Eds.), Tongkat Ali, Kachip Fatimah & Pegaga New

Dimensions in Complementary Healthcare. Proceedings of the Seminar on Medicinal Plants, 21-21 Aug. 2002, Forest Research Institute Malaysia, Kuala Lumpur (in Malay).

Kour, K., Sharma, N., Chandan, B.K., Koul, S., Sangwan, P.L. and Bani, S. (2010). Protective effect of *Labisia pumila* on stress-induced behavioral, biochemical, and immunological alterations. *Planta Med.* [Epub. ahead of print]

Latiff, A.(1997). Medicinal and aromatic plants of Malaysia: approaches to exploitation and conservation. In: Kamaruddin, M.S., Natesh, S., Asiah, O., Azizol, A.K. (Eds.), Proceedings of the Medicinal and Aromatic Plants of Malaysia: Strategies and Technologies for Conservation, 29–30 September, 1997, Kuala Lumpur, Malaysia, pp. 20–31.

Lee, Suan., Chua, Norliza., Abdul, Latiff., Sze Yean, Lee., Chew Tin, Lee., Mohamad Roji, Sarmidi and Ramlan, Abdul Aziz. (2011). Flavonoids and phenolic acids from *Labisia pumila* (Kacip Fatimah). *Food Chemistry*, **127(3)**: 1186-1192.

Mannerals, L., Fazliana, M. and Wan Nazaimoon, W. M. (2010). Beneficial metabolic effects of the Malaysian herb *Labisia pumila* var. *alata* in a rat model of polycystic ovary syndrome. *J. Ethnopharmacol.*, **127(2)**: 346 – 351.

Nazaimoon, W.M.W. (2002). Estrogenic and androgenic *activities* of Kacip Fatimah (*Labisia pumila* var. *alata* and var. *pumila*). Project summary.

Norhaiza, M., Maziah, M. and Hakiman, M. (2009). Antioxidative properties of leaf extracts of a popular Malaysian herb, *Labisia pumila*. *J. Med Plants Res.*, **3(4):** 217 -223.

Norlela, S., Nor Azmi, K. N., Hazlina, N.H., Azidah, A.K., Siti Harnida, M.I., Mustafa, N., Ming, W., Khalid, B.A.K., Wan Mohd, W.B., Letchumanan, G.R. and Wan Nazaimon, W.M. (2004). Study of Kacip Fatimah. (http: //research.ukm.my/ppp/penerbitan/saripenyelidikan/2004/2004rh1.htm)

Pandey, A., Bani, S., Sangwan, P. and Koul, S. (2010). Selective Th1 upregulation by ethyl acetate fraction of *Labisia pumila*. *J Ethnopharmacol.* [Epub ahead of print]

Pandey, A., Kour, K., Bani, S., Singh, G., Latief, R., Youssouf, M.S., Koul, S., Gupta, B.D. and Qazi, G.N. (2008). Effects of aqueous extract of *Labisia pumila* on immune profile of pregnant rats. *Journal of Tropical Medicinal Plants*, **9:** 360–364.

Qazi, Ghulam Nabi., Bani, Sarang., Kaul, Anpurna., Pandey, Anjali., Kour, Kiranjeet., Koul, Surrinder., Gupta, Bishan Dutt., Sangwan, Pyrelal., Raina, Ravinder Kumar and Manickavasagar, Rajendran. (2009). Immunopotentiating Composition from *Labisia pumila* extract. United States Patent Application 20100303933.

Runi, S. P. (2001). Studies on medicinal plant in Sarawak. In Chang *et al.* (eds.) *Towards Bridging Science and Herbal Industry*. Forest Research Institute of Malaysia (FRIM), Kuala Lumpur. pp. 112-119.

Sapna, Shrikumar and Ravi,T.K. (2007). Approaches towards development and promotion of herbal drugs. *Pharmacognosy reviews,* **1(1):** 180-184.

Shahrim *et al.,* 2006. The *in vitro* Rodent Micronucleus Assay of Kacip Fatimah *(Labisia pumila)* extract. *Tropical Biomedicine,* **23**: 214-219.

Singh, G.D., Ganjoo, M., Youssouf, M.S., Koul, A., Sharma, R., Singh, S., Sangwan, P.L., Koul, S., Ahamad, D.B. and Johri, R.K. (2009). Sub-acute toxicity evaluation of an aqueous extract of *Labisia pumila,* a Malaysian herb. *Food Chem Toxicol.,* **47(10):** 2661-2665.

Stone, B.C. (1988). Notes on the genus *Labisia lindl* (Myrsinaceae). *Malayan Nature Journal,* **42:** 43–51.

Van der Voort, M. E. (1998). An inventory of wild-harvested plants in the Otter Creek Wilderness Area of the Monongahela National Forest, West Virginia. M.S. thesis. Morgantown, WV.

Wan Ezumi, M.F., Amrah, S.S., Suhaimi, A. and Mohsin, S. (2007). Evaluation of the female reproductive toxicity of aqueous extract of *Labisia pumila* var. *alata* in rats. *Indian J Pharmacol.,* **39:** 30-32.

Wan Ezumi, Mohd Fuad., Siti Amrah, Sulaiman., Mohamad Nazrul, Islam., Mohd Suhaimi, Abdul Wahab., Syed Mohsin and Sahil, Jamalullail. (2005). Evaluation of the teratogenicity of aqueous extract of *Labisia pumila* var. *alata* in rats. *Malaysian Journal of Medical Sciences,* **12(2):** 13-21.

Wan Ezumi, S. *et al.* (2006). Evaluation of the female reproductive toxicity of the aqueous extract of *Labisia pumila* var. *alata* in rats. *Indian Journal of Pharmacology,* **38**: 355-356.

Waxler, N.E. (1988). Morrison Plural medicine in India and Srilanka: do ayurvedic and westron medical practices offer. *Soc. Sci. Med.,* **27**: 531-544.

Zaizuhana, S., Puteri, J., Noor, M.B., Noral'ashikin, Y., Muhammad, H., Rohana, A.B. and Zakiah, I. (2006). The *in vivo* rodent micronucleus assay of Kacip Fatimah *(Labisia pumila)* extract. *Trop Biomed.,* **23(2):** 214-219.

Zakaria, M. and Mohd, M.A. (1994). Traditional Malay medicinal plants. *Penerbit Fajar Bakti Sdn. Bhd;* Kuala Lumpur, Malaysia. pp.8.

Medicinal Plants: Phytochemistry, Pharmacology and Therapeutics Vol. 2 (2012) *Pages* **97–127**
Editor-in-Chief: **V.K. Gupta**
Published by: **DAYA PUBLISHING HOUSE, NEW DELHI**

7

Jeju Seaweeds Inhibit Proinflammatory Cytokines, iNOS, and COX-2 Expression in Macrophage RAW Cells

Eun-Jin YANG[1], Sang-Suk KIM[2], Gi-Ok KIM[3,4], Nam Ho LEE[1,2,4] and Chang-Gu HYUN[1,3,4*]

ABSTRACT

Various seaweed species are used in traditional medicine worldwide. Despite the fact that seaweeds are frequently used in the practice of human health, little is known regarding the role of seaweed in the context of inflammation. Therefore, this study aimed to investigate the influence of Jeju seaweeds on the mouse macrophage line RAW 264.7 under lipopolysaccharide (LPS) stimulation. Ethyl acetate extracts obtained from 7 different kinds of Jeju seaweeds were screened for inhibitory effects on proinflammatory mediators. Our results revealed that extracts from Laurencia intricata, Leathesia marina, Chondrus crispus, Lomentaria hakodatensis, Colpomenia sinuosa, Scytosiphon gracilis and Polyopes affinis potently inhibited LPS-induced nitric oxide (NO) (IC_{50} values for these 7 seaweeds were: 37.3, 30.5, 36.4, 22.3, 23.4, 18.1, and 24.5 μg/mL, respectively) and prostaglandin E_2 (PGE_2) (IC_{50} values 141.0, 50.4, 12.2, 10.5, 16.5, 10.4, and 27.6 μg/mL, respectively) production. Consistent with these findings, the 7 seaweeds also reduced the LPS-induced expressions of inducible

1 Jeju Seaweed Industry Development Agency, Cheju National University, Jeju 690-756, Korea

2 Department of Chemistry, Cheju National University, Jeju 690-756, Korea

3 Bio-Convergence Center, Jeju Technopark, Jeju 690-121, Korea

4 Cosmetic Science Center, Cheju National University, Jeju 690-756, Korea

* *Corresponding author*: E-mail: cghyun@jejutp.or.kr, Tel: +82-64-720-2931; Fax: +82-64-720-2901.

Analysis of Total Phlorotannin

The total phlorotannin content in the seaweed extracts was determined by the Folin-Ciocalteu colorimetric method (Huang *et al.*, 2005; López-Vélez *et al.*, 2003). Briefly, we added 550 μL of distilled water/Folin-Ciocalteu solution (10:1, v/v) to 50 μL of diluted extract (1 mg/mL of ethanol). After 3 min, 200 μL of 2 M sodium carbonate (Na_2CO_3) and 300 μL of distilled water were added. After 1 h standing at laboratory temperature, the absorbance was measured at 725 nm. The total phlorotannin content was calculated as a phloroglucinol equivalent from the calibration curve of phloroglucinol standard solutions (concentration range, 0–1.0 mg/mL). All measurements were conducted in triplicate.

Cell Culture and Viability

Murine RAW 264.7 macrophages were cultured in Dulbecco's modified Eagle's medium (DMEM) supplemented with 10 per cent fetal bovine serum, 100 U/mL penicillin, and 100 μg/mL streptomycin, all from GIBCO (Grand Island, NY, USA), in an incubator at 37 °C in a humidified atmosphere of 95 per cent air and 5 per cent CO_2. Cell viability was determined by the 3-(4,5-dimethylthiazol-2-yl)-2,5-diphenyltetrazolium bromide (MTT) assay. RAW 264.7 cells were cultured in 96-well plates for 18 h, followed by treatment with various concentrations (12.5, 25, 50, or 100 μg/mL) of the EtOAc fraction of Jeju seaweeds. After 24-h incubation, MTT was added to the medium for 4 h. Finally, the supernatant was removed, and formazan crystals were dissolved in DMSO. Absorbance was measured at 540 nm. The percentage of cells showing cytotoxicity was determined relative to the control group.

Determination of NO Concentration

The determination of NO concentration in the Jeju seaweed extracts was determined based on the method of Yang *et al.* (2010a and 2010b) as follows. RAW 264.7 cells (5×10^5 cells/well) were incubated on 24-well dishes for 18 h with 1 μg/ml of LPS and various concentrations (12.5, 25, 50, or 100 μg/mL) of the EtOAc fraction of Jeju seaweeds. The presence of nitrite, a stable oxidized product of NO, was determined in cell-culture media by a modified Griess method. The culture supernatant (100 μL) was mixed with the same volume of Griess reagent (1 per cent sulfanilamide and 0.1 per cent N-[1-naphthyl]-ethylenediamine dihydrochloride in 5 per cent phosphoric acid) for 10 min, and the absorbance was measured at 540 nm.

Measurement of PGE_2 and Cytokine Assays

PGE_2 and cytokines were measured using a previously described method with slight modifications (Yang *et al.*, 2010a,b,c,d). RAW 264.7 cells were cultured in 24-well plates for 18 h, followed by treatment with LPS in the presence of various concentrations (12.5, 25, 50, or 100 μg/mL) of the EtOAc fraction of Jeju seaweeds. After 24-h incubation, PGE_2 in the culture supernatants was measured using an enzyme-linked immunosorbent assay (ELISA) kit. The amounts of TNF-α and IL-6 in the cell-culture supernatant and in serum were measured using an ELISA kit (R&D, Minneapolis, MI). RAW 264.7 cells were plated on a 12-well cell-culture plate at a density of 2.5×10^5 cells and incubated with various concentrations of seaweed extracts (12.5, 25, 50, or 100 μg/mL) in 1 μg/mL LPS for 24 h. The culture supernatant was collected and assayed according to the manufacturer's instructions to determine the amounts of TNF-α and IL-6 released from the cells.

Statistical Analysis

All the results were expressed as mean ± S.E. Each experiment was repeated at least 3 times. Statistical significances were compared between each treated group and analyzed by Student's *t*-test. Data with $p < 0.05$ were considered statistically significant.

Results

Effects of Jeju Seaweed Extracts on LPS-induced NO Production and Cell Viability

Since the overproduction of NO is harmful and results in various inflammatory and autoimmune diseases, pharmacological interference with the NO production cascade offers promising strategies for therapeutic intervention in inflammatory disorders (Yoon *et al.*, 2009c; Yoon *et al.*, 2009d; Yoon *et al.*, 2010c; Yoon *et al.*, 2010d; Yoon *et al.*, 2010e). Therefore, we first investigated the effect of Jeju seaweed extracts on NO synthesis in activated macrophages. Marine macrophage RAW 264.7 cells can induce iNOS transcription and protein synthesis, and subsequent NO production following LPS stimulation alone. This cell system is thus an excellent model for evaluating topical agents and for screening potential inhibitors of the pathways that induce iNOS and NO production.

In this study, which aimed to identify natural products that possess anti-inflammatory activity, we prepared 80 per cent ethanol crude extracts from 7 native seaweeds from Jeju Island, Korea. The evaporated EtOH extract was partitioned with ethyl acetate. All ethyl acetate seaweed fractions were dissolved in 80 per cent ethanol and diluted with sterile water to normalise the concentration of the test sample. The Griess reaction, a spectrophotometric determination for nitrite, was carried out to quantify the nitrite levels in the conditioned medium of RAW 264.7 cells treated with LPS. The final concentration of ethanol in the culture media was 0.1 per cent, and this concentration of ethanol was demonstrated to have no effect on the assay systems.

Table 7.1 shows the inhibitory activity by seaweed extracts toward NO production by LPS-activated macrophages. All extracts showed greater than 50 per cent inhibition of NO production at a concentration of 50 μg/mL in the culture medium. Among these 7 extracts, 4 extracts–*i.e.* those from *Lomentaria hakodatensis*, *Colpomenia sinuosa*, *Scytosiphon gracilis* and *Polyopes affinis*–showed the most potent inhibition in a concentration-dependent manner (Figure 7.1). Their IC_{50} values were 22.3, 23.4, 18.1, and 24.5 μg/mL, respectively. As shown in Figure 7.1, the numbers of viable activated macrophages were not significantly altered by the 7 extracts as determined by MTT assays, thus indicating that the inhibition of NO synthesis by the seaweed extracts did not occur due to cytotoxicity and cell death, but involved other mechanisms.

Table 7.1. Inhibitory effect of Jeju seaweeds on the production of pro-inflammatory mediators.

Specimen Number	*Scientific Names*	*IC50 (μg/mL)*				*Phlorotannin Contents*
		NO	*PGE_2*	*IL-6*	*TNF-α*	*(μg/mL)*
JBR261	*Lomentaria hakodatensis* Yendo	22.3	10.5	32.3	48.3	43.5
JBR276	*Laurencia intricata* Lamouroux	37.3	141.0	62.9	116.0	49.2
JBR351	*Colpomenia sinuosa* (Mertens *ex* Roth) Derbès and Solier	23.4	15.51	73.6	44.9	43.5
JBR359	*Leathesia marina* (Lyngbye) Decaisne	30.5	50.4	46.3	33.5	42.0
JBR512	*Scytosiphon gracilis* Kogame	18.11	10.4	17.0	31.9	61.5
JBR514	*Chondrus crispus* Stackhouse	36.4	12.2	31.9	43.8	45.2
JBR519	*Polyopes affinis* (Harvey) Kawaguchi and Wang	24.5	27.6	23.8	31.8	56.3

The presence of nitrite, as a stable oxidized product of NO, was determined in cell-culture media by a modified Griess method. The amount of PGE_2, TNF-α, and IL-6 in the cell-culture supernatant and in serum was measured using an ELISA kit. RAW 264.7 cells incubated with various concentrations of seaweed extracts (12.5, 25, 50, or 100 μg/mL). Cell viability was determined by MTT assay.

Effects of Jeju Seaweed Extracts on LPS-induced PGE_2 Production

COX is a key enzyme catalyzing the rate-limiting step in the biosynthesis of prostaglandins from arachidonic acid. Growing evidence indicates that COX-2 plays a key role in several biological processes, such as inflammation and tumorigenesis. Thus, the targeted inhibition of COX-2 is a promising approach for inhibiting inflammation and carcinogenesis. Therefore, we next examined the effects of Jeju seaweed extracts on PGE_2 production in LPS-stimulated RAW 264.7 macrophages. When the macrophages were stimulated with LPS (1 μg/mL) for 24 h, the levels of PGE_2 increased in the culture medium. As shown in Figure 7.2, all seaweed samples (*Laurencia intricata*, *Leathesia marina*, *Chondrus crispus*, *L. hakodatensis*, *C. sinuosa*, *S. gracilis*, and *P. affinis*) suppressed the LPS-induced PGE_2 production, exhibiting IC_{50} values of 141.0, 50.4, 12.2, 10.5, 16.5, 10.4, and 27.6 μg/mL, respectively. They also inhibited LPS-induced PGE_2 production in a dose-dependent manner (Figure 7.2).

Effects of Jeju Seaweed Extracts on LPS-induced Expression of iNOS and COX-2 Proteins

Western blot analyses were performed to determine whether the inhibitory effects of Jeju seaweed extracts on the proinflammatory mediators NO and PGE_2 were related to the modulation of iNOS and COX-2 expression. We did not detect iNOS and COX-2 proteins or *m*RNA in non-stimulated RAW 264.7 cells. However, iNOS and COX-2 protein levels were markedly upregulated by LPS, an effect that was inhibited by co-treatment with Jeju seaweed extracts (Figures 7.3 and 7.4). On the other hand, Jeju

Figure 7.1. Effect of Jeju seaweed extracts on nitric oxide production in LPS-stimulated RAW 264.7 cells.

The cells were stimulated with 1 μg/mL of LPS alone or with a combination of LPS and various concentrations (12.5, 25, 50, or 100 μg/mL) of seaweed varieties JBR261 (A), JBR276 (B), JBR351 (C), JBR359 (D), JBR512 (E), JBR514 (E), and JBR519 (F) for 24 h. Nitric oxide production was determined by the Griess reagent method. Cell viability was determined using the 24-h culture of cells stimulated with LPS (1 μg/mL) in the presence of each sample. The data represent the mean ± SD of triplicate experiments. *$p < 0.05$; **$p < 0.01$ vs. LPS alone.

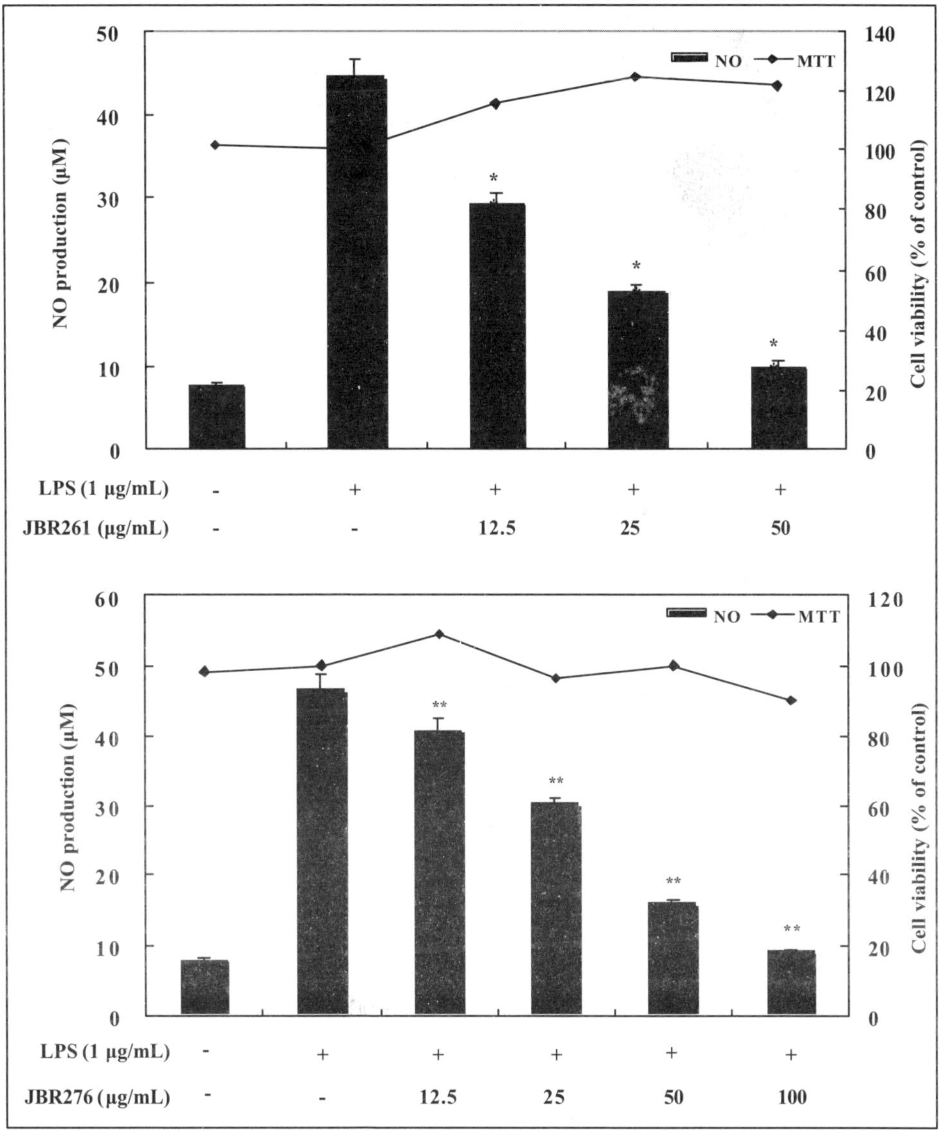

Contd...

Figure 7.1–*Contd...*

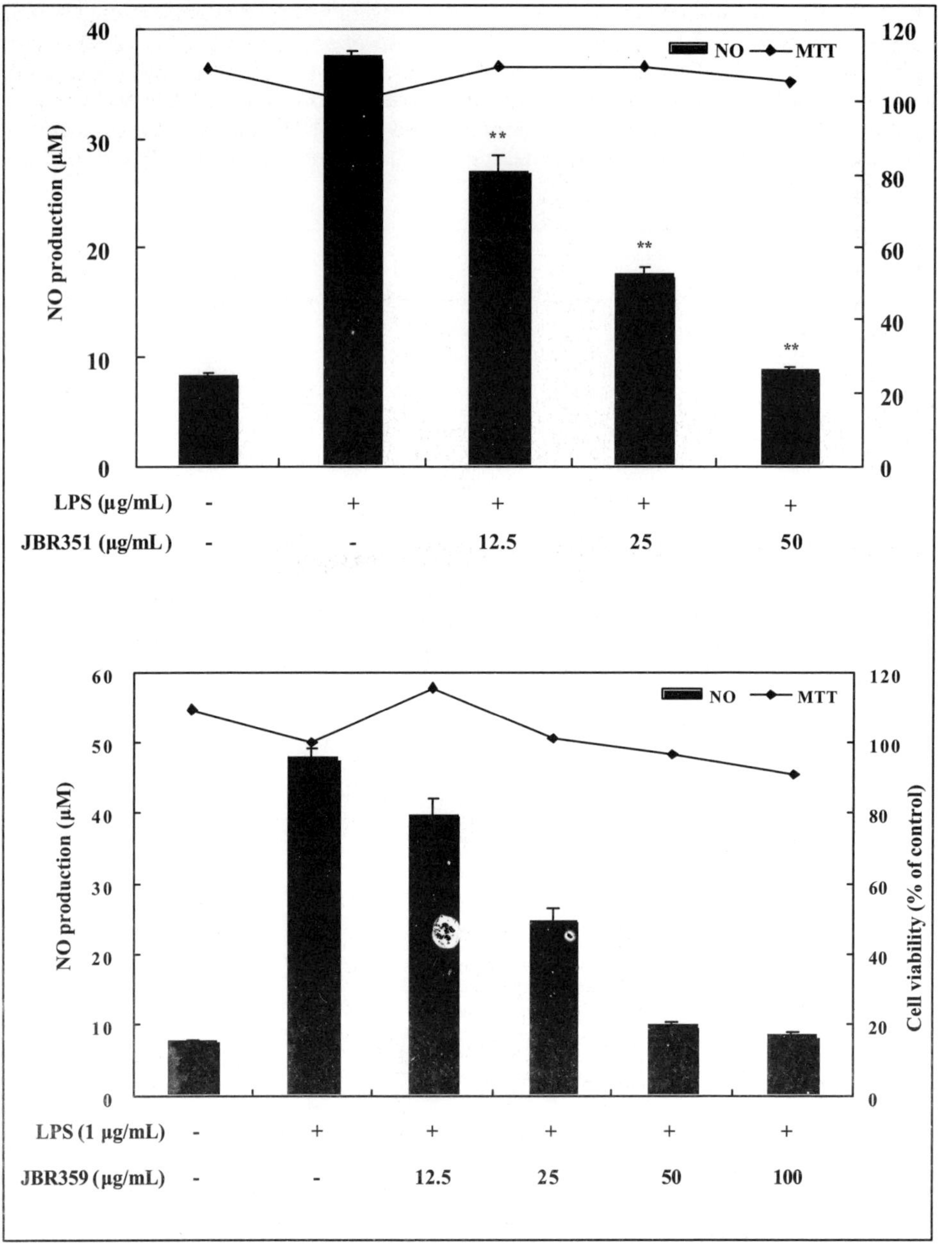

Contd...

Figure 7.1–*Contd...*

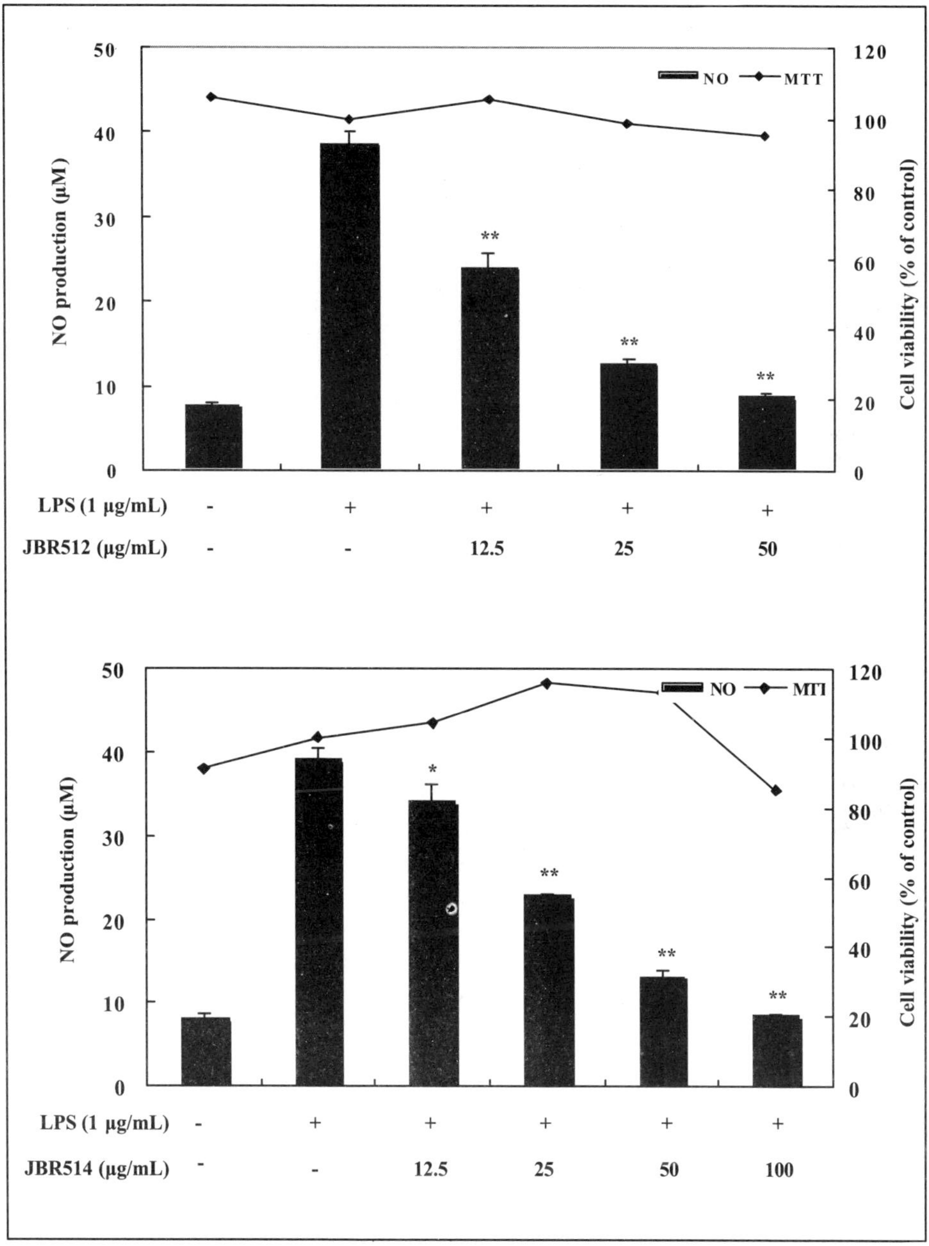

Contd...

Figure 7.1–*Contd...*

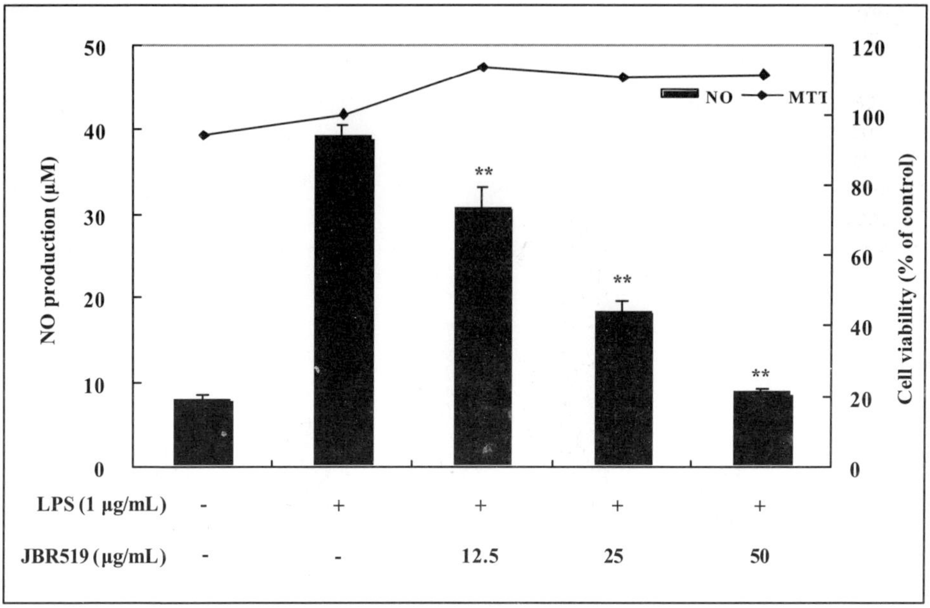

seaweed extracts did not affect the expression of β-actin, a housekeeping gene. In general, these results indicate that the inhibitory effects of Jeju seaweed extracts on LPS-induced NO and PGE_2 production are the result of the suppression of iNOS and COX-2.

Effects of Jeju Seaweed Extracts on LPS-induced TNF-α and IL-6 Production

Inflammation is activated on appropriate extracellular stimulation, most often by stress or proinflammatory cytokines, including TNF-α and IL-6, and by bacterial components including LPS through Toll-like receptors. Since the Jeju seaweed extracts potently inhibited the proinflammatory mediators, we further investigated their effects on LPS-induced IL-6 and TNF-α release by enzyme immunoassay. After 24-h incubation with both LPS (1 μg/mL) and solvent fractions of seaweed (12.5, 25, 50, or 100 μg/mL), remarkable inhibition of TNF-α and IL-6 release was noted. As shown in Figures 7.5 and 7.6, extracts from *L. intricata*, *L. marina*, *C. crispus*, *L. hakodatensis*, *C. sinuosa*, *S. gracilis*, and *P. affinis* inhibited the production of IL-6 and TNF-α in a dose-dependent manner. Furthermore, the *S. gracilis* fraction significantly decreased the levels of IL-6 and TNF-α production with IC_{50} values of 17.0 and 31.9 μg/mL, respectively.

Figure 7.2. Effect of Jeju seaweed extracts on PGE_2 production in LPS-stimulated RAW 264.7 cells.

The cells were stimulated with 1 µg/mL of LPS alone or with a combination of LPS and various concentrations (12.5, 25, 50, or 100 µg/mL) of JBR261 (A), JBR276 (B), JBR351 (C), JBR359 (D), JBR512 (E), JBR514 (E), and JBR519 (F) for 24 h. PGE_2 produced and released into the culture medium was assayed by the ELISA method. The data represent the mean ± SD of triplicate experiments. $^*p < 0.05$; $^{**}p < 0.01$ vs. LPS alone.

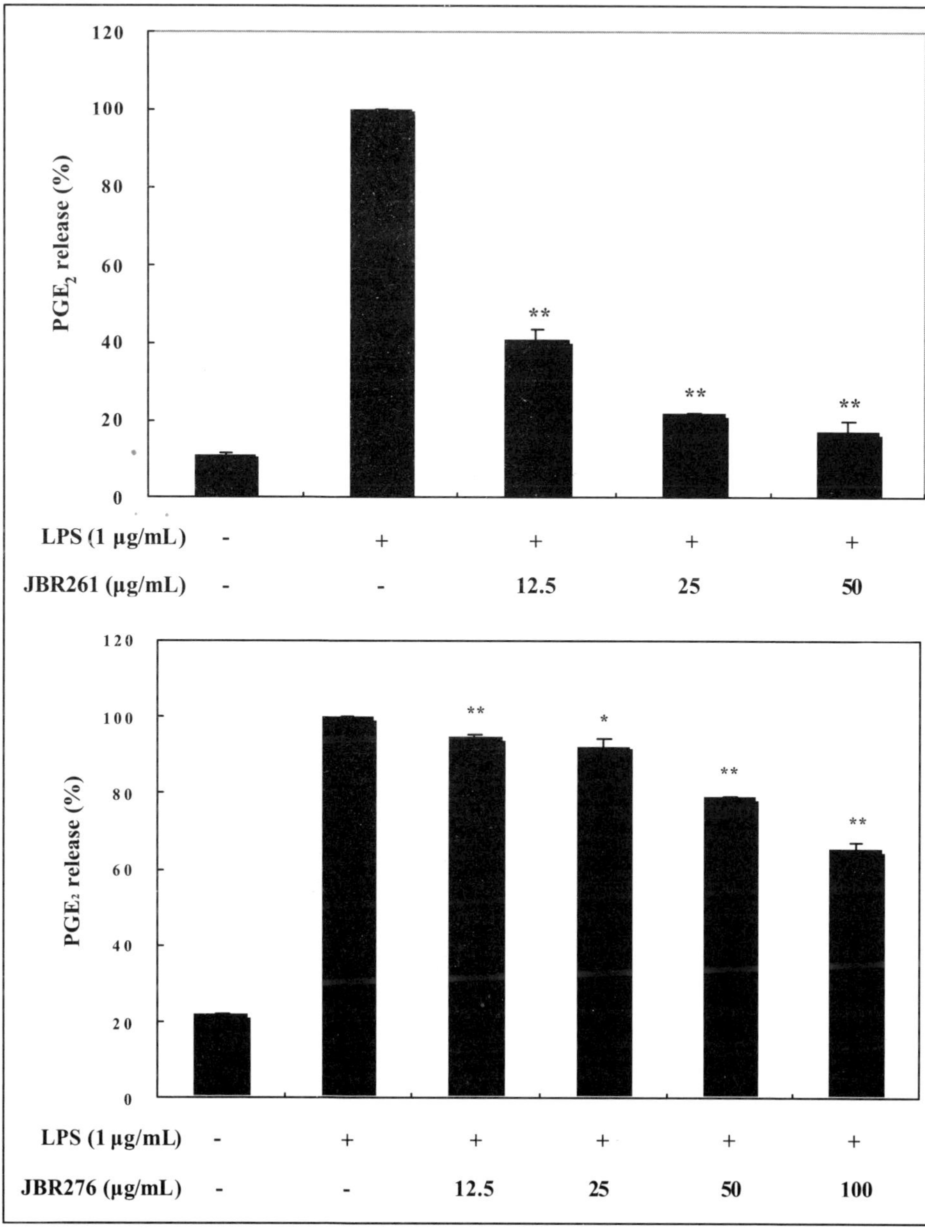

Contd...

Figure 7.2–*Contd...*

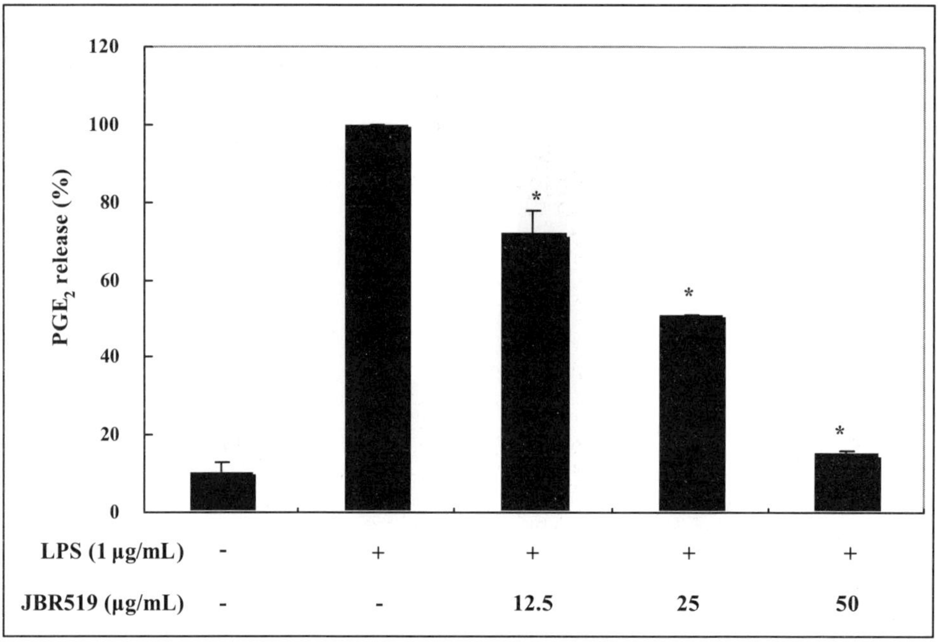

Phlorotannin Contents of Jeju Seaweed Extracts

Phlorotannins are aromatic secondary plant metabolites, widespread in seaweeds associated with nutritional, anti-inflammatory, and antioxidant properties. Therefore, the total phlorotannin contents of 7 seaweed extracts were assessed. As shown in Table 7.1, the phlorotannin contents were as follows: *L. intricate*, 49.2 μg/mg; *L. marina*, 42.0 μg/mg; *C. crispus*, 45.2 μg/mg; *L. hakodatensis*, 43.5 μg/mg; *C. sinuosa*, 43.5 μg/mg; *S. gracilis*, 61.5 μg/mg; and *P. affinis*, 56.3 μg/mg. *S. gracilis* showed the highest phlorotannin content (>60 μg/mg). These results were consistent with the higher inhibition efficacy of *S. gracilis* toward NO, PGE_2, IL-6, and TNF-α production.

Discussion

Marine natural products provide a rich source of chemical diversity that can be used to design and develop new and potentially useful therapeutic agents (Blunt *et al.*, 2009; Usami, 2009; Yang *et al.*, 2010a; Yang *et al.*, 2010c). Certain marine products have been reported to exhibit anti-tumor (Bae, 2007; Rocha *et al.*, 2007), antibacterial (González *et al.*, 2001; Devi *et al.*, 2008), and anti-inflammatory effects (Dang *et al.*, 2008; Khan *et al.*, 2008; Kang *et al.*, 2008). The present study was undertaken to elucidate the pharmacological and biological effects of Jeju seaweed extracts on the production of inflammatory mediators in macrophages.

Figure 7.3. Effect of Jeju seaweed extracts on the activation of iNOS in LPS-stimulated RAW 264.7 cells.

RAW 264.7 cells (5.0 × 10^5 cells/mL) were stimulated with LPS (1 μg/mL) in Jeju seaweed extracts (12.5, 25, 50, and 100 μg/mL) for 24 h. Whole-cell lysates (25 μg) were prepared, and the protein lysates were subjected to 10 per cent SDS-PAGE; the expressions of iNOS and β-actin were determined by western blotting. The figure is representative of 3 similar experiments. The Jeju seaweed extract fractions were prepared as described in the Materials and Methods section.

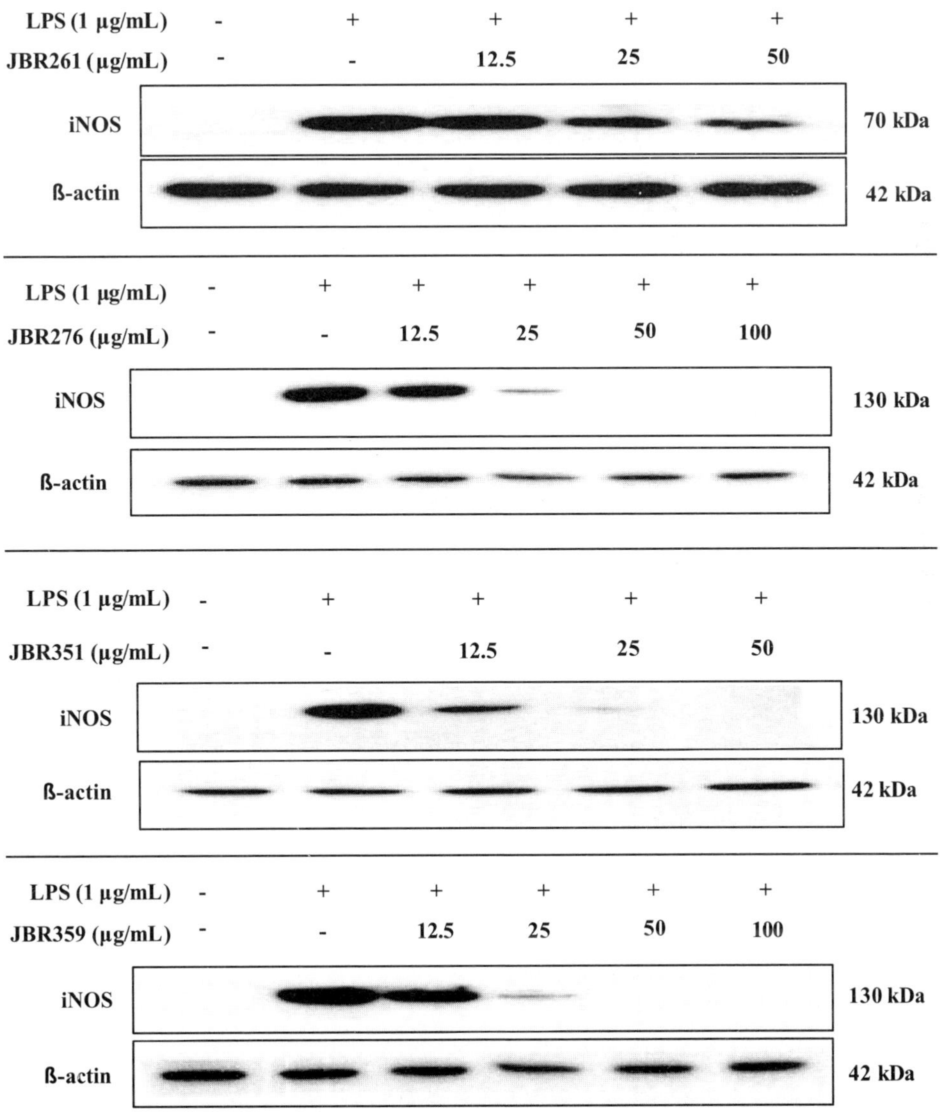

Contd...

Figure 7.3–*Contd...*

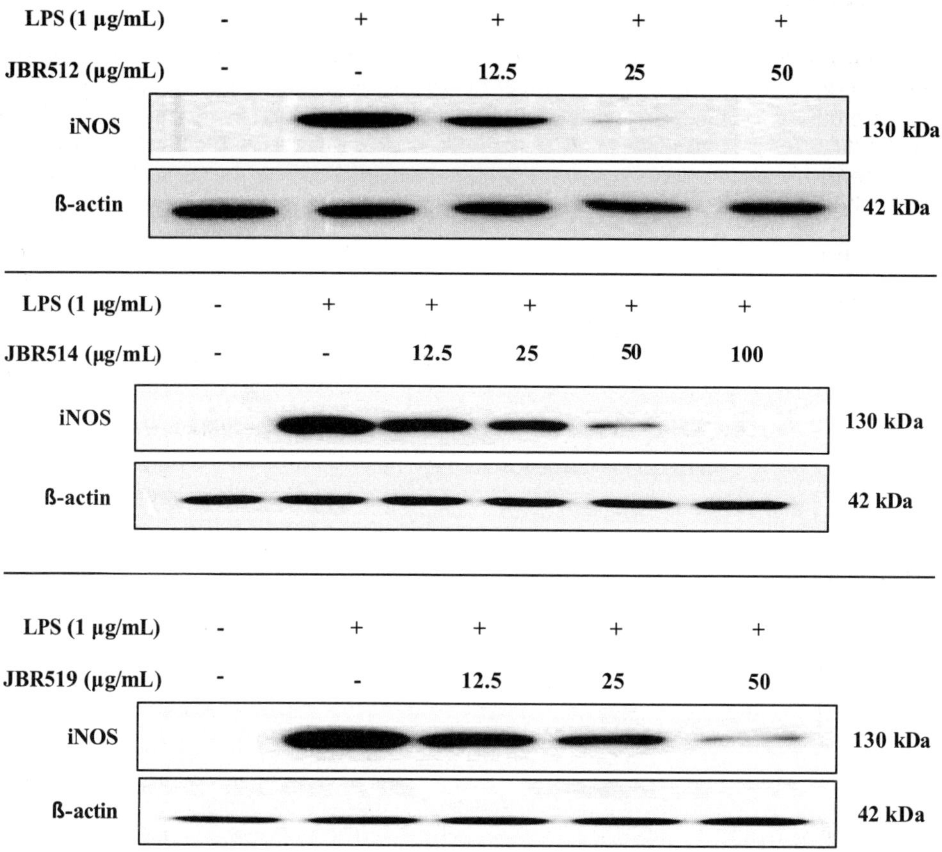

The proinflammatory cytokines PGE_2 and NO, which are produced by activated macrophages, play critical roles in inflammatory diseases such as sepsis and arthritis (Ci *et al.*, 2010; Cuzzocrea, 2006; Silverman, 2009). Hence, the inhibition of these proinflammatory cytokines or of iNOS and COX-2 expression in inflammatory cells offers a new therapeutic strategy for the treatment of inflammation. RAW 264.7 marine macrophage cells are an example of inflammatory cells that actively participate in inflammatory responses by releasing proinflammatory cytokines (TNF-α, IL-1β and IL-6) and inflammatory factors (NO and PGE_2); these factors subsequently recruit additional immune cells to the sites of infection or tissue injury. Interestingly, the production of these inflammatory molecules by macrophages can be induced in response to LPS stimulation. Therefore, the inhibitors of these inflammatory molecules have been considered as anti-inflammatory drug candidates for alleviating a variety of disorders caused by the activation of macrophages. Thus, RAW 264.7 macrophages

Figure 7.4. Effect of Jeju seaweed extracts on the activation of COX-2 in LPS-stimulated RAW 264.7 cells

RAW 264.7 cells (5.0×10^5 cells/mL) were stimulated with LPS (1 μg/mL) in Jeju seaweed extracts (12.5, 25, 50, and 100 μg/mL) for 24 h. Whole-cell lysates (25 μg) were prepared, and the protein lysates were subjected to 10 per cent SDS-PAGE; the expressions of iNOS and β-actin were determined by western blotting. The figure is representative of 3 similar experiments. The Jeju seaweed extract fractions were prepared as described in the Materials and Methods section.

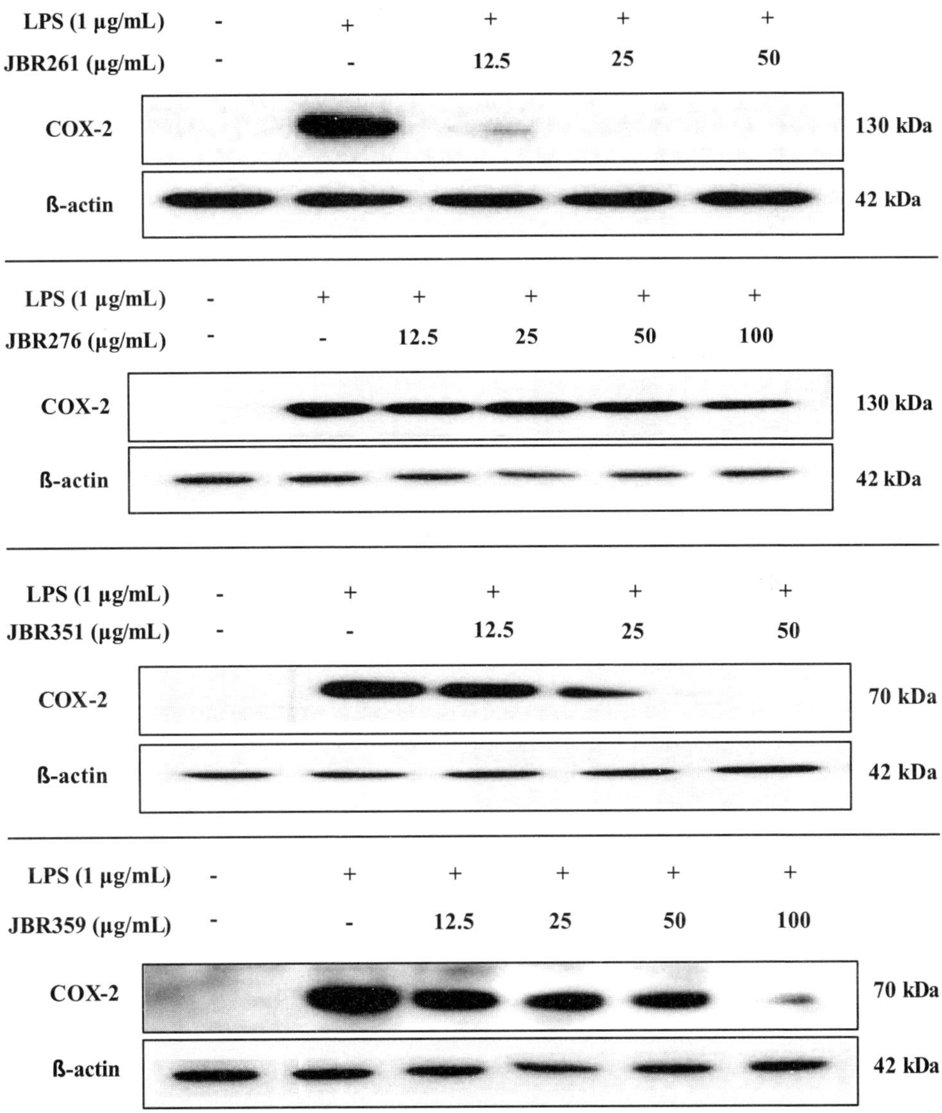

Contd...

Figure 7.4—*Contd...*

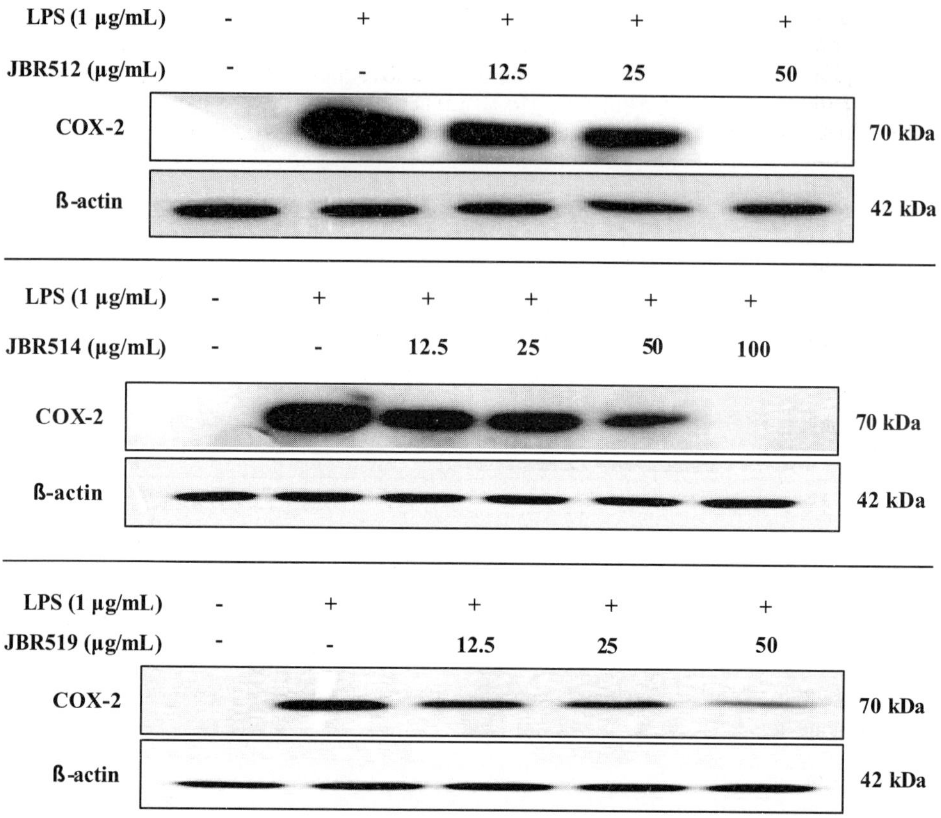

provide us with an excellent model for anti-inflammatory drug screening and for subsequently evaluation of the inhibitors of the pathways that lead to the induction of proinflammatory enzymes and to the production of proinflammatory cytokines (Jung *et al.,* 2010).

In order to validate the use of Jeju seaweed extracts as an anti-inflammatory drug in traditional Korean medicine, we have previously investigated the effects of Jeju seaweed extracts on the production of NO and PGE_2 in LPS-activated RAW 264.7 macrophages (Yang *et al.,* 2010c; Yang *et al.,* 2010d). In the present study, we additionally found that 7 types of Jeju seaweed extracts inhibited PGE_2 and NO production in macrophage cells, wherein the inhibition probably occurs at transcriptional and/or translational levels, as evidenced by dose-dependent reduction in protein expression.

It has been reported that cytokines such as TNF-α, IL-6, and IL-1β have proinflammatory effects both *in vitro* and *in vivo*. Moreover, TNF-α production is crucial

Figure 7.5. Effect of Jeju seaweed extracts on TNF-*a* production in LPS-stimulated RAW 264.7 cells

The cells were stimulated with 1 μg/mL of LPS alone or with a combination of LPS and various concentrations (12.5, 25, 50, or 100 μg/mL) of JBR261 (A), JBR276 (B), JBR351 (C), JBR359 (D), JBR512 (E), JBR514 (E), and JBR519 (F) for 24 h. TNF-α produced and released into the culture medium was assayed by the ELISA method. The data represent the mean ± SD of triplicate experiments. *$p < 0.05$; **$p < 0.01$ vs. LPS alone.

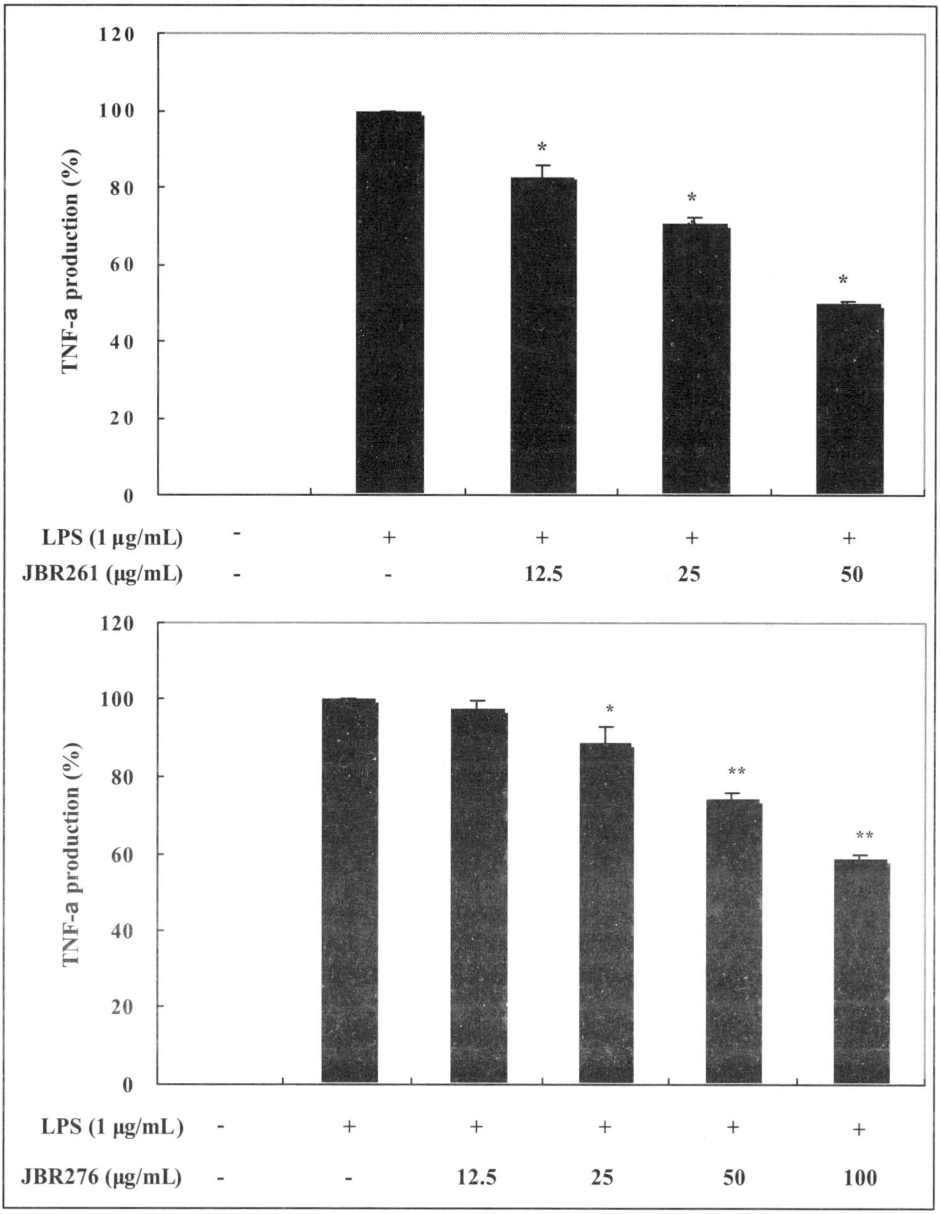

Contd...

Figure 7.5–*Contd...*

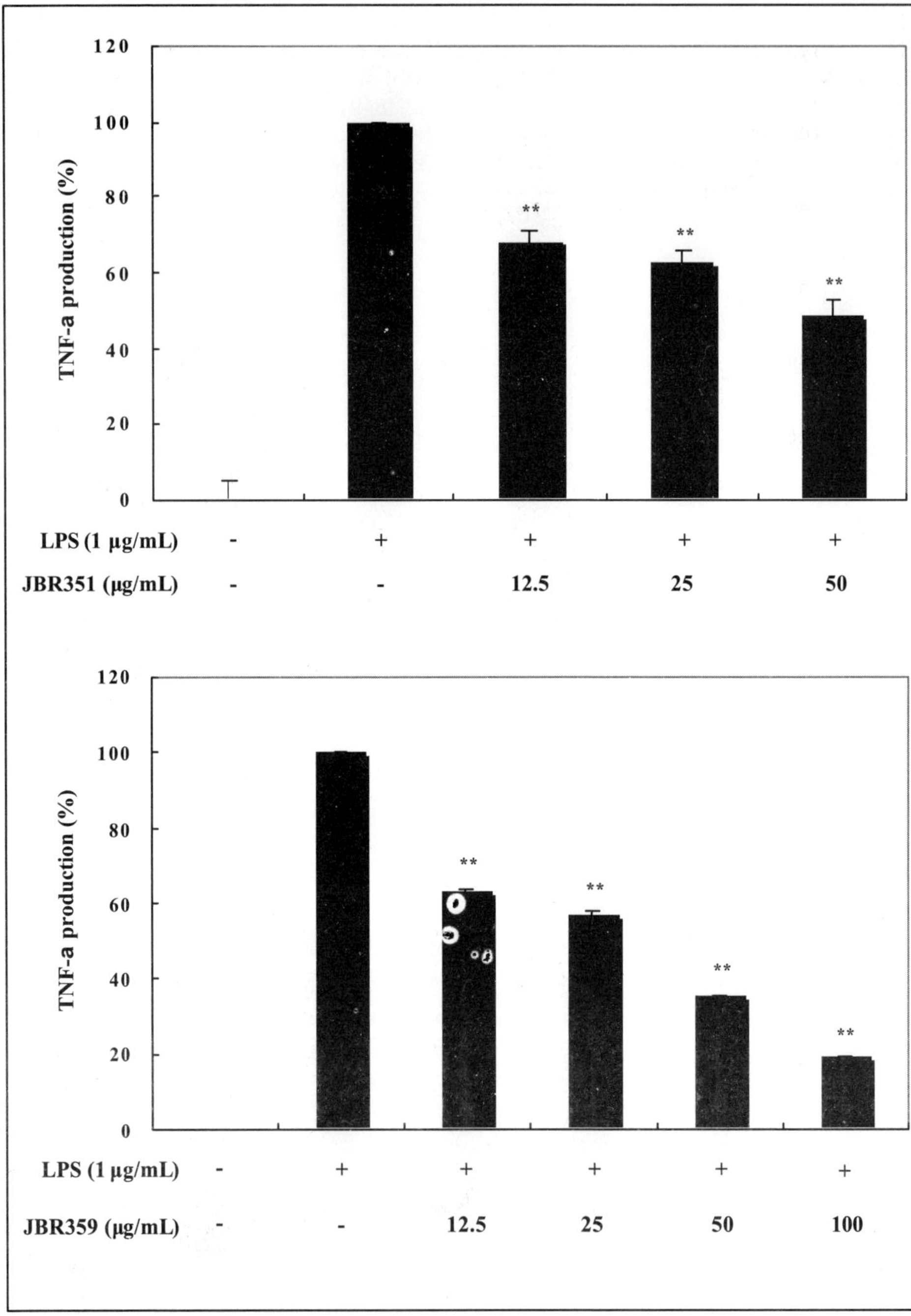

Contd...

Figure 7.5–*Contd...*

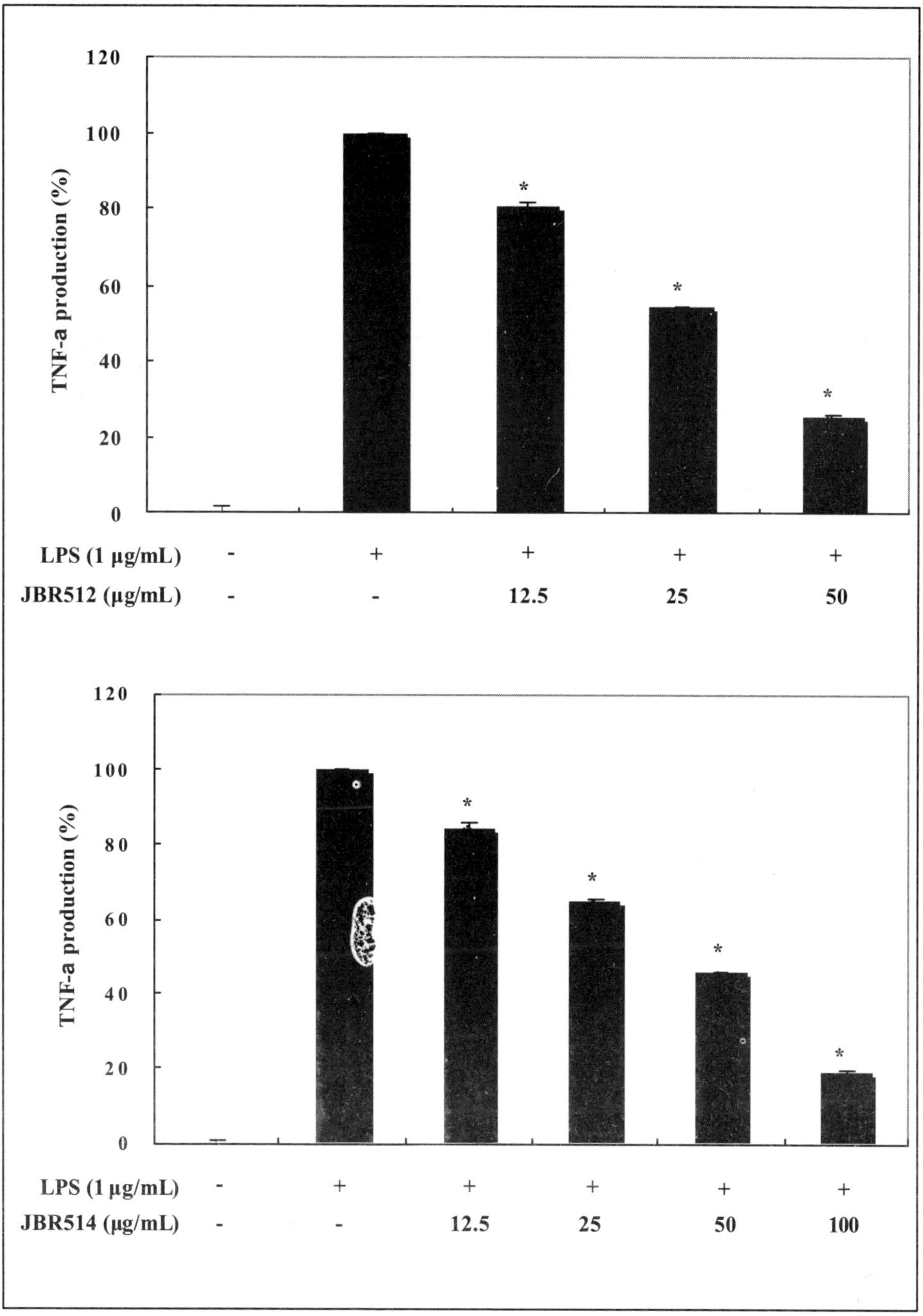

Contd...

Figure 7.5–*Contd...*

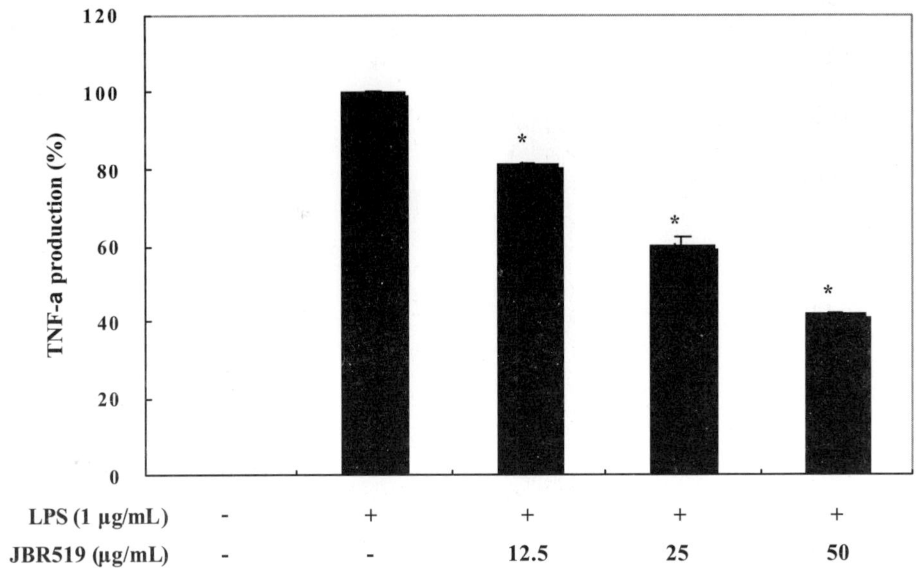

to the synergistic induction of NO synthesis in IFN-γ- and/or LPS-stimulated macrophages. TNF-α elicits a number of physiological effects such as septic shock, inflammation, cachexia, and cytotoxicity, while IL-6 is believed to be an endogenous mediator of LPS-induced fever (Feldmann, 2008; Ding *et al.*, 2009; Kim and Bachmann, 2009; Sugita, 2009; Yoon *et al.*, 2010e). In the present study, we demonstrated that Jeju seaweed extracts also significantly inhibited TNF-α and IL-6 production in a concentration-dependent manner.

NF-κB is known to play a critical role in the regulation of cell survival genes and to coordinate the expression of proinflammatory enzymes and cytokines, such as iNOS, COX-2, TNF-α, and IL-6 (Edwards *et al.*, 2009; Wong and Tergaonkar, 2009; Yoon *et al.*, 2010e). Hence, we hypothesized that the inhibitory effects of Jeju seaweed extracts on the production of NO, PGE_2, TNF-α, and IL-6 probably occurred via the NF-κB signaling pathway. However, we cannot exclude the inhibition of other transcription factors, since it is possible that another mechanism, such as MAPKs signaling, plays critical roles in the regulation of cell growth and differentiation and in the control of cellular responses to cytokines and stressors (Kang *et al.*, 2008).

In conclusion, our observations suggest that Jeju seaweed extracts have strong anti-inflammatory properties that could inhibit LPS-stimulated inflammation-associated gene expression. These effects may be exerted by the blocking of NF-κB activation

Figure 7.6. Effect of Jeju seaweed extracts on IL-6 production in LPS-stimulated RAW 264.7 cells

The cells were stimulated with 1 μg/mL of LPS alone or with a combination of LPS and various concentrations (12.5, 25, 50, or 100 μg/mL) of JBR261 (A), JBR276 (B), JBR351 (C), JBR359 (D), JBR512 (E), JBR514 (E), and JBR519 (F) for 24 h. IL-6 produced and released into the culture medium was assayed by the ELISA method. The data represent the mean ± SD of triplicate experiments. $^{*}p < 0.05$; $^{**}p < 0.01$ vs. LPS alone.

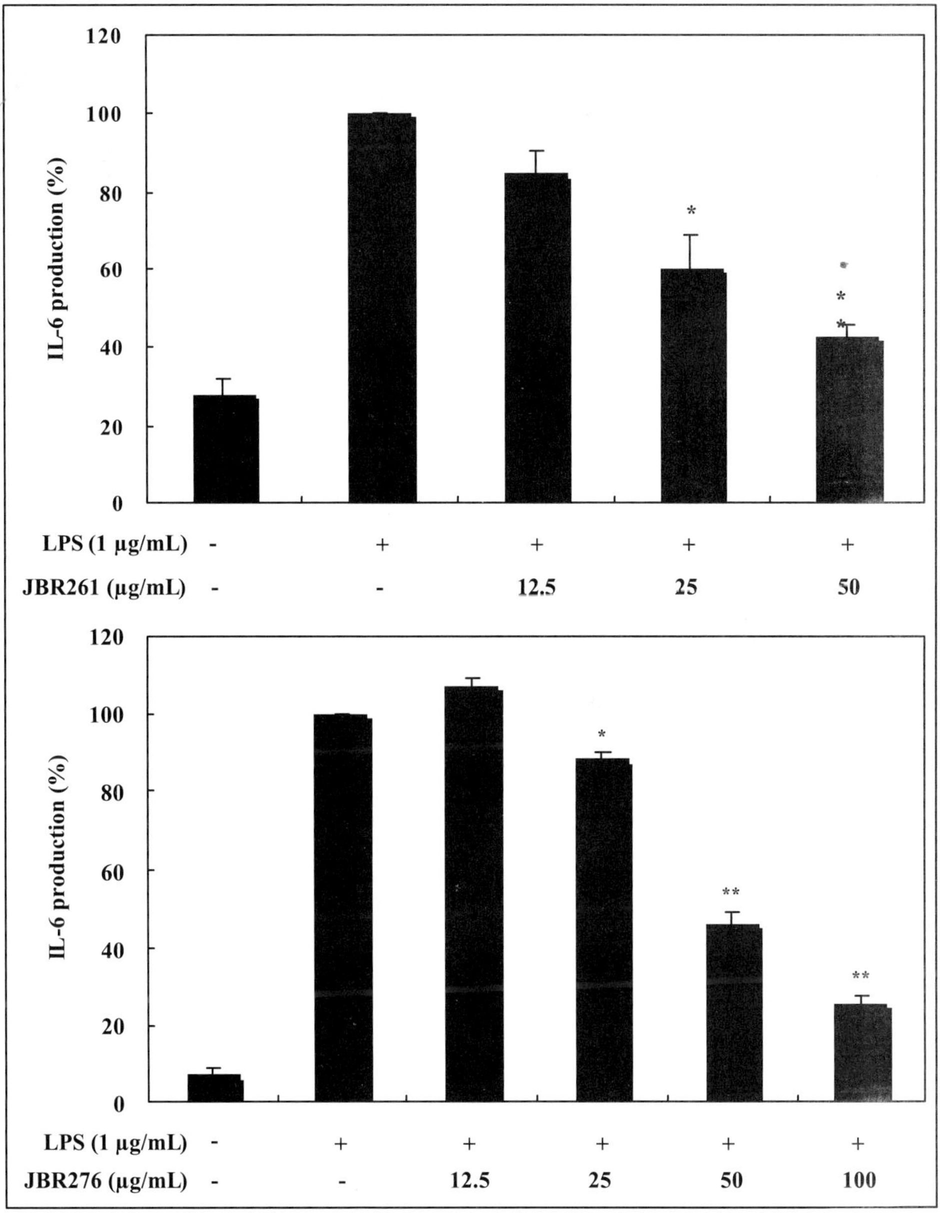

Contd...

Figure 7.6–*Contd...*

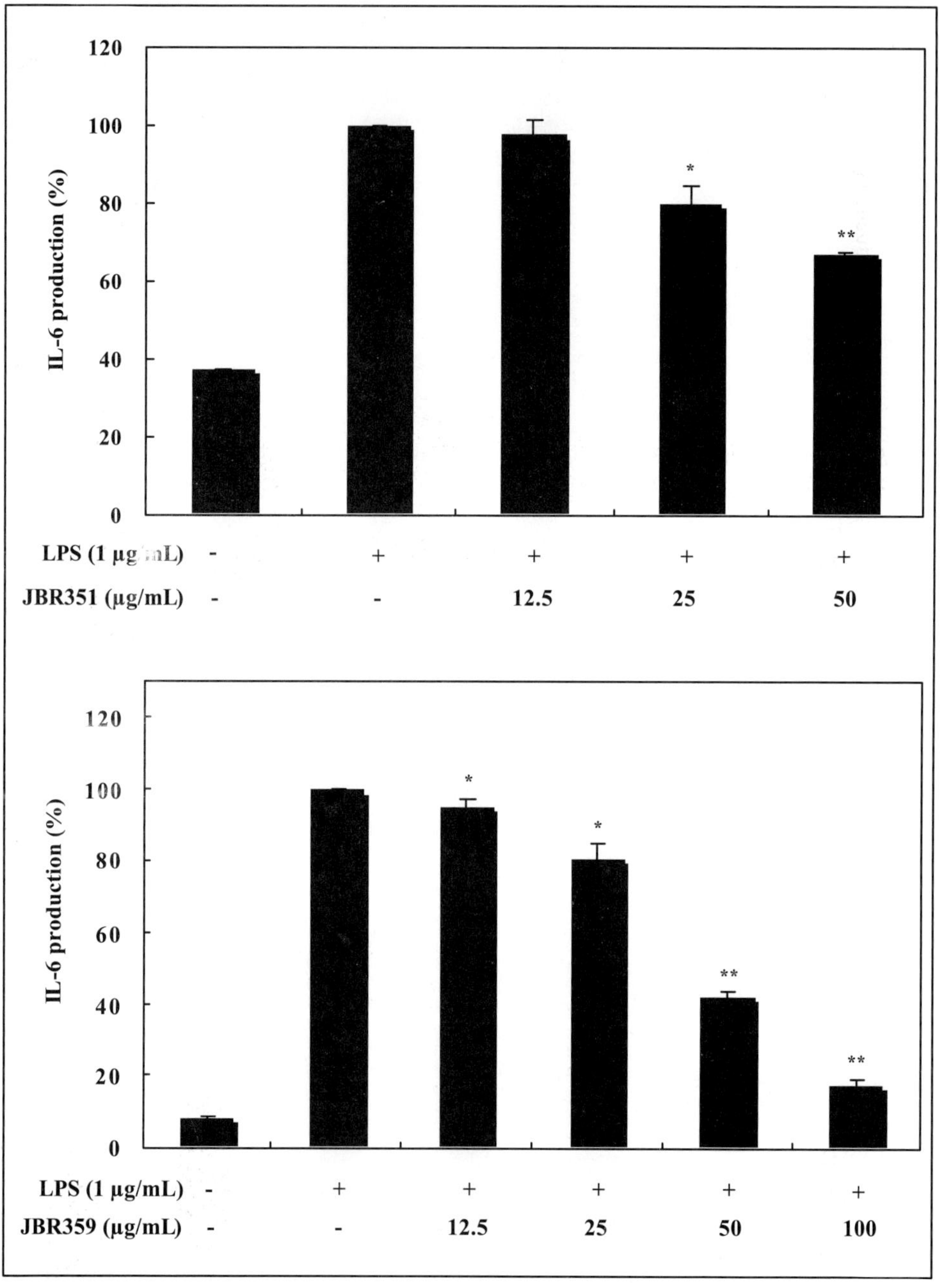

Contd...

Figure 7.6–*Contd...*

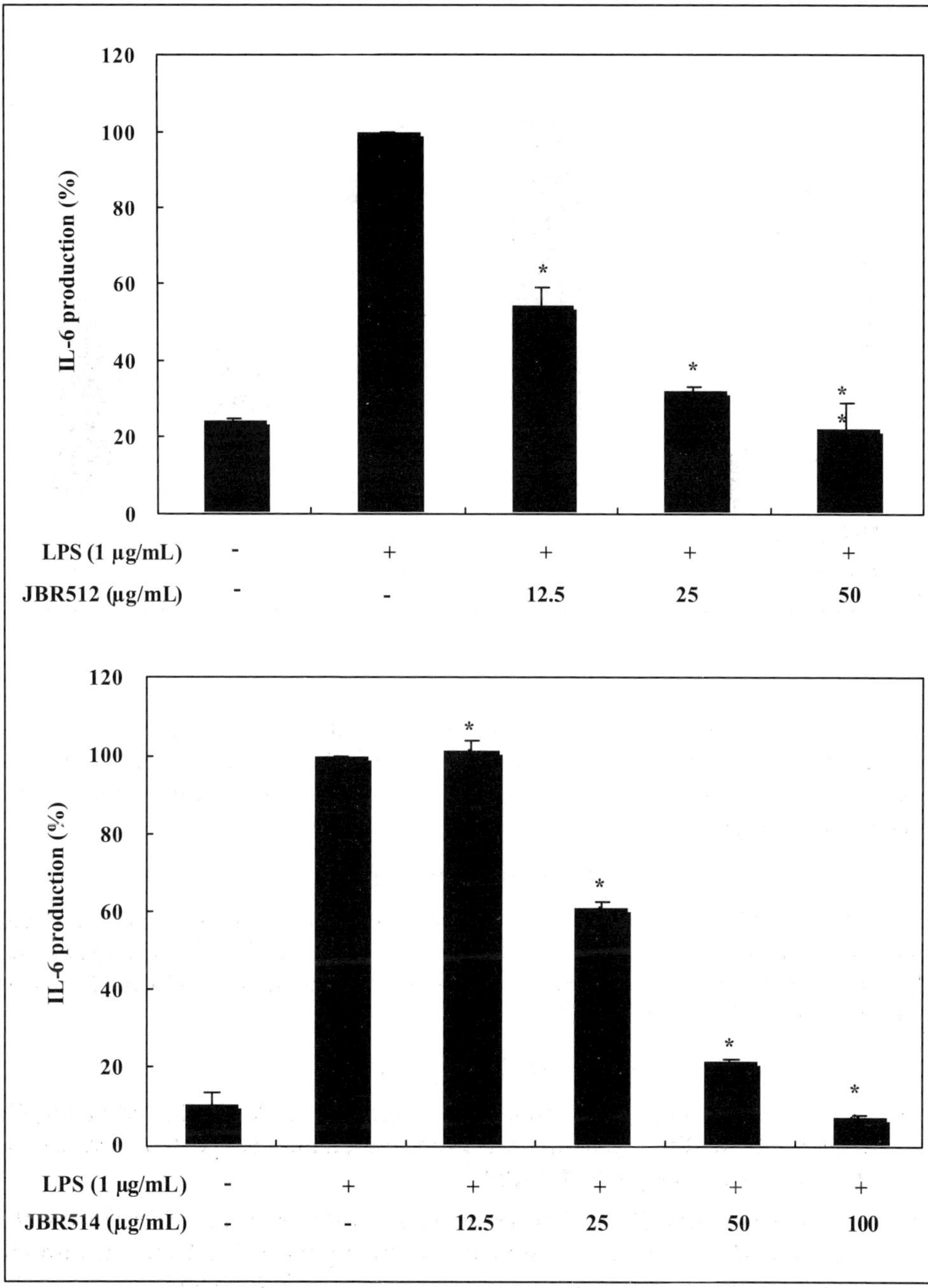

Contd...

Figure 7.5–*Contd...*

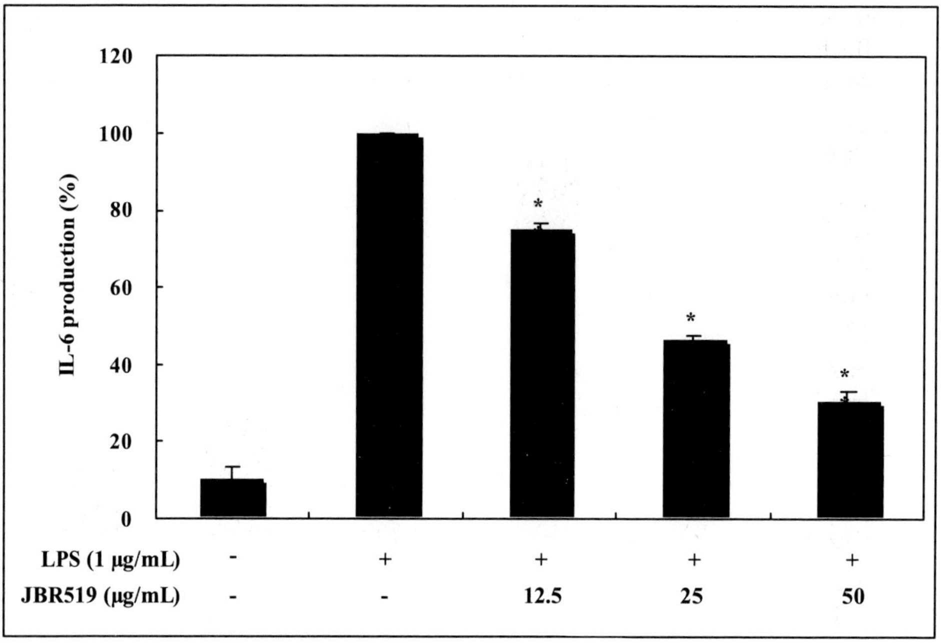

and/or the phosphorylation of MAPK pathways; these mechanisms need to be investigated further. Thus, the anti-inflammatory effects and low cytotoxicity of these seaweed extracts suggest potential therapeutic applications in the regulation of the inflammatory response.

Acknowledgments

This research was partially supported by Programs for the Regional Strategic Industries, the Regional Innovation System (JEJU SEA-GREEN PROJECT) and the Regional Technology Innovation (RTI04-02-07), which are managed by the Ministry of Knowledge and Economy, Korea.

References

Adorini, L., Amuchastegui, S., Corsiero, E., Laverny, G., Le Meur, T., and Penna, G. (2007). Vitamin D receptor agonists as anti-inflammatory agents. *Expert Review of Clinical Immunology*, **3**: 477-489.

Bae, S.J., and Choi, Y.H. (2007). Methanol extract of the seaweed *Gloiopeltis furcata* induces G2/M arrest and inhibits cyclooxygenase-2 activity in human hepatocarcinoma HepG2 cells. *Phytotherapy Research*, **21**: 52-57.

Blunt, J.W., Copp, B.R., Hu, W.P., Munro, M.H., Northcote, P.T., and Prinsep, M.R. (2009). Marine natural products. *Natural Product Reports*, **26**: 170-244.

Calabrese, V., Cornelius, C., Rizzarelli, E., Owen, J.B., Dinkova-Kostova, A.T., and Butterfield, D.A. (2009). Nitric oxide in cell survival: a janus molecule. *Antioxidants and Redox Signaling*, **11**: 2717-2739.

Chakraborti, A.K., Garg, S.K., Kumar, R., Motiwala, H.F., Jadhavar, P.S. Progress in COX-2 inhibitors: a journey so far. *Current Medicinal Chemistry*, **17**: 1563-1593.

Chang, Y.C., Li, P.C., Chen, B.C., Chang, M.S., Wang, J.L., Chiu, W.T., and Lin, C.H. (2006). Lipoteichoic acid-induced nitric oxide synthase expression in RAW 264.7 macrophages is mediated by cyclooxygenase-2, prostaglandin E_2, protein kinase A, p38 MAPK, and nuclear factor-kappaB pathways. *Cellular signaling*, **18**: 1235-1243.

Choi, E.Y., Hwang H.J., and Nam, T.J. (2010). Protective effect of a polysaccharide from *Hizikia fusiformis* against ethanol-induced cytotoxicity in IEC-6 cells. *Toxicology in vitro*, **24**: 79-84.

Choi, E.Y., Hwang H.J., Kim, I.H., and Nam, T.J. (2009). Protective effects of a polysaccharide from *Hizikia fusiformis* against ethanol toxicity in rats. *Food and Chemical Toxicology*, **47:** 134-139

Choi, H.J., Eun, J.S., Park, Y.R., Kim, D.K., Li, R., Moon, W.S., Park, J.M., Kim, H.S., Cho, N.P., Cho, S.D., and Soh, Y. (2008). Ikarisoside A inhibits inducible nitric oxide synthase in lipopolysaccharide-stimulated RAW 264.7 cells via p38 kinase and nuclear factor-kappaB signaling pathways. *European Journal of Pharmacology*, **601**: 171-188.

Ci, X., Ren, R., Xu, K., Li, H., Yu, Q., Song, Y., Wang, D., Li, R., and Deng, X. (2010). Schisantherin A exhibits anti-inflammatory properties by down-regulating NF-kappaB and MAPK signaling pathways in lipopolysaccharide-treated RAW 264.7 cells. *Inflammation*, **33**: 126-136.

Cuzzocrea, S. (2006). Role of nitric oxide and reactive oxygen species in arthritis. *Current Pharmaceutical Design*, **12**: 3551-3570.

Dang, H.T., Lee, H.J., Yoo, E.S., Shinde, P.B., Lee, Y.M., Hong, J., Kim, D.K., and Jung, J.H. (2008). Anti-inflammatory constituents of the red alga *Gracilaria verrucosa* and their synthetic analogues. *Journal of natural products*, **71**: 232-240.

De Benedetti, F. (2009). Targeting interleukin-6 in pediatric rheumatic diseases. *Current Opinion in Rheumatology*, **21**: 533-537.

Devi, K.P., Suganthy, N., Kesika, P., and Pandian, S.K. (2008). Bioprotective properties of seaweeds: in vitro evaluation of antioxidant activity and antimicrobial activity against food borne bacteria in relation to polyphenolic content. *BMC Complementary and Alternative Medicine*, **8**: 38.

Ding, C., Cicuttini, F., Li, J., and Jones, G. (2009). Targeting IL-6 in the treatment of inflammatory and autoimmune diseases. *Expert Opinion on Investigational Drugs*, **18**: 1457-1466.

Edwards, M.R., Bartlett, N.W., Clarke, D., Birrell, M., Belvisi, M., and Johnston, S.L. (2009). Targeting the NF-kappaB pathway in asthma and chronic obstructive pulmonary disease. *Pharmacology and Therapeutics*, **121**: 1-13.

Esposito, E., and Cuzzocrea, S. (2009). TNF-alpha as a therapeutic target in inflammatory diseases, ischemia-reperfusion injury and trauma. *Current Medicinal Chemistry*, **16**: 3152-3167.

Feldmann, M. (2008). Many cytokines are very useful therapeutic targets in disease. *Journal of Clinical Investigation*, **118**: 3533-3536.

Fitzpatrick, B., Mehibel, M., Cowen, R.L., and Stratford, I.J. (2008). iNOS as a therapeutic target for treatment of human tumors. *Nitric Oxide*, **19**: 217-224.

Fonseca, J.E., Santos, M.J., Canhão, H., and Choy, E. (2009). Interleukin-6 as a key player in systemic inflammation and joint destruction. *Autoimmunity Reviews*, **8**: 538-542.

González del Val, A., Platas, G., Basilio, A., Cabello, A., Gorrochategui, J., Suay, I., Vicente, F., Portillo, E., Jiménez del Río, M., Reina, G.G., and Peláez, F. (2001). Screening of antimicrobial activities in red, green and brown macro-algae from Gran Canaria (Canary Islands, Spain). *International Journal of Microbiology*, **4**: 35-40.

Huang, D., Ou, B., and Prior, R.L. (2005). The chemistry behind antioxidant capacity assays. *Journal of Agricultural and Food Chemistry*, **53**: 1841-1856.

Hwang, H.J., Kim I.H., and Nam, T.J. (2008). Effect of a glycoprotein from *Hizikia fusiformis* on acetaminophen-induced liver injury. *Food and Chemical Toxicology*, **46**: 3475-3481.

Iyer, J.P., Srivastava, P.K., Dev, R., Dastidar, S.G., and Ray, A. (2009). Prostaglandin E_2 synthase inhibition as a therapeutic target. *Expert Opinion on Therapeutic Targets*, **13**: 849-865.

Jung, H.W., Mahesh, R., Park, J.H., Boo, Y.C., Park, K.M., and Park, Y.K. (2010). Bisabolangelone isolated from *Ostericum koreanum* inhibits the production of inflammatory mediators by down-regulation of NF-kappaB and ERK MAP kinase activity in LPS-stimulated RAW264.7 cells. *International Immunopharmacology*, **10**: 155-162.

Kang, J.Y., Khan, M.N., Park, N.H., Cho, J.Y., Lee, M.C., Fujii, H., and Hong, Y.K. (2008). Antipyretic, analgesic, and anti-inflammatory activities of the seaweed *Sargassum fulvellum* and *Sargassum thunbergii* in mice. *Journal of Ethnopharmacology*, **116**: 187-190.

Kang, O.H., Chae, H.S., Choi, J.G., Oh, Y.C., Lee, Y.S., Kim, J.H., Seung, M.J., Jang, H.J., Bae, K.H., Lee, J.H., Shin, D.W., and Kwon, D.Y. (2008). Ent-pimara-8(14),15-dien-19-oic acid isolated from the roots of *Aralia cordata* inhibits induction of inflammatory mediators by blocking NF-kappaB activation and mitogen-activated protein kinase pathways. *European Journal of Pharmacology*, **601**: 179-185.

Kanwar, J.R., Kanwar, R.K., Burrow, H., and Baratchi, S. (2009). Recent advances on the roles of NO in cancer and chronic inflammatory disorders. *Current Medicinal Chemistry*, **16**: 2373-2394.

Khan, M.N., Choi, J.S., Lee, M.C., Kim, E., Nam, T.J., Fujii, H., and Hong, Y.K. (2008). Anti-inflammatory activities of methanol extracts from various seaweed species. *Journal of Environmental Biology*, **29**: 465-469.

Kim, J.H., Bachmann, R.A., Chen, J. (2009). Interleukin-6 and insulin resistance. *Vitamins and Hormones*, **80**: 613-633.

Kim, J.Y., Kim, D.S., Yang, E.J., Yoon, W.J., Baik, J.S., Lee, W.J., Lee, N.H., and Hyun, C.G. (2009a). Green alga *Ulva pertusa* inhibits nitric oxide and prostaglandin-E_2 formation in murine macrophage RAW 264.7 cells. *Journal of Applied Biological Chemistry*, **52**: 38-40.

Kim, J.Y., Park, S.J., Yun, K.J., Cho, Y.W., Park, H.J., and Lee, K.T. (2008a). Isoliquiritigenin isolated from the roots of *Glycyrrhiza uralensis* inhibits LPS-induced iNOS and COX-2 expression via the attenuation of NF-kappaB in RAW 264.7 macrophages. *European Journal of Pharmacology*, **584**: 175-184.

Kim, K.N., Ham, Y.M., Moon, J.Y., Kim, M.J., Kim, D.S., Lee, W.J., Lee, N.H., and Hyun, C.G. (2009b). *In vitro* cytotoxic activity of *Sargassum thunbergii* and *Dictyopteris divaricata* (Jeju seaweeds) on the HL-60 tumour cell line. *International Journal of Pharmacology*, **5**: 298-306.

Kim, M.M., Rajapakse, N., and Kim, S.K. (2009c). Anti-inflammatory effect of *Ishige okamurae* ethanolic extract via inhibition of NF-kappaB transcription factor in RAW 264.7 cells. *Phytotherapy Research*, **23**: 628-634.

Leonard, B.E. (2007). Inflammation, depression and dementia: are they connected? *Neurochemical Research*, **32**: 1749-1756.

López-Vélez, M., Martínez-Martínez, F., and Del Valle-Ribes, C. (2003). The study of phenolic compounds as natural antioxidants in wine. *Critical Reviews in Food Science and Nutrition*, **43**: 233-244.

Murakami, A. (2009). Chemoprevention with phytochemicals targeting inducible nitric oxide synthase. *Forum of nutrition*, **61**: 193-203.

O'Connor, D.M., and O'Brien, T. (2009). Nitric oxide synthase gene therapy: progress and prospects. *Expert Opinion on Biological Therapy*, **9**: 867-878.

Radovits, B.J., Kievit, W., and Laan, R.F. (2009). Tumour necrosis factor-alpha antagonists in the management of rheumatoid arthritis in the elderly: a review of their efficacy and safety. *Drugs and Aging*, **26**: 647-664.

Rocha, F.D., Soares A.R., Houghton P.J., Pereira R.C., Kaplan M.A., and Teixeira V.L. (2007) Potential cytotoxic activity of some Brazilian seaweeds on human melanoma cells. *Phytotherapy Research*, **21**: 170-175.

Silverman, R.B. (2009). Design of selective neuronal nitric oxide synthase inhibitors for the prevention and treatment of neurodegenerative diseases. *Accounts of Chemical Research*, **42**: 439-451.

Uðar-Cankal, D., and Ozmeric, N. (2006). A multifaceted molecule, nitric oxide in oral and periodontal diseases. *Clinica Chimica Acta*, **366**: 90-100.

Usami, Y. (2009). Recent synthetic studies leading to structural revisions of marine natural products. *Marine Drugs,* **7**: 314-330.

Wang, D., and Dubois, R.N. (2010). The role of COX-2 in intestinal inflammation and colorectal cancer. *Oncogene,* **29**: 781-788.

Wong, E.T., and Tergaonkar, V. (2009). Roles of NF-kappaB in health and disease: mechanisms and therapeutic potential. *Clinical Science,* **116**: 451-465.

Yang, E.J., Ham, Y.M., Kim, D.S., Kim, J.Y., Hong, J.P., Kim, M.J., Moon, J.Y., Lee, W.J., Lee, N.H., and Hyun, C.G. (2010a). *Ecklonia stolonifera* inhibits lipopolysaccharide-induced production of nitric oxide, prostaglandin E_2, and proinflammatory cytokines in RAW264.7 macrophages. *Biologia,* **65**: 362-371.

Yang, E.J., Kim, J.G., Kim, J.Y., Kim, S.C., Lee, N.H., and Hyun, C.G. (2010b) Anti-inflammatory effect of chitosan oligosaccharides in RAW 264.7 cells. *Central European Journal of Biology,* **5**: 95-102.

Yang, E.J., Moon, J.Y., Kim, M.J., Kim, D.S., Kim, C.S., Lee, W.J., Lee, N.H., and Hyun, C.G. (2010c). Inhibitory effect of Jeju endemic seaweeds on the production of pro-inflammatory mediators in mouse macrophage cell line RAW 264.7. *Journal of Zhejiang University SCIENCE B,* **11**: 315-322.

Yang, E.J., Moon, J.Y., Kim, M.J., Kim, D.S., Lee, W.J., Lee, N.H., and Hyun, C.G. (2010d). Anti-inflammatory effect of *Petalonia binghamiae* in LPS-induced macrophages is mediated by suppression of iNOS and COX-2. *International Journal of Agriculture and Biology,* **12**: 754-758.

Yang, E.J., Moon, J.Y., Lee, J.S., Koh, J., Lee, N.H., and Hyun, C.G. (2010e). *Acanthopanax koreanum* fruit waste inhibits lipopolysaccharide-induced production of nitric oxide and prostaglandin E_2 in RAW 264.7 macrophages. *Journal of Biomedicine and Biotechnology,* **2010**: 715739.

Yen, G.C., Duh, P.D., Huang, D.W., Hsu, C.L., and Fu, T.Y. (2008). Protective effect of pine (*Pinus morrisonicola* Hay.) needle on LDL oxidation and its anti-inflammatory action by modulation of iNOS and COX-2 expression in LPS-stimulated RAW 264.7 macrophages. *Food and Chemical Toxicology,* **46**: 175-185.

Yoon, W.J., Ham, Y.M., Kim, K.N., Park, S.Y., Lee, N.H., Hyun, C.G., and Lee, W.J. (2009a). Anti-inflammatory activity of brown alga *Dictyota dichotoma* in murine macrophage RAW 264.7 cells. *Journal of Medicinal Plants Research,* **3**: 1-8.

Yoon, W.J., Ham, Y.M., Kim, S.S., Yoo, B.S., Moon, J.Y., Baik, J.S., Lee, N.H., and Hyun, C.G. (2009b). Suppression of proinflammatory cytokines, iNOS, and COX-2 expression by brown algae *Sargassum micracanthum* in RAW 264.7 Macrophages. *EuAsian Journal of Biology,* **3**: 130-143.

Yoon, W.J., Ham, Y.M., Lee, W.J., Lee, N.H., and Hyun, C.G. (2010a). Brown alga *Sargassum muticum* inhibits proinflammatory cytokines, iNOS, and COX-2 expression in macrophage RAW 264.7 cells. *Turkish Journal of Biology,* **34**: 25-34.

Yoon, W.J., Ham, Y.M., Yoo, B.S., Moon, J.Y., Koh, J., and Hyun, C.G. (2009c). *Oenothera laciniata* inhibits lipopolysaccharide induced production of nitric oxide, prostaglandin E_2, and proinflammatory cytokines in RAW264.7 macrophages. *Journal of Bioscience and Bioengineering,* **107**: 429-438.

Yoon, W.J., Kim, D.S., Yang, E.J., Moon, J.Y., Kim, M.J., Lee, W.J., Lee, N.H., and Hyun, C.G. (2010b). Inhibitory effects of *Enteromorpha prolifera* on the production of nitric oxide, prostaglandin E_2, and pro-inflammatory cytokines in RAW 264.7 cells. *Latin American Journal of Pharmacy,* **29**: 165-170.

Yoon, W.J., Kim, S.S., Oh, T.H., Lee, N.H., and Hyun, C.G. (2009d). *Abies koreana* essential oil inhibits drug-resistant skin pathogen growth and LPS-induced inflammatory effects of murine macrophage. *Lipids,* **44**: 471-476.

Yoon, W.J., Lee, N.H., and Hyun, C.G. (2010c). Limonene suppresses lipopolysaccharide-induced production of nitric oxide, prostaglandin E_2, and pro-inflammatory cytokines in RAW 264.7 macrophages. *Journal of Oleo Science,* **59**: 415-421.

Yoon, W.J., Moon, J.Y., Kang, J.Y., Kim, G.O., Lee, N.H., and Hyun, C.G. (2010d). *Neolitsea sericea* essential oil attenuates LPS-induced inflammation in RAW 264.7 macrophages by suppressing NF-κB and MAPK activation. *Natural Product Communications,* **5**: 1311-1316.

Yoon, W.J., Moon, J.Y., Song, G., Lee, Y.K., Han, M.S., Lee, J.S., Ihm, B.S., Lee, W.J., Lee, N.H., and Hyun, C.G. (2010e). *Artemisia fukudo* essential oil attenuates LPS-induced inflammation by suppressing NF-kappaB and MAPK activation in RAW 264.7 macrophages. *Food and Chemical Toxicology,* **48**: 1222-1229.

Zhou, H.Y., Shin, E.M., Guo, L.Y., Youn, U.J., Bae, K.H., Kang, S.S., Zou, L.B., and Kim, Y.S. (2008). Anti-inflammatory activity of 4-methoxyhonokiol is a function of the inhibition of iNOS and COX-2 expression in RAW 264.7 macrophages via NF-κB, JNK and p38 MAPK inactivation. *European Journal of Pharmacology,* **586**: 340-349.

Zhou, L., and Zhu, D.Y. (2009). Neuronal nitric oxide synthase: structure, subcellular localization, regulation, and clinical implications. *Nitric Oxide,* **20**: 223-230.

Medicinal Plants: Phytochemistry, Pharmacology and Therapeutics Vol. 2 (2012) *Pages* **129–146**
Editor-in-Chief: **V.K. Gupta**
Published by: **DAYA PUBLISHING HOUSE, NEW DELHI**

8

Mining of Novel Antifungal Proteins from Medicinal Plants

Modhumita Dasgupta[1*]

ABSTRACT

Antifungal proteins and polypeptides have been isolated from diverse groups of organisms, including plants, fungi, bacteria, insects, and animals. The mechanisms of action of these proteins are as varied as their sources and include fungal cell wall polymer degradation, membrane channel and pore formation, damage to cellular ribosomes, inhibition of DNA synthesis and inhibition of cell cycle. The mode of action of many proteins remains unknown and is a subject of active research. In plants, antifungal proteins or pathogenesis related (PR) proteins have been extensively reviewed in crop plants and currently comprise 17 families of induced proteins. Reports on characterization of PR proteins from plants of pharmacological significance are limited. The present report demonstrates the identification and characterization of non-race specific, broad spectrum PR proteins showing toxicity against phytopathogens from Plumbago capensis, Andrographis paniculata, Acorus calamus (AcPOX) and Withania somnifera (Wsl). This chapter highlights a new dimension to the utilization of the untapped genetic resources for novel peptides.

Keywords: Chitin binding, Hyphal inhibition, Lectin, Medicinal plants, Pathogenesis-related proteins, Peroxidase.

Introduction

Plants require a broad range of defence mechanisms to effectively combat invasion by microbial pathogens and possess both preformed and inducible mechanisms to

1 Division of Plant Biotechnology, Institute of Forest Genetics and Tree Breeding, Forest Campus, R.S. Puram, Coimbatore – 641 002, India

* *Corresponding author*: E-mail: ghoshm@icfre.org; modhumitaghosh@hotmail.com

resist pathogen entry. Some of the responses are constitutive and pathogen non-specific, but a majority of them are induced after recognition of the pathogen. However, they have orchestrated defense mechanisms which are either preformed or induced during a stress. The inducible defense responses include hypersensitive cell death (Levine *et al.*, 1994), production of phytoalexins (Kuc and Rush, 1985), induction of oxidative burst (Baker and Orlandi, 1995), lignification (Ride, 1986), cross-linking of wall glycoprotein (Bradley *et al.* 1992) and accumulation of Pathogenesis-Related (PR) proteins (Velazhahan *et al.*, 1998; 2000).

PR-proteins are a group of extracellular proteins that are induced by different phytopathogens such as fungi, bacteria and viruses, fungal elicitors and certain chemicals such as salicylic acid, polyacrylic acid and 2,6-dichloroisonicotinic acid (Uknes *et al.*, 1992). The recognized PR proteins have been extensively reviewed (Broekaert *et al.*, 2000) and currently comprise 17 families of induced proteins (van Loon *et al.*, 2006) including four families of chitinases (Graham and Sticklen, 1994), one each of 1,3-glucanases (Simmons, 1994; Leubner-Metzger and Meins, 1999), proteinase inhibitors (Mosolov *et al.*, 2001), one specific peroxidase (Kawano, 2003), PR-1 family with unknown biochemical properties (Niderman *et al.*, 1995), the thaumatin-like PR-5 family (Trudel *et al.*, 1998), the birch allergen Betv1-related PR-10 family (McGee *et al.*, 2001), defensins (Thomma *et al.*, 2002), lipid-transfer proteins (LTPs) (García-Olmedo *et al.*, 1995), thionins (Bohlmann and Apel, 1991; Peligrini and Franco, 2005) and other proteins including 2S storage albumins (Terras *et al.*, 1993) and Ribosome inactivating proteins (RIPs) (Nielsen and Boston, 2001). The roles of PR proteins, their classification, mechanism of action, role in defence mechanisms and generation of transgenics with increased resistance have been extensively reviewed (Selitrennikoff, 2001; Punja, 2001; De Lucca *et al.*, 2005).

However, most of the reports on purification and characterization of antifungal proteins are limited to crop plants. The present paper demonstrates an alternate source of novel antifungal proteins/peptides from plants known for their pharmaceutical properties.

Materials and Methods

Plant Material

The medicinal plants used for isolation of antifungal proteins included *Plumbago capensis, Andrographis paniculata, Acorus calamus* and *Withania somnifera*. Young leaves of *Plumbago capensis* Thunb. and *Andrographis paniculata* (Burm. F.) Wall. Ex Nees were collected from germplasm collection assembled at botanical garden at the Institute of Forest Genetics and Tree Breeding, Coimbatore, India. Rhizomes of *Acorus calamus* were obtained from Munnar, Iddukki district and Tropical Botanical Garden and Research Institute, Palode, Kerala, India. The rhizomes were propagated and maintained in vermiculite (grade 3), coir pith and river sand (1:1:1 ratio) under shade conditions. Seeds of *Withania somnifera* obtained from Regional Forest Research Institute, Andhra Pradesh Forest Department, Rajahmundry, Andhra Pradesh, India were germinated and maintained in polybags containing sand, red soil and celrich (commercial organic manure, SPIC India Ltd, India) in ratio 2:1:0.1.

Fungal Culture

The fungal isolates of *Rhizoctonia solani* (*Phyllanthus* isolate), *Fusarium moniliforme* (rice isolate), *Macrophomina phaseolina* (blackgram isolate) and *Trichosporium vesiculosum* (*Casuarina* isolate) were grown and maintained in potato dextrose agar medium.

Purification of Antifungal Proteins

The protein fraction showing antifungal activity was purified from the total proteins through series of purification steps including selective precipitation, gel filtration, ion exchange chromatography and affinity chromatography. The purification steps employed for each species varied due to the nature of the metabolites present in the plant species and the category of antifungal proteins targeted for purification.

Purification of Antifungal Proteins from Selected Medicinal Plants

In *Plumbago capensis*, total protein was extracted from young leaves in ice cold extraction buffer (10mM NaH_2PO_4; 15mM Na_2HPO_4; 100mM KCl; 2mM EDTA and 1mM PMSF) at 1:3 w/v for 2 hours at 4°C. The extract was clarified by centrifugation and the supernatant was subjected to sequential precipitation with ammonium sulphate at 30 per cent and 75 per cent relative precipitation for 1 hour at room temperature. The final pellet was pooled and desalted by gel filtration using Sephadex G50 column. The total proteins were fractionated through Superdex 75 (HR 10/30) pre packed gel filtration column (GE Healthcare, Piscataway, NJ, USA) using Fast Protein Liquid chromatography system (GE Healthcare, Piscataway, NJ, USA) using 0.1M ammonium acetate pH 5.0 (Ghosh *et al.*, 2002). The peak giving fractions were pooled and freeze- dried. The freeze- dried samples were suspended in sterile water and stored at -20°C until further use.

Similarly, in *Andrographis paniculata*, total proteins were extracted from leaves in ice cold extraction buffer containing 50mM sodium acetate (pH 5.2), 1mM ascorbic acid, 0.5mM PMSF and 0.5 per cent polyvinyl polypyrrolidone and the supernatant was subjected to 30 per cent ammonium sulphate precipitation. The protein pellets were desalted using sephadex G50 column and subjected to cation exchange chromatography using carboxy methyl cellulose (CMC) as matrix. The pre swollen CMC sorbent was equilibrated with 50mM ammonium acetate, pH 3.7 prior to loading the total protein. Proteins were eluted with 100mM ammonium acetate, pH 3.7 and peak giving fractions were pooled, freeze-dried and suspended in sterile water and desatted using microcon (Millipore) column with membrane nominal molecular weight limit [NMWL] of 3000 Daltons (Ghosh *et al.*, 2004). The desalted protein fractions were stored at –20°C until further use.

The total proteins from *Acorus calamus* were isolated from leaves of 25 day to 30 day old sprouting. The leaf tissues were homogenized in buffer containing 25mM sodium phosphate, pH 7.0, 250mM NaCl, 10mM EDTA, 5mM ß-mercaptoethanol, 1mM PMSF and 1.5 per cent PVPP. The extract was clarified and centrifuged twice to remove the debris. The pellet was discarded and the supernatant was subjected to selective precipitation by adjusting the pH to 4.6 with glacial acetic acid. The precipitated protein was discarded after centrifugation at 10,000rpm for 10 minutes at 4°C and the supernatant was passed through pre-packed desalting columns with exclusion limit of 5,000Da (Bangalore Genei Ltd., India) for buffer exchange. Protein sample was loaded and allowed to drain completely followed by elution of the proteins using 50mM sodium acetate buffer, pH 4.6. The crude sample was further purified through cation exchange chromatography using HiTrap SP FF column in the Fast Protein Liquid Chromatography (FPLC) system (GE Healthcare, Piscataway, NJ, USA). Proteins were eluted with NaCl gradient of 50mM sodium acetate pH 4.6 (0 to 1M NaCl) and the peak giving fractions were pooled and dialyzed. The proteins present in the fractions were precipitated with four volumes of ice-cold acetone after incubation for 20 minutes at –80°C. The proteins were pelleted, air dried and dissolved in 50mM sodium phosphate buffer, pH 7.0. The fractions were subsequently purified by gel filtration using superose 12 10/300 GL column in the FPLC system and protein fractions were eluted 50mM sodium phosphate, pH 7.0 with 15mM NaCl. Peak giving fractions were pooled, desalted and concentrated using Microsep centrifugal device (Pall life sciences, Ann Arbor, MI, USA) with 3000Da cut off membrane (Ghosh, 2006).

In *Withania somnifera*, modifications were made to purify the antifungal proteins. The leaf tissues were homogenized in liquid nitrogen and extracted in three volumes of phosphate buffer, pH 7.0 (25mM Na_2PO_4; 250 mM NaCl; 10mM EDTA; 1mM PMSF; 1.5 per cent PVPP; 0.2 per cent activated charcoal and 100mM ascorbic acid) and the supernatant was subjected to 60 per cent ammonium sulfate precipitation. The protein pellet was dissolved in 50mM sodium phosphate buffer, pH 7.0 and desalted by diafiltration using Microsep centrifugal device (Pall life sciences, Ann Arbor, MI, USA). Total proteins were fractionated twice by gel filtration using sepharose 6B column (Sigma Aldrich Ltd., USA) column and superose 12 10/300 GL column using FPLC system (GE Healthcare, Piscataway, NJ, USA). In both columns, the proteins were eluted using 50mM sodium phosphate buffer, pH 7.0. Finally the protein fractions were subjected to affinity chromatography using concanavalin A sepharose column (Sigma Aldrich Ltd., USA) and eluted with a gradient of methyl –D- mannopyranoside (0 – 0.5M) in binding buffer. The eluted fractions were pooled, concentrated and desalted by diafiltration (Ghosh, 2009).

The concentrations of purified proteins isolated from all four species were determined using Bradford's reagent (Sigma Aldrich Ltd., USA) (Bradford, 1976).

In vitro Bioassay of Purified Proteins

The *in vitro* bioassay of the purified fractions against phytopathogens was conducted by hyphal extension inhibition assay and microtitre plate assay (Ghosh *et al.*, 2006). The protein treated hyphae from *A. calamus* and *W. somnifera* were subjected to morphological analysis using light microscopy and scanning electron microscopy (Ghosh, 2006; 2009).

Characterization of Purified Protein

The molecular weight of the purified proteins was determined by native/SDS PAGE using standard molecular weight markers (Bangalore Genei Ltd, India) as described by Laemmli (1970) and stained with Ezee blue gel stainer (Bangalore Genei Ltd, India) or silver nitrate.

The pI of the purified proteins was determined by isoelectric focusing in IEF 3 – 9 precast gel using the Phast automated electrophoretic system (GE Healthcare, Piscataway, NJ, USA) using broad range (pH 3 – 10) IEF marker (GE Healthcare, Piscataway, NJ, USA) as standard. The gels were stained with Ezee blue gel stainer (Bangalore Genei Ltd, India) or silver nitrate.

The proteins purified from *A. calamus* and *W. somni*fera were additionally characterized by peptide sequencing. The purified protein was separated on a 12 per cent SDS-PAGE and stained with Ezee Blue gel stainer (Bangalore Genei Ltd, India). Gel plugs containing protein spots were subjected to automated tryptic digestion on a ProGest Workstation (Genomic Solutions, Ann Arbor, MI). Mass spectroscopic peptide separation and sequencing was carried out on Applied Biosystems QSTAR PULSARi™ quadrupole time of flight mass spectrometer coupled to an Amersham Ettan™ MDLC nano HPLC workstation (Applied Biosystems, CA, USA). TOFms spectra were collected between the mass range 100-2000 amu throughout the gradient elution and precursor ion selection and product ion spectra were generated using Applied Biosystems BioAnalyst™ software's fully automated switching and acquisition procedures. Only multiple charged precursor ion species were selected for fragmentation and peptide sequencing (Ghosh, 2006; 2009).

Comparison of Purified Antifungal Protein Activity with Standard Proteins

The antifungal protein from *A. calamus* was compared with a standard horseradish peroxidase (HRP) through *in vitro* hyphal extension inhibition assay. 1mg of HRP dissolved in sterile water was loaded on sterile disc along with 15 µg of the purified peroxidase from *A. calamus* (*AcPOX*). A control (C) with sterile water was also maintained. In *W. somnifera*, 1 mg of standard lectins including concanavalin A, phytohemagglutinin and wheat germ agglutinin (Bangalore Genei Ltd., India) were dissolved in 50ml of sterile distilled water and tested for their toxicity against *T. vesiculosum* using *in vitro* hyphal extension inhibition bioassay. 8 µg purified protein was also loaded to compare the efficacy of the *Withania* protein with standard lectins (Ghosh, 2009).

Results

The total proteins from *P. capensis* fractionated into four major peaks after gel filtration in superdex 75 column. All the fractions were tested for their antifungal activity against *M. phaseolina*. The second fraction was found to inhibit the spore germination and hyphal extension of *M. phaseolina* at concentrations of 15 µg/100 µl at 72 hours incubation (Figure 8.1). The molecular weight of the protein constituent in the second fraction was determined to be approximately 20 KDa.

In *Andrographis paniculata*, cation exchange chromatography generated three peaks which were tested for their antifungal activity. The first fraction inhibited the spore germination and hyphal extension of major pathogens like *M. phaseolina*, *A. flavus* and *T. vesiculosum* at concentrations of 15mg ml^{-1}, 24mg ml^{-1} and 10 mg ml^{-}

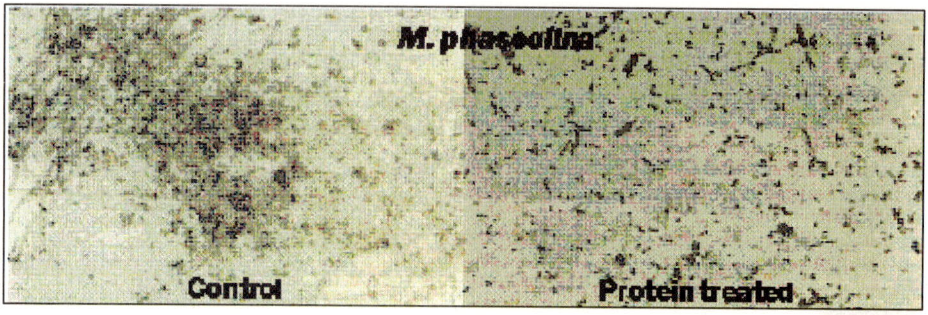

Figure 8.1. *In vitro* bioassay of antifungal protein from *P. capensis* against *M. phaseolina.*

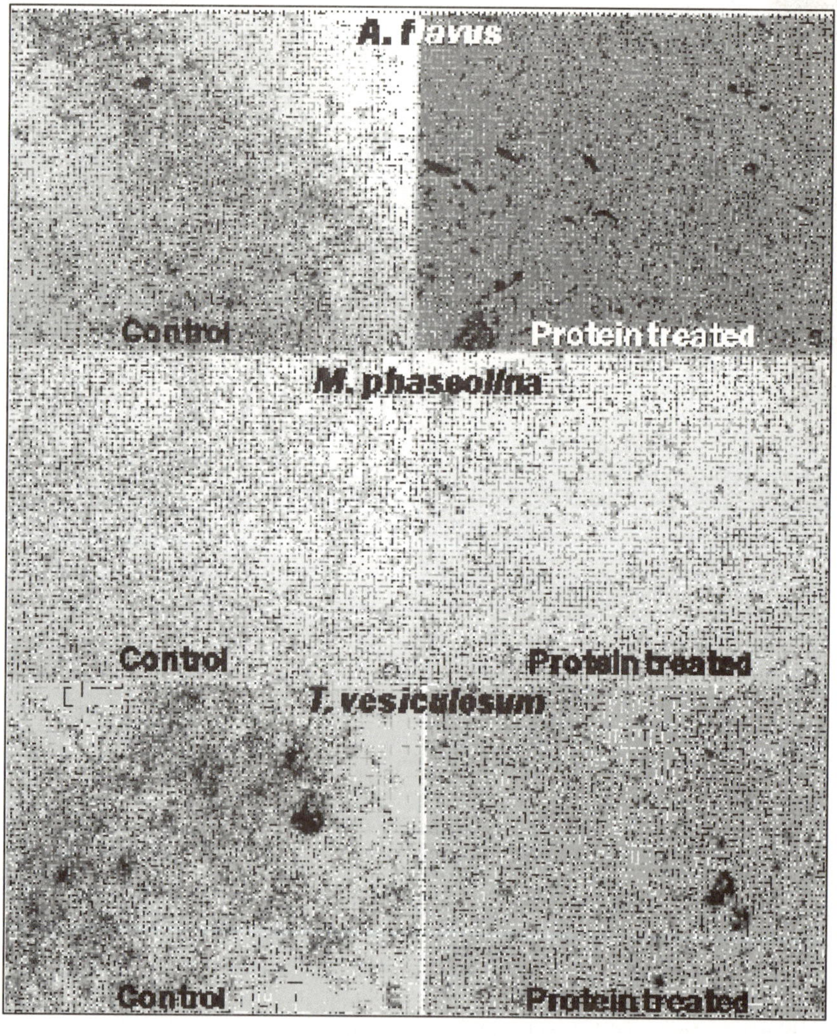

Figure 8.2. *In vitro* bioassay of antifungal protein from *A. paniculata* against phytopathogens.

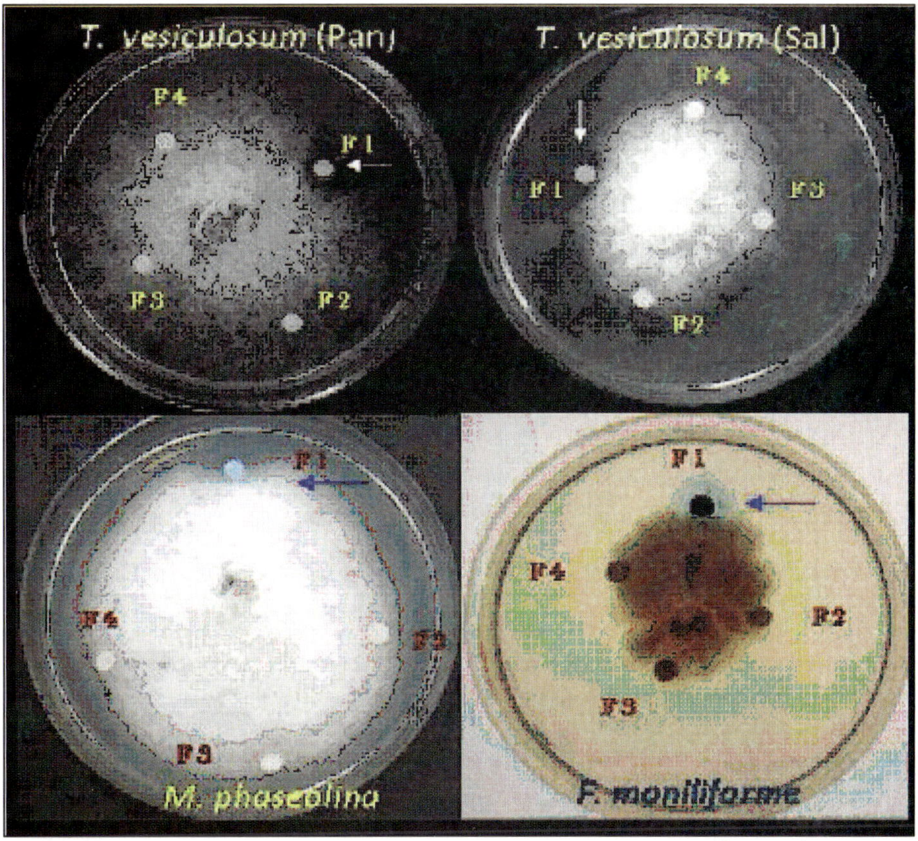

Figure 8.3. Hyphal extension inhibition assay of antifungal peroxidase from *Acorus calamus* (*AcPOX*) against phytopathogens.

[1] respectively (Figure 8.2). The molecular mass of the protein component in the first fraction was determined in 12 per cent native PAGE using standard markers, to be approximately 39.5 KDa.

The total leaf protein extracted from *A. calamus* was purified through cation exchange chromatography followed by gel filtration using superose 12 10/300 GL column. Four peak giving fractions were obtained and fraction 1 showed antifungal activity inhibiting the pathogen, *T. vesiculosum, M. phaseolina* and *F. moniliforme* at concentrations of 8 μg, 10 μg and12 μg respectively (Figure 8.3). The microtitre plate assay indicated that the purified protein caused stunted growth of hyphae with abnormal swelling in both isolates of *T. vesiculosum* and *M. phaseolina*. In *F. moniliforme*, an increased hyphal branching was observed along with stunted growth after 48 hours of protein treatment (Figure 8.4). The purified protein from fraction 1 had a molecular weight of approximately 32 KDa and pI was approximately 7.93.

The purified protein was subjected to tryptic digestion followed by LC MSMS. The digest generated 10 peptide fragments of which six were unique fragments with

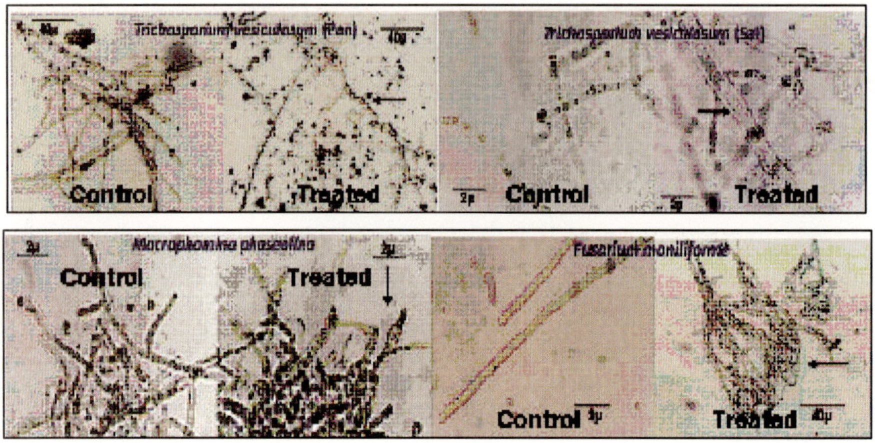

Figure 8.4. Morphological difference of *AcPOX* treated hyphase of phytopathogens.

sequence coverage of 37 per cent with putative bacterial-induced peroxidase from *Oryza sativa* (japonica cultivar-group) (Accession number BAD61674). The peptides matched the full length of the sequence including N-terminal and C-terminal region of the *Oryza* bacterial-induced peroxidase sequences. The blastp search also revealed the similarity of the peptide sequence with putative bacterial induced peroxidases from rice with accession numbers BAD61674, BAD61677, BAD61671 with similarity percentages of 49 per cent, 42 per cent and 41 per cent respectively (Figure 8.5).

The comparative analysis of the peroxidase purified from *A. calamus* (*AcPOX*) with standard HRP revealed a clear zone of inhibition around *AcPOX* treated discs, while no inhibition was exhibited by HRP (Figure 8.6).

The antifungal protein from *W. somnifera* was purified by gel filtration and fractionated four peaks, which were tested for antifungal activity. The second peak with antifungal activity was purified through affinity chromatography. The fraction showed a distinct zone of inhibition at a concentration of 7µg against *T. vesiculosum*. This fraction also inhibited *F. moniliforme* and *M. phaseolina* at a concentration of 9µg and *R. solani* at 11µg concentration (Figure 8.7).

The purified protein was separated on a precast SDS PAGE and presence of a single band was observed at approximately 30 KDa revealing the monomeric nature of the protein. The pI of the purified protein was determined to be approximately 4.0. The protein was further characterized by peptide mass fingerprinting using LC MSMS. The digest generated four unique peptide fragments with sequence coverage of 21 per cent and 20 per cent with concanavalin A lectin from *Canavalia ensiformis* with PDB accession number 1DQ4B and 1DQ2A respectively (Figure 8.8).

The SEM studies conducted in the present study revealed a distinct cell wall adhesion in protein treated hyphae, when compared to water treated hyphae, suggesting a probable binding of the *Withania* lectin to the cell wall components of the pathogen (Figures 8.9 a and b). Morphological changes in the fungal vesicles were also observed in the treated hyphae (Figures 8.9 c and d).

```
BAD61674      1   MPAPPPLAAVSARRCSGPHRPPR 23
BAD61677      1   ----------------------- 23
BAD61671      1   ----------------------- 23
AcPOX             MPAPPPLAAVSARRCSGPHRPPR

BAD61674     80   RSCPATVSCADVLALAARDAVAMLSGPSWGVLLGRKDSLTAS IDMANKDLPNPKDSLAEL  139
BAD61677    123   RSCPATVSCADVLALAARDAVAMLGGPSWGVLLGRKDSLTAS IDMAKEDLPNPKDSLAEL  182
BAD61671    123   RSCPATVSCADVLALAARDAVAMLGGPSWGVLLGRKDSLAARMDMANKDLPRPTDSLAEL  182
AcPOX             -SCPATVSCADVLALAAR---------------------------------------

BAD61674    140   IRMFEKNGLDERDLTALSGAHTVGMAHDCKNYDDRIYSRVGQGGDSIDPSFAAQRRQECE  199
BAD61677    183   IRMFKEHDLDERDLTALSGAHTVGMAHDCKNYDDRIYSRVGQGGDSIDPSFAALRRQECE  242
BAD61671    183   IRMFKENNLDERDLTALSGAHTVGRTH SCEHYEERIYSLVGQGGDSIDPSFAAQRRQECE 242
AcPOX             ------NGLDERDLTALSGAHTVGMAHDCK---------VGQGGDSIDPSFAAQR----

BAD61674    200   QKHGNATAPFDERTPAKFDNAYYIDLLARRGLLTSDQELYTQGCETGDLVKTYAMNGDVF 259
BAD61677    243   QKHDKATAPFDERTPAKFDNAYYVDLLARRGLLTSDQELYTQGCQTGDLVKTYAMNGDVF 302
BAD61671    243   QKHGNATAPFDERTPAKFDNAYYVDLLARRGLLTSDQELYTQGCETGDLVKTYAMNGDVF 302
AcPOX             ----------------- FDNAYYI DL L A R--------------------------

BAD61674    260   FADFVRAMVKMGNIRPKHWWTPAEVR  285
BAD61677    303   FADFTRAMVKMGNIRPKHWWTPAEVR  328
BAD61671    303   FADFARAMVKMGNIRPKHWWTPTEVR  328
AcPOX             ------AMVKMGNIRPKHWWTPAEVR
```

Figure 8.5. Similarity of peroxidase sequence from *A. calamus* (*AcPOX*) with putative bacterial-induced peroxidases from *Oryza sativa*.

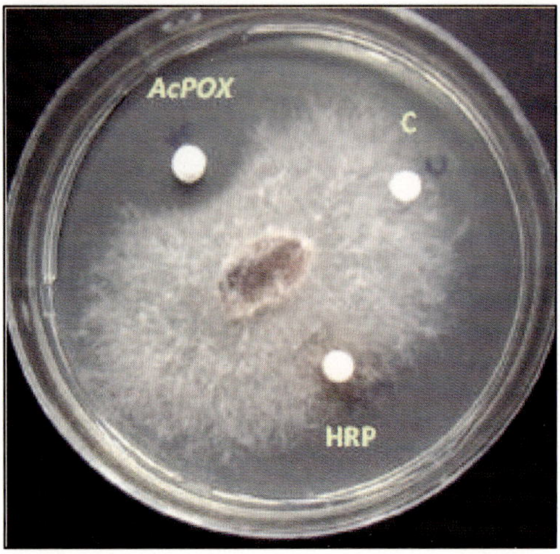

Figure 8.6. Comparison of antifungal efficacy of (*AcPOX* with standard horse radish peroxidase (HRP).

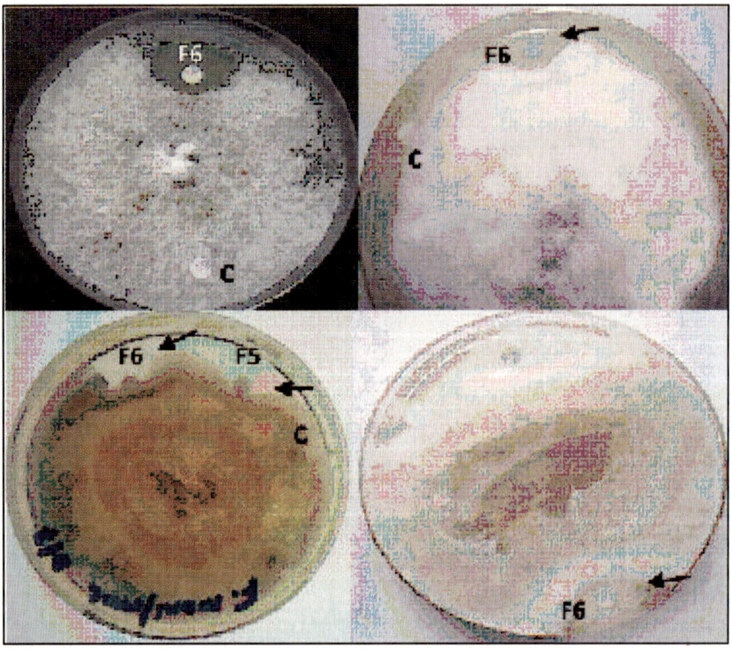

Figure 8.7. Hyphal extension inhibition assays of antifungal lectin from *Withania somnifera* against phytopathogens.

The antifungal nature of the purified lectin from *Withania* (*Wsl*) was compared with standard lectins through *in vitro* assay. Standard lectins like concanavalin A from jack bean, phytohemagglutinin from *Phaseolus vulgaris* and wheat germ

1DQ4B	1 ADTIVAVELDTYPNTDIGDPSYPHIGIDIKSVRSKKTAKWNMQNGKVGTAHIIYNSVDKR 60
1DQ2A	1 ADTIVAVELDTYPNTDIGDPSYPHIGIDIKSVRSKKTAKWNMQNGKVGTAHIIYNSVDKR 60
WSP	--VGTAHIIYNSVDKR
IDQ4B	61 LSAVVSYPNADSATVSYDVDLDNVLPEWVRVGLSASTGLYKETNTILSWSFTSKLKSNST 120
IDQ2A	61 LSAVVSYPNADSATVSYDVDLDNVLPEWVRVGLSASTGLYKETNTILSWSFTSKLKSNST 120
WSP	------------------------------------VGLSASTGLYKETNTILSWSFTSK----------
IDQ4B	121 HETNALHFMFNQFSKDQKDLILQGDATTGTDGNLELTRVSSNGSPQGSSVGRALFYAP 178
IDQ2A	121 HETNALHFMFNQFSKDQKDLILQGDATTGTDGNLELTRVSSNGSPQGSSVGRALFYAP 178
WSP	--
IDQ4B	179 VHIWESSAVVASFEATFTFLIKSPDSHPADGIAFFISNIDSSIPSGSTGRLLGLFPDAN 237
IDQ2A	179 VHI WESSAVVASFEATFTFLIKSPDSHPADGIAFFISNIDSSIPSGSTGRLLGLFPDAN 237
WSP	---LLGLFPDAN

Figure 8.8. Similarity of lectin sequence from *W. somnifera* (WSP) with concanavalin A lectin from *Canavalia ensiformis.*

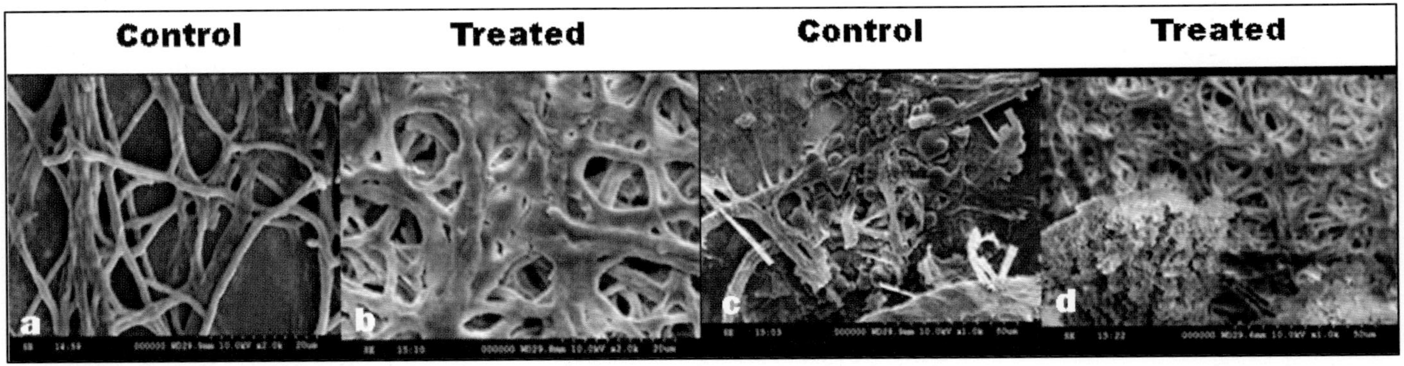

Figure 8.9. Hyphal morphology studies of lectin treated *Trichosporium vesiculosum* using SEM.

agglutinin from *Triticum vulgaris* showed no antifungal activity at 1mg concentration, while a clear zone of inhibition was observed with *Wsl* (Figure 8.10).

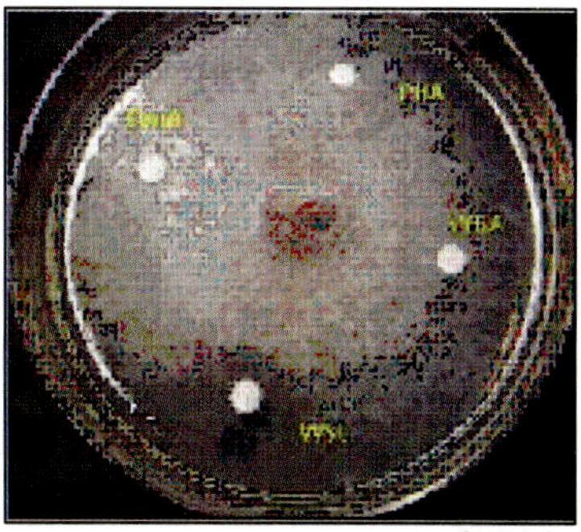

Figure 8.10. Comparison of antifungal efficacy of *W. somanifera* lectin (WSL) with standard lectins.

Discussion

In recent years low molecular weight proteins and peptides with antibacterial/ antifungal activity have been characterized from medicinal plants. A novel antifungal protein, designated chrysancorin, was isolated from seeds of *Chrysanthemum coronarium* var. *spatiosum* with molecular mass of 13.4 KDa (Wang *et al.*, 2001). A 35 KDa protein similar to chitinase was purified from the roots of sanchi ginseng, *Panax notoginseng* which also exhibited anticancer and anti HIV activities (Lam and Ng, 2002). Two structurally different chitin-binding proteins were isolated from bark and leaves of the spindle tree (*Euonymus europaeus*) with potent antifungal activity (Van den Bergh *et al.*, 2004). Phaseococcin, a 5422 Da antifungal protein with antiproliferative and anti-HIV-1 reverse transcriptase activities was purified from small scarlet runner beans (*Phaseolus coccineus* 'Minor') (Ngai and Ng, 2005) while from red beans (*Phaseolus angularis*), a 7.1 KDa defensin like protein with antifungal and antiproliferative activity was reported (Ma *et al.*, 2009). An antifungal protein, *Psc-AFP*, with molecular mass of 18 kDa, was isolated from a traditional Chinese herb, malaytea scurfpea (*Psoralea corylifolia*) with peptide sequence similarity to trypsin inhibitors (Yang *et al.*, 2006). A heat stable protein of 7.8 kDA designated as *LJAMP1* was purified from seeds of the medicinal herb *Leonurus japonicas* and introduced into tobacco. Transgenic tobacco showed enhanced resistance to the fungal pathogen *Alternaria alternata* and bacterial pathogen *Ralstonia solanacearum* (Yang *et al.*, 2007). A 5907 Da antifungal peptide was purified and characterized from kale seeds (*Brassica alboglabra*). The peptide exhibited pronounced thermostability and pH stability and possessed both antifungal and anticancer properties (Lin and Ng, 2008). In the present study antifungal proteins were purified from four medicinal herbs, *P. capensis*, *A. paniculata*, *A. calamus* and *W. somnifera*. Two proteins from *A. calamus* and *W. somnifera* were further characterized by peptide sequencing and were identified as peroxidase and lectin from *A. calamus* and *W. somnifera* respectively.

In vitro studies have indicated that peroxidases in presence of H_2O_2 inhibit the growth of fungi (Yang and Anderson, 1999; Joseph *et al.*, 1998). However, few reports have suggested the antifungal nature of specific peroxidases in absence of H_2O_2 including reports from wheat (Caruso *et al.*, 2001), french bean legume (Ye and Ng, 2002), *Hibiscus esculentus* and *Vigna sinensis ssp. sesquipedalis* (Joseph *et al.*, 1998) and *Acorus calamus* as demonstrated in the present study (Ghosh, 2006). The increased efficacy of the protein in comparison to standard peroxidase was also demonstrated. This study indicates the role of peroxidase in first line defence in plants against invading pathogens.

Plant lectins are proteins with sugar-binding properties, whose biological role in the plant is ill-defined (Etzler, 1986; Chrispeel and Raikhel, 1991; Giovanini *et al.*, 2007). Only a few lectins with antifungal properties are reported to have a role in first line defense. *Urtica dioica* agglutinin (UDA) from the stinging nettle and hevein from the *Hevea brasiliensis*, are low molecular weight, monomeric chitin-binding lectins that possess antifungal properties *in vitro* (Broekaert *et al.*, 1989; Van Parijs *et al.*, 1991). Antifungal lectin were also reported from potato tubers (Gozia *et al.*, 1993), *Gastrodia elata* (gastrodianin) (Hu *et al.*, 1988; Xu *et al.*, 1998), *Phaseolus vulgaris* (Ye *et al.*, 2001), *Astragalus mongholicus* (Yan *et al.*, 2005) and *Pisum sativum* (Sitohy *et al.*, 2007). The present study also demonstrates the antifungal nature of acidic lectin from *W. somnifera* (Ghosh, 2009).

Till date, plant sciences have contributed to drug development through the discovery of bioactive compounds that are used to treat infections or other diseases, such as the anti-inflammatory aspirin or the anticancer agent taxol. Possibly, proteins and peptides are the next hallmark in the contribution of medicinal plants to biological sciences.

Acknowledgements

I express my gratitude to Dr. Bill Simons, Senior Experimental Officer, University of Durham School of Biological and Biomedical Sciences, Durham, UK for LC- MS MS Analysis and Dr. S.S. Madhavendra, Scientist, Indian Institute of Chemical Technology, Hyderabad, India for SEM studies of fungal hyphae. I acknowledge the Department of Biotechnology and Indian Council of Forestry Research and Education, Government of India for providing financial grant to conduct the research work.

References

Baker, C.J., and Orlandi, E.W. (1995). Active oxygen in plant/pathogen interactions. *Annu. Rev. Phytopathol.*, **33**: 299-321.

Bohlmann, H., and Apel, K. (1991). Thionins. *Annual Review of Plant Physiology and Plant Molecular Biology*, **42**: 227-240.

Bradford, M.M. (1976). A rapid and sensitive for the quantitation of microgram quantitites of protein utilizing the principle of protein-dye binding. *Analytical Biochemistry*, **72:** 248-254.

Bradley, D.J., Kjellbom, P., and Lamb, C.J. (1992). Elicitor- and wound-induced oxidative cross-linking of a proline-rich plant cell wall protein: A novel, rapid defense response. *Cell*, **70**: 21-30.

Broekaert, W.F., Van Parijs, J., Leyns, F., Joos, H., and Peumans, W.J. (1989). A Chitin-Binding Lectin from Stinging Nettle Rhizomes with Antifungal Properties. *Science*, **245**: 1100 – 1102.

Broekaert, W.F., Terras, F.R.G., and Cammue, B.P.A. (2000). Induced and preformed antimicrobial. *In*: Ed. By Slusarenko, A.J., Fraser, R.S.S., and van Loon, L.C., Mechanisms of resistance in plant diseases, Kluwer, Dordrecht, p. 371.

Caruso, C., Chilosi, G., Leonardi, L., Bertini, L., Margo, P., Buonocore, V., and Caporale, C. (2001). A basic peroxidase from wheat kernel with antifungal activity. *Phytochemistry*, **58**: 743 – 750.

Chrispeel, M.J., and Raikhel, N.V. (1991). Lectins, lectin genes and their role in plant defense. *Plant Cell*, **3**: 1–9.

De Lucca, A.J., Cleveland, T.E., and Wedge, D.E. (2005). Plant-derived antifungal proteins and peptides. *Can. J. Microbiol.*, **51**: 1001 – 1014.

Etzler, M.E. (1986). Distribution and function of plant lectins. *In*: The Lectins: Properties, Functions, and Applications in Biology and Medicine, Ed. By Liener, *I.E.*, and Sharon, N. Academic Press, New York, pp. 371-435.

García-Olmedo, F., Molina, A., Segura, A., and Moreno, M. (1995). The defensive role of nonspecific lipid-transfer proteins in plants. *Trends Microbiol.*, **3**: 72-74.

Ghosh, M., Thangamani, D., Thapliyal, M., Yasodha, R., and Gurumurthi, K. (2002). Purification of a 20 KD antifungal protein from *Plumbago capensis*- a medicinal plant. *JMAPS*, **24**: 16- 18.

Ghosh, M., Thangamani, D., Thapliyal, M., Yasodha, R., and Gurumurthi, K. (2004). Isolation of *Andrographis paniculata* leaf protein with antifungal property. *Acta Phytopathologica et Entomologica Hungarica*, **39**: 377- 381.

Ghosh, M. (2006). Antifungal Properties of Haem Peroxidase from *Acorus calamus. Annals of Botany*, **98**: 1145-1153.

Ghosh, M. (2009). Purification of a lectin-like antifungal protein from the medicinal herb, *Withania somnifera. Fitoterapia*, **80**: 91 – 95.

Giovanini, M.P., Saltzmann, K.D., Puthoff, D.P., Gonzalo, M., Ohm, H.W., and Williams, C.E. (2007). A novel wheat gene encoding a putative chitin-binding lectin is associated with resistance against Hessian fly. *Molecular plant pathology*, **8**: 69-82.

Gozia, O., Ciopraga, J., Bentia, T., Lungu, M., Zamfirescu, I., Tudor, R., Roseanu, A., and Nitu, F. (1993). Antifungal properties of lectin and new chitinases from potato tubers. *C R Acad Sci III.*, **316**: 788-792.

Graham, L.S., and Sticklen, M.B. (1994). Plant chitinases. *Can. J. Bot.* **72**: 1057 – 1083.

Hu, Z., Yang, Z., and Wang, J. (1988). Isolation and partial characterization of an antifungal protein from *Gastrodia elata* corm. *Acta Bot. Yunnan*, **10**: 373–380.

Joseph, L.M., Koo, T.T., and Man, W.S. (1998). Antifungal effects of hydrogen peroxide and peroxidase on spore germination and mycelial growth of *Pseudocercospora* species. *Can. J. Bot.*, **76**: 2119 – 2124.

Kawano, T. (2003). Roles of the reactive oxygen species-generating peroxidase reactions in plant defence and growth induction. *Plant Cell Rep.*, **21**: 829 – 837.

Kuc, J., and J.S. Rush. (1985). Phytoalexins. *Arch. Biochem. Biophys.*, **236**: 455-472.

Laemmli, U.K. (1970). Cleavage of structural proteins during the assembly of the head of bacteriophage T4. *Nature,* **227**: 680-685.

Lam, S.K., and Ng, T.B. (2002). Pananotin, a potent antifungal protein from roots of the traditional chinese medicinal herb *Panax notoginseng*. *Planta Med.*, **68**: 1024-1028.

Leubner-Metzger, G., and Meins, F. (1999). Functions and regulation of plant β-1,3-glucanases (PR-2). *In*: Pathogenesis-related proteins in plants, Ed. By Datta, S.K., and Muthukrishnan, S., CRC Press, Boca Raton, Florida, pp.49-76.

Levine, A., Pennell, R.I., Alvarez, M.E., Palmer, R., and Lamb, C. (1996). Calcium-mediated apoptosis in a plant hypersensitive disease resistance response *Curr. Biol.,* **6**: 427-437.

Lin, P., and Ng, T.B. (2008). A novel and exploitable antifungal peptide from kale (*Brassica alboglabra*) seeds. *Peptides,* **29**: 1664-1671.

Ma, D.Z., Wang, H.X., and Ng, T.B. (2009). A peptide with potent antifungal and antiproliferative activities from Nepalese large red beans. *Peptides,* **30**: 2089-2094.

McGee, J.D., Hamer, J.E., and Hodges, T. K. (2001). Characterization of a PR-10 pathogenesis-related gene family induced in rice during infection with *Magnaporthe grisea. Mol. Plant Microbe Interac.,* **14**: 877 – 886.

Mosolov, V.V., Grigor'eva, L.I., and Valueva, T.A. (2001). Plant proteinase inhibitors as multifunctional proteins (Review). *Applied Biochemistry and Microbiology,* **37**: 545-551.

Ngai, P.H.K., and Ng, T.B. (2005). Phaseococcin, an antifungal protein with antiproliferative and anti-HIV-1 reverse transcriptase activities from small scarlet runner beans. *Biochem. Cell Biol.,* **83**: 212–220.

Niderman, T., Genetet, I., Bruyere, T., Gees, R., Stintzi, A., Legrand, M., Fritig, B., and Mosinger, E. (1995). Significance of inducible defense-related proteins in infected plants. *Annu. Rev. Phytopathol.,* **44**: 135–162.

Nielsen, K., and Boston, R. (2001). Ribosome – inactivating proteins: A plant perspective. *Annual Review of Plant Physiology and Plant Molecular Biology,* **52**: 785-816.

Peligrini, P.B., and Franco, O.L. (2005). Plant γ-thionins: Novel insights on the mechanism of action of a multi-functional class of defence proteins. *The International Journal of Biochemistry and Cell Biology,* **37**: 2239–2253.

Punja, Z.K. (2001). Genetic engineering of plants to enhance resistance to fungal pathogens–a review of progress and future prospects. *Can. J. Plant Pathol.,* **23**: 216–235.

Ride, J.P. (1986). Induced structural defenses in plants. *In*: Natural Antimicrobial Systems in Plants and Animals, Ed. By Gould, G.W., Rhodes-Roberts, M.E., Charnley, A.K., Cooper, R.M. and Board, R.G. Bath University Press, Bath, UK, pp. 159-165.

Selitrennikoff, C.P. (2001). Antifungal proteins. *Applied and Environmental Microbiology*, **67**: 2883 – 2894.

Simmons, C.R. (1994). The physiology and molecular biology of plant 1,3-ß-Dglucanases and 1,3;1,4-ß-D-glucanases. *Crit. Rev. Plant Sci.*, **13**: 325- 387.

Sitohy, M., Doheim, M., and Badr, H. (2007). Isolation and characterization of a lectin with antifungal activity from Egyptian *Pisum sativum* seeds. *Food Chemistry*, **104**: 971–979.

Terras, F.R.G., Schoofs, H.M.E., Thevissen, K., Osborn, R.W., Vanderleyden, J., Cammue, B.P.A., and Broekaert, W.F. (1993). Synergistic enhancement of the antifungal activity of wheat and barley thionins by radish and oilseed rape 2S albumins and by barley trypsin inhibitors. *Plant Physiol.*, **103**: 1311–1319.

Thomma, B.P.H.J., Cammue, B.P.A., and Thevissen, K. (2002). Plant defensins. *Planta*, **216**: 193–202.

Trudel, J., Grenier, J., Potvin, C., and Asselin, A. (1998). Several thaumatin-like proteins bind to b-1,3-glucans. *Plant Physiol.*, **118**: 1431–1438.

Uknes, S., Mauch-Mani, B., Moyer, M., Potter, S., Williams, S., Dincher, S., Chandler, D., Slusarenko, A., Ward E., and Ryals, J. (1992). Acquired Resistance in *Arabidopsis*. *The Plant Cell.*, **4**: 645-656.

Van den Bergh, K.P., Rougé, P., Proost, P., Coosemans, J., Krouglova, T., Engelborghs, Y., Peumans, W.J., and Van Damme, E.J. (2004). Synergistic antifungal activity of two chitin-binding proteins from spindle tree (*Euonymuseuropaeus* L.). *Planta*, **219**: 221-232.

van Loon, L.C., Rep, M., and Pieterse, C.M.J. (2006). Significance of inducible defense-related proteins in infected plants. *Annu. Rev. Phytopathol.*, **44**: 135–162.

Van Parijs, J., Broekaert, W.F., Goldstein, I.J., and Peumans, W.J. (1991). Hevein: an antifungal protein from rubber-tree (*Hevea brasiliensis*) latex. *Planta*, **183**: 258-262.

Velazhahan, R., Cole, K.C., Anuratha, C.S., and Muthukrishnan, S. (1998). Induction of thaumatin-like proteins (TLPs) in *Rhizoctonia solani* – infected rice and characterization of two new cDNA clones. *Physiol. Plant*, **102**: 21-28.

Velazhahan, R., Samiyappan, R., and Vidhyasekaran, P. (2000). Purification of an elicitor-inducible antifungal chitinase from suspension-cultured rice cells. *Phytoparasitica*, **28**: 131-139.

Wang, H., Ye, X.Y., and Ng, T.B. (2001). Purification of chrysancorin, a novel antifungal protein with mitogenic activity from garland chrysanthemum seeds. *Biol Chem.*, **382**: 947-51.

Xu, Q., Liu, Y., Wang, X., Gu, H., and Chen, Z. (1998). Purification and characterization of a novel antifungal protein from *Gastrodia elata*. *Plant Physiol. Biochem.*, **36**: 899–905.

Table 9.3. Effect of aqueous leaf extract of *M. lucida* on white blood cells (WBC) count of rats infected with *T. brucei brucei.*

	WBC Count (× 10^9/L)
Group A: Not Infected and not treated (normal control)	4,200±2.01
Group B: Infected but not treated (negative control)	14,400±7.07[a]
Group C: Infected and treated with *M. lucida.*	12,400±9.62[a]
Group D: Not infected but treated with *M. lucida*	4,000±2.00[a]

a: Mean value significantly different from the control at P < 0.05.

Table 9.4. Effect of aqueous leaf extract of *M. lucida* on red blood cell (RBC) count of rats infected with *T. brucei brucei.*

	RBC Count(× 10^{12}/L)
Group A	3.10±0.01
Group B	2.05±0.16[a]
Group C	2.45±0.71[a]
Group D	3.50±0.25[a]

a: Mean value significantly different from the control at P < 0.05.

Table 9.5. Effect of aqueous leaf extract *of M. lucida* on haemoglobin concentration of rats infected with *T. brucei brucei.*

	Haemoglobin Concentration (g/dl)
Group A	8.0±0.04
Group B	6.0±0.42[a]
Group C	7.5±0.21[a]
Group D	9.0±0.56[a]

a: Mean value significantly different from the control at P < 0.05.

respectively on 11th day. This implies that *M. lucida* may contain some toxic component that contributed to the 50 per cent mortality in groups C and D. Nwaorgu (1981), reported histopathologic changes after *T.brucei brucei* infection, manifesting as lesions in various tissues and organs, anemia, emaciation and eventually death. Trypanosomes were observed in the infected rats from the 3rd day post infection. There was reduction in percentage parasitemia in group C from a maximum of 27.3 per cent on day 10 to 6.5 per cent on day 14 post infection. However, the level of parasitemia in group B increased progressively up to day 14 post infection. This result showed that aqueous leaf extract of *M. lucida* contain active antitrypanosomal agent against *T. brucei brucei*. Carver (1973), reported that a 50 per cent reduction in parasitemia is an indication of significant activity of a trypanocide. This is also consistent with the result of Asuzu *et al*. (1990), that demonstrated significant reduction in the level of parasitemia with intraperitoneal and oral administration of *M. lucida* leaf extract. Also the best trypanocidal activity was obtained when treatment with extract commenced simultaneously with trypanosome inoculation. The initial increase in the level of parasitemia in group C could be attributed to inadequate dose of the extract administered orally or enzymatic inactivation of active compounds in the gut or reduced absorption from the gut or a combination of all the above factors, Mann *et al.* (2008). All the infected rats showed progressive signs of weakness and reduction in weight. The initial increase in the level of parasitemia could also be attributed to the variant surface glycoprotein (VCG) coat of the parasite which makes them elusive to host immune system and chemotherapy (Vickerman, 1985).

WBC count was found to be highest in group B, followed by group C. This is consistent with normal body response to infection, as WBCs are primary body defense against infection. (Vickermann *et al.,* 1969). RBC count was found to be lowest in group B followed by group C, however, microscopic examination of blood film revealed marked red cell changes with hypochromia, microcytosis, and fragmented cells. These features are in keeping with trypanosome infection (Nwaorgu *et al.,* 1981).

There was a high haemoglobin concentration in group C and D; 7.5 g/dl and 9.0g/dl respectively; when compared with 6.0g/dl for control. This beneficial effect on haemoglobin concentration can be used to correct the anaemia induced by trypanosome infection. This is in agreement with the report of Asuzu *et al.* (1990), that *M. lucida* leaf extract increases packed cell volume and haemoglobin concentration.

Conclusions

The results obtained from this study provides evidence that aqueous extract of *M. lucida* possess trypanocidal activity and can also correct anaemia induced by Trypanosomiasis. Further investigations are needed to identify and isolate the active agent(s) in *M. lucida.*

References

Adewunmi, C.O., and Adesogan, E.K. (1984). Anthraquinone and oruwacin from *M. lucida* as possible agents in fasciolasis and schistosomiasis control. *Fitoterapia,* **55:** 259-263.

Aldhous, P. (1994). Fighting parasites on a shoe string. *Science,* **264**: 1857-1859.

Asuzu, I.U., and Chineme, C.N. (1990). Effects of *Morinda lucida* leaf extract on *T. brucei brucei* infected mice. *J. Ethnopharmacol.,* **30:** 307-3133.

Atawodi, S.E., Ameh, D.A., Ibrahim, S., Andrew J.N., Nzelibe, H.C., Onyike, E., Anigo, K.M., and Sallau, A.B. (2002). Indigenous knowledge system for treatment of trypsnosomiasis in Kaduna State of Nigeria. *J. Ethnopharmacol.,* **79:** 279-282.

Carver, R. (1973). Chemotherapy of Helminthiasis. Pergamon Press Vol 1: 101-115.

Dacie, J.V., and Lewis, S.M. (1991). Practical haematology, 7th (ed.) ELBS, Churchill Livingstone, England, pp 37-85.

Gbile, Z.O. (1986). Ethnobotany, Taxonomy and Conservation of medicinal plants in: The state of medicicnal plants in Nigeria. OAU Press. 13-29.

Herbert, W.J., and Lumsden, W.H. (1976). *Trypanosoma brucei*: A rapid 'matching' method for estimating the host parasitemia. *Exp. Prasitol.,* **40:** 427-431.

Kuzoe, F.A.S. (1993). Current situation of African Trypanosomiasis. *Acta Tropica.,* **54:** 153-162.

Mann, A., Gbate, M., Nda Umar, A. (2003). Medicinal economic plants of Nupe land. Jube-Evans Books and Publications, Bida, Niger State, Nigeria. p. 276.

Nwaorgu, O., and Iwuala, M.O.E. (1981). Studies on the histopathology of *T. brucei* in albino rats. *Nig. J. Parasitol.,* **2(1):** 15-27.

Onyeyili, R.A., and Egwu, G.O. (1995). Chemotherapy of African Trypanosomiasis: A historical review. *Protozool. Abstr.,* **5:** 229-243.

Vickermann, K. (1985). Antigenic variations in African trypanosomes in: "Parasites of the immunized host, mechanism of survival''. Cibal Foundation, Amsterdam. 53-80.

Vickermann, K., and Barry, J. (1973). Cell biology of *Trypanosoma cruzi*. *Int. Rev. Cytol.,* **86:** 197-203.

World Health Organisation (WHO). Chemotherapy of African Trypanosomiasis. WHO *Technical Report Series,* **601**: 32-40.1980

World Medical Association; American Physiological Society (2002). Guilding Principles for research involving animals and human beings. *Am. J. Physiol. Regul. Integr. comp. Physiol.,* **283(2):** R281-3.

Medicinal Plants: Phytochemistry, Pharmacology and Therapeutics Vol. 2 (2012) *Pages* **155–181**
Editor-in-Chief: **V.K. Gupta**
Published by: **DAYA PUBLISHING HOUSE, NEW DELHI**

10

Therapeutic Potential of Saptaparna, *Alstonia scholaris* in the Treatment of Cancer: Preclinical Evaluation in Ehrlich Ascites Carcinoma Model

Ganesh Chandra Jagetia[1*]

ABSTRACT

Despite spending billions of dollars for drug development for cancer treatment, the mortality rates have not come down than it was fifty years ago. Therefore, it is necessary to search newer paradigms that could be of great help in the treatment of cancer. The exploration of medicinal plants for their anticancer activity may provide the desired treatment modality. The anticancer activity of various doses of hydroalcoholic extract of Alstonia scholaris R. Br. (ASE) belonging to family Apocynaceae was studied in Ehrlich ascites carcinoma (EAC) tumor bearing Swiss albino mice. The safety evaluation of this extract in normal mice revealed that ASE was non-toxic up to a dose of 2 g/kg body weight after oral administration, whereas the non-toxic dose for intraperitoneal administration was 700 mg/kg. The daily administration of various doses of ASE into the tumor bearing mice caused a dose dependent remission of EAC tumor and the maximum tumor regression was observed for 480 mg/kg body weight ASE. However, this dose exhibited some toxic manifestations, therefore the next lower dose of 420 mg/kg was considered as the best dose, where 33.33 per cent of the animals survived up to 120 days post-tumor-cell inoculation as against no survivors in the saline treated control group. All the ASE treated animals that survived up to 120 days were disease free and healthy. Administration of cyclophosphamide, the positive control increased the tumor free survivors up to 30 days, where approximately 17 per cent animals did survive, however, it failed to prolong the survival and all animals succumbed to death by 40 days. ASE treatment

1 Department of Zoology, Mizoram University, Tanhril, Aizawl – 796 004, Mizoram, India

* *Corresponding author*: E-mail: gc.jagetia@gmail.com / gc.jagetia@aol.in

help of a hand club. The plant material was then extracted with 85 per cent ethyl alcohol in a Soxhlet apparatus extensively for 3 days. The cooled liquid extract was concentrated by evaporating its liquid contents, with an approximate yield of 28 per cent. Henceforth, the extract of *Alstonia scholaris* will be called as ASE.

Animal Care and Handling

The animal care and handling was done according to the guidelines set by the World Health Organization, Geneva, Switzerland and the INSA (Indian National Science Academy, New Delhi, India). Ten to twelve weeks old female Swiss albino mice weighing 30 to 36 g were selected from an inbred colony maintained under the controlled conditions of temperature (23 ± 2°C), humidity (50±5 per cent) and light (14 and 10 h of light and dark, respectively). The animals had free access to the sterile food and water. Four animals were housed in a polypropylene cage containing sterile paddy husk (procured locally) as bedding throughout the experiment.

Tumor Model

Ehrlich ascites carcinoma (EAC) procured from the Cancer Research Institute (ACTREC), Mumbai, India, was maintained and propagated by serial intraperitoneal transplantation of EAC cells in an aseptic environment. 10^6 viable EAC cells were injected intraperitoneally into each animal in an aseptic condition and the day of tumor inoculation was considered as day 0.

Preparation of Drug and Mode of Administration

The ASE was dissolved in 100 ml of ethanol and diluted with the normal sterile saline (SPS) containing 0.5 per cent carboxymethyl cellulose (CMC) as per the requirement. The SPS, ASE or cyclophosphamide (CPA) was administered in the tumor bearing mice intraperitoneally.

Acute Toxicity Studies

The acute toxicity of the ASE was determined according to Prieur *et al.* (1972) and Ghosh (1984). Briefly, the animals (non tumor bearing) were allowed to fast by withdrawing the food and water for 18 h. The fasted animals were divided into several groups of 10 each. Each group of animals was injected with 600, 800, 900, 1000, 1100, 1200, 1300 and 1400 mg/kg body weight (b. wt.) of ASE intraperitoneally. The animals were provided with food and water immediately after the drug administration. Mortality of the animals was recorded up to 14 days post drug treatment.

Selection of Optimum Dose

The dose of ASE was selected following the standard protocol recommended by the National Service Centre of Cancer Chemotherapy, CCNSC, USA (Geran *et al.*, 1972). Twenty-four hours after the tumor inoculation, the animals were divided into the following groups:

SPS Control

The animals of this group received 0.3 to 0.36 ml of sterile physiological saline (SPS) containing 0.5 per cent carboxymethyl cellulose once daily, consecutively for 9 days.

CPA Control

This group of animals was injected once daily with 25 mg/kg b. wt. of the freshly prepared CPA dissolved in sterile saline containing 0.5 per cent carboxymethyl cellulose (CMC) consecutively for 9 days and served as the positive control.

ASE Group

The animals of this group were injected with 30, 60, 90, 120, 180, 240, 300, 360, 420, 480, 540, and 600 mg/kg ASE once daily, consecutively for 9 days.

Stage Specific Evaluation

The tumors were inoculated and allowed to grow for 1, 3, 6, 9, 12 and 15 days and for reasons of clarity these days have been designated as stage I, II, III, IV, V and VI, respectively. The tumor bearing animals of these stages were divided into the following groups:

ASE Group

The animals of this group were administered once daily with 420 mg/kg ASE (the best dose) for nine consecutive days at I, II, III, IV, V or VI stage of tumor development.

CPA Group

This group of animals received 25 mg/kg b. wt. of cyclophosphamide in a similar fashion and served as concurrent positive control.

In vitro to In vivo Studies

A separate experiment was carried out to investigate the early and delayed cell death after EAC treatment, where the EAC cells were collected aseptically from the peritoneum of a 7 day old tumor, washed in sterile PBS followed by serum free RPMI medium. The cells were resuspended in the serum free RPMI medium at a density of 10^7cells/ml in several culture flasks. The cells were treated with 30, 36, 42, 48, 54 or 60 µg/ml of ASE or 100 µg/ml echitamine chloride (ECL) with occasional shaking. The cultures were incubated at 37°C for 6 h in an atmosphere of 5 per cent CO_2 and 95 per cent air in a CO_2 incubator.

The immediate cytotoxic effect of ASE and ECL was evaluated by using the trypan blue dye exclusion test. Briefly, 4 h after the drug/s exposure the cells were washed in sterile PBS and the cell viability was determined using trypan blue dye exclusion test using a hemocytometer under an inverted transmitted light microscope (Leitz, Wetzlar, Germany). The number of viable and dead cells were scored and expressed as percent live cells. The delayed cell death or the reproductive cell death was determined by injecting 10^6 viable EAC cells exposed to ASE or ECL in normal healthy mice as described earlier.

The animals of all the experiments were monitored regularly for alteration in body weight, signs of toxicity and mortality. The weight of animals was recorded every third day up to 30 days after tumor inoculation in all the groups. A 33 per cent of drug related deaths or a weight loss of 5 g per mouse was considered as an index of toxicity (Geran *et al.*, 1972). The animal survival was monitored daily up to 120 days, since the survival of animals up to 120 days is roughly equivalent to 5 years survival in man (Nias, 1990). The tumor response was assessed on the basis of median survival time and tumor free survival. The median survival time (MST), and the average survival time (AST) were calculated from the animals dying within 120 days and those surviving 120 days were excluded from the calculation. The MST and AST was calculated as follows:

$$MST = \frac{\text{First death} + \text{Last death in the group}}{2}$$

$$AST = \frac{\text{Sum of animal death on different days}}{\text{Number of animals}}$$

The increase in median life span (per cent IMLS) and increase in average life span (per cent IALS) were also calculated using the following formulae:

$$IMLS = \frac{\text{MST of treated mice} - \text{MST of control}}{\text{MST of control}} \times 100$$

$$IALS = \frac{\text{AST of treated mice} - \text{AST of control}}{\text{AST of control}} \times 100$$

Biochemical Estimations

A separate experiment was carried out to estimate glutathione and lipid peroxidation in the tumor cells. The animals were inoculated with tumor cells as described above and the tumor was allowed to grow for six days. On the seventh day, the tumor bearing animals were divided into the following groups:

SPS Control

The animals of this group received 0.3 to 0.36 ml of SPS containing 0.5 per cent CMC.

CPA Control

This group of animals was injected once with 25 mg/kg b. wt. of freshly prepared CPA dissolved in sterile saline containing 0.5 per cent CMC.

ASE Group

The animals of this group were administered with a single injection of 240 or 420 mg/kg b. wt. of the ASE dissolved in sterile saline containing 0.5 per cent CMC.

Four animals from each group were sacrificed at 1.5, 3, 6, 9 12, 18 or 24 h after the drug administration. The tumor cells were aspirated in aseptic condition and were washed with SPS thrice. The cells were counted under the inverted microscope and 1 x 10^7 cells were sonicated (Virsonic, USA) and processed for the estimation of glutathione and lipid peroxidation assays as follows:

Glutathione (GSH)

GSH content was measured by the method of Moron*et al.* (1979). Briefly, proteins were precipitated by 25 per cent TCA, centrifuged and the supernatant was collected.

The supernatant was mixed with 0.2 M sodium phosphate buffer pH 8.0 and 0.06 mM DTNB and incubated for 10 minutes at room temperature. The absorbance of the sample/s was read against the blank at 412 nm in a UV-Visible double beam spectrophotometer (Shimadzu UV-260, Shimadzu Corp., Tokyo, Japan) and the GSH concentration was calculated from the standard curve.

Lipid Peroxidation (LOO)

LOO was measured by the method of Beuege and Aust (1978). Briefly, the homogenate was mixed with TCA-TBA-HCl and heated for 15 min in a boiling water bath. After centrifugation the absorbance was recorded at 535 nm using a UV-Visible double beam spectrophotometer (Shimadzu UV-260, Shimadzu Corp, Japan). The lipid peroxidation has been expressed as MDA in nmol per 10^7 cells. LOO in the sample was determined against the standard curve of TMP (1,1,3,3-tetramethoxy propane).

Statistical Analysis

The statistical significance between the treatments was determined using the "Z" test for the survival studies, whereas the student's 't' test was used for the cytotoxicity and biochemical studies. All the data are expressed as mean ± SEM (standard error of the mean).

Results

Acute Toxicity Studies

The administration of different doses *viz.*, 600, 800 and 900 mg/kg b. wt. of ASE did not induce any mortality during the whole observation period. However, a further increase in the ASE dose up to 1000 mg/kg b. wt. caused a 20 per cent reduction in the survival of mice. An increase in the dose of ASE up to 1200 mg/kg b. wt. resulted in a 50 per cent reduction in the survival of mice and was considered as LD50 dose. A further increase in the administration dose up to 1300 mg/kg resulted in 80 per cent death of the animals and 100 per cent mortality was observed at 1400 mg/kg and thereafter up to a dose of 1500 mg/kg b. wt. of ASE, the last dose evaluated.

Selection of Optimum Dose

There was no spontaneous regression of tumors in the mouse transplanted with the EAC cells and the animals exhibited a constant weight gain and increase in the volume due to tumor cell multiplication and growth (Figure 10.1). The MST of tumor bearing mouse was found to be approximately 19 and an AST of 18 days, respectively in the SPS treated group (Table 10.1).

Administration of one day old tumors with 30, 60, 90, 120, 180, 240, 300, 360, 420, 480, 540 or 600 mg/kg ASE or 25 mg/kg CPA inhibited the weight gain in all the treatment groups, indicating arrest of tumor cell proliferation and growth (Figure 10.1). However, administration of 480, 540 and 600 mg/kg was accompanied with toxic side effects like ruffling of hair, sluggishness and lacremation in the recipients and none of the animals treated with 600 mg/kg group (½ of LD_{50}) survived beyond day 6 post-tumor inoculation (Figure 10.1). The administration of 30 or 60 mg/kg ASE did not

Table 10.1. Effect of drug treatment schedule on the median survival time (MST) and average survival time (AST) of the EAC mice.

		MST	*IMLS*	*AST*	*IALS*	*Percent Survival (Day)* 30	60	90	120
Dose selection	SPS	19	–	18	–	0	0	0	0
	CPA 25	29	57.89	28	55.8	16.66	0	0	0
	ASE 30	18	–	18	0.6	0	0	0	0
	ASE 60	18.5	–	18.7	4.3	0	0	0	0
	ASE 90	21.5	13.15	20.5	14	0	0	0	0
	ASE 120	25	31.6	25.6	42.3	0	0	0	0
	ASE 180	26	36.8	25.7	43.3	0	0	0	0
	ASE 240	32.5	71.05	29.6	64.6	25	0	0	0
	ASE 300	35.5	86.8	34.9	94.3	66.66[c]	0	0	0
	ASE 360	48.5	155.3	49.4	174.9	100[d]	41.66[b]	16.66	16.66
	ASE 420	53.5	181.6	55.4	208.1	100[d]	50[b]	33.33[a]	33.33[a]
	ASE 480	65.5	244.7	64.3	257.7	100[d]	75[d]	75[d]	41.66[b]
	ASE 540	10	–	9.3	–	0	0	0	0
	ASE 600	4.5	–	4	–	0	0	0	0
Stages of tumor	ASE I	53.5	181.6	55.4	208.1	100[d]	50[b]	33.33[a]	33.33[a]
	CPA 1	29	57.9	28	55.8	16.66	0	0	0
	ASE II	47	147.4	40.4	124.8	91.66[d]	66.66[c]	25[a]	16.66
	CPA II	26.5	39.5	26.3	46.6	8.33	0	0	0
	ASE III	42	121	37	106	66.66[c]	33.33[a]	16.66	0
	CPA III	24	26.3	23.1	28.5	0	0	0	0
	ASE IV	33	73.7	29.7	65.1	25	0	0	0
	CPA IV	21.5	13	21.1	17.4	0	0	0	0
	ASE V	23	21	23.4	30.3	8.33	0	0	0
	CPA V	19	–	18.9	5.3	0	0	0	0
	ASE VI	20	5.3	19.7	9.9	0	0	0	0
	CPA VI	18.5	–	18.2	1.6	0	0	0	0
In vitro to *in vivo* studies	ASE 00	19.5	–	18.4	–	0	0	0	0
	ASE 24	20	2.6	19.8	7.6	0	0	0	0
	ASE 30	21.5	10.2	21.3	15.8	0	0	0	0
	ASE 36	23.5	20.5	25	35.9	0	0	0	0
	ASE 42	27	38.5	27.7	50.5	0	0	0	0
	ASE 48	30	53.8	29.8	62	10	0	0	0
	ASE 54	32	64.1	32	74	20	0	0	0
	ASE 60	39	100	40.3	117	40[a]	0	0	0
	ECL 100	25	28.2	24.4	32.6	0	0	0	0

P: a < 0.05; b p < 0.001; c 0.002; d 0.0001 (compared with SPS).

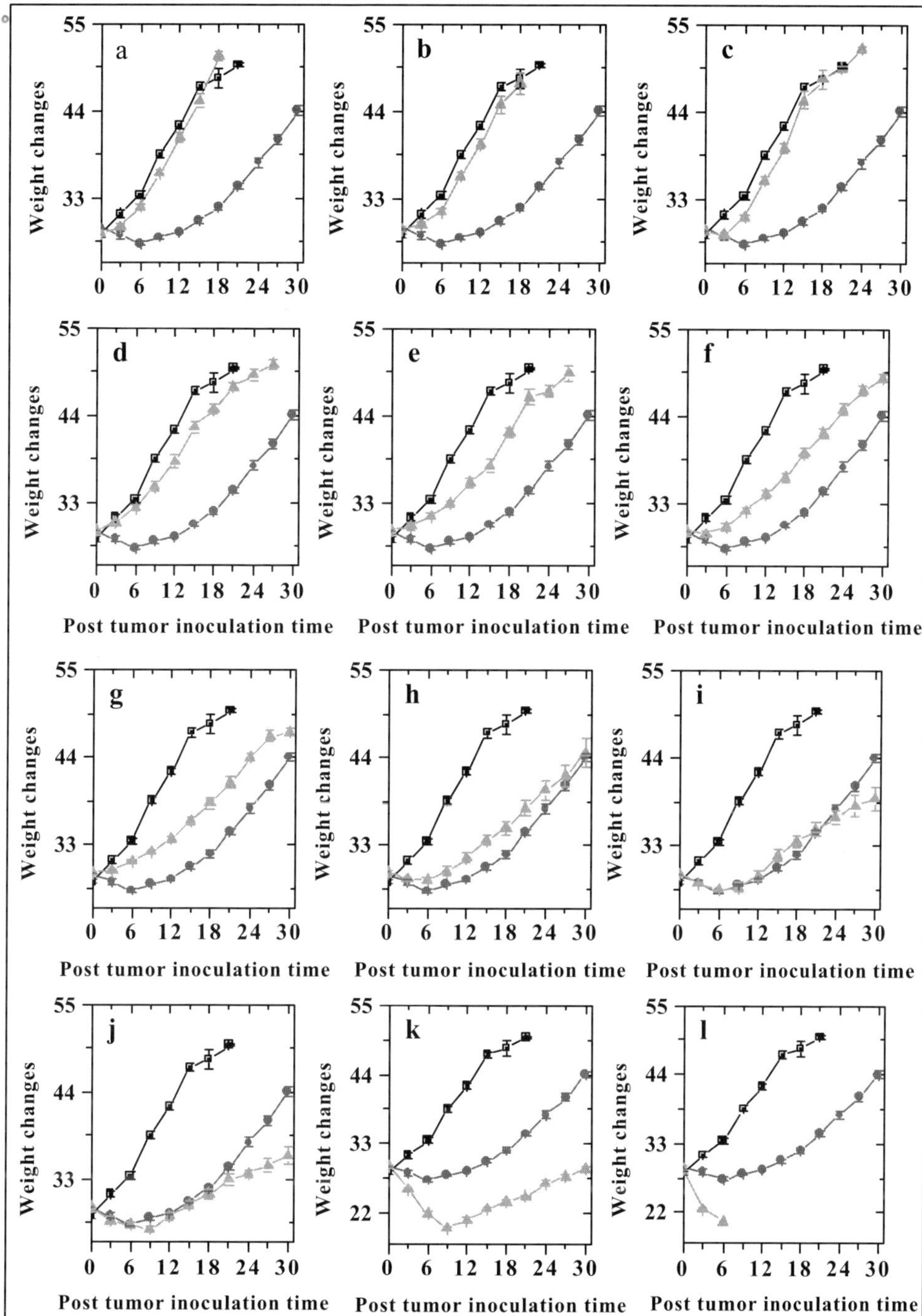

Figure 10.1. Alterations in the weight changes in the Ehrlich ascites carcinoma bearing mice treated with SPS (closed squares), 25 mg/kg CPA (closed circles) and *Alstonia scholaris* (triangles). a: 30, b: 60, c: 90, d: 120, e: 180, f: 240, g: 300, h: 360, i: 420, j: 480, k: 540 and l: 600 mg/kg.

Treatment of mice with 420 mg/kg ASE at various stages of tumor development resulted in an increase in the MST up to 53.5, 47, 42, 33, 23 and 20 days and AST to 55.4, 40.4, 37, 29.7, 23.4 and 19.7 at stage I, II, III, IV, V or VI, respectively, when compared with the CPA treatment (Figures 10.4a, b). The ASE treatment caused an elevation in the IMLS and IALS depending on the stage of the tumor development. The IMLS and IALS declined depending on the treatment stage and the lowest values were observed for stage VI. The IMLS of 181.6, 147.4, 121, 73.7, 21 and 5.3 per cent while the IALS of 208, 124.8, 105.9, 65.1, 30.3 and 9.9 per cent was found for stage I, II, III, IV, V and VI, respectively (Table 10.1).

The administration of ASE was superior than CPA as 41.7, and 16.7 per cent survivors were observed at the end of 120 days for stage I and III, respectively, whereas no survivors were reported for the CPA group. The IMLS was 3.1, 3.7, 4.6 and 5.6 folds greater for stage I, II, III, IV, V and VI, respectively and the IALS was elevated by 3.7, 2.7, 3.7, 3.7, 5.7 and 6.3 folds for stage I to VI, respectively, when compared with concurrent CPA group (Table 10.1).

In vitro to In vivo Studies

Exposure of cells to PBS in vitro for 4 h did not induce any adverse effect on the cell viability and a maximum number of viable cells were observed in the PBS treated group (99.5 per cent). However, the exposure of EAC cells to 100 mg/ml of ECL, the positive control resulted in approximately 21 per cent reduction in the viable cells. Treatment of EAC cells to different concentrations of ASE resulted in a concentration dependent reduction in the cell viability (Figure 10.5a). The exposure of EAC cells to 24, 30 and 36 µg/ml ASE caused a gradual decrease in the cell viability, where 98, 95 and 87 per cent viability was observed. A further increase in the drug dose up to 42 µg/ml caused an abrupt decline in the viable cell population, where only 75 per cent viable cells were observed (Table 10.2). A 39 per cent reduction in the viable cell population was observed after treatment of EAC cells with 60 mg/ml ASE, where the cell viability reached a nadir of 61 per cent (Table 10.2).

The inoculation of the SPS treated EAC cells into the healthy mice (non tumor bearing) exhibited a constant weight gain due to the tumor cell multiplication and growth as was observed for the other experiments (Figure 10.6). The MST was found to be 19.5 and 18.4 days respectively for this group (Figure 10.5b). The exposure of EAC cells to 100 µg/ml of ECL resulted in a MST and AST of 25 and 24.4 days, and the IMLS and IALS also increased up to 28.2 and 32.6 per cent, respectively (Table 10.1).

Table 10.2. Cytotoxic effect of various doses of ASE and 100 µg/ml ECL on the HeLa cells.

Dose (µg/ml)	*% Viable Cells*
SPS	99.5±0.35
ASE 24	98.8±0.45
ASE 30	95.0±0.71
ASE 36	87.1±0.68 [a]
ASE 42	75.2±0.57 [b]
ASE 48	69.3±0.61 [c]
ASE 54	65.2±0.59 [c]
ASE 60	61.4±0.65 [c]
ECL	79.6±0.72 [b]

p: a $p < 0.05$; b $p < 0.01$, c $p < 0.001$ (Compared with SPS)

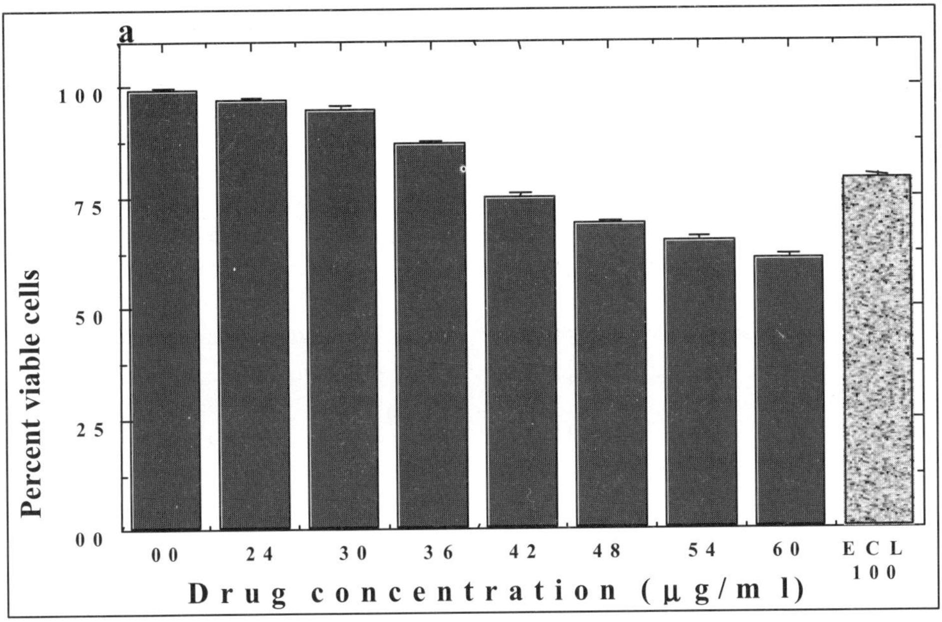

Figure 10.5a. Effect of various concentrations of ASE and 100 μg/ml of ECL on the cytotoxicity of EAC cells *in vitro.*

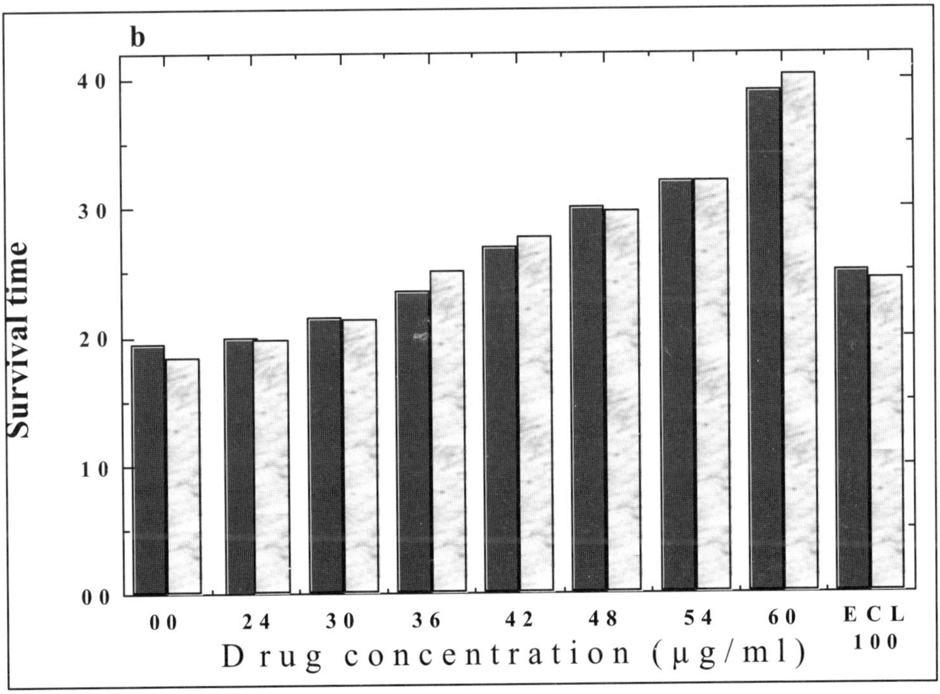

Figure 10.5b. Alterations in the median survival (MST) and average survival time (AST) of the mice inoculated with EAC cells after treatment with various concentrations of ASE and 100 μg/ml of ECL *in vitro* and then injected to animals. Solid bars: MST, mottled bars: AST.

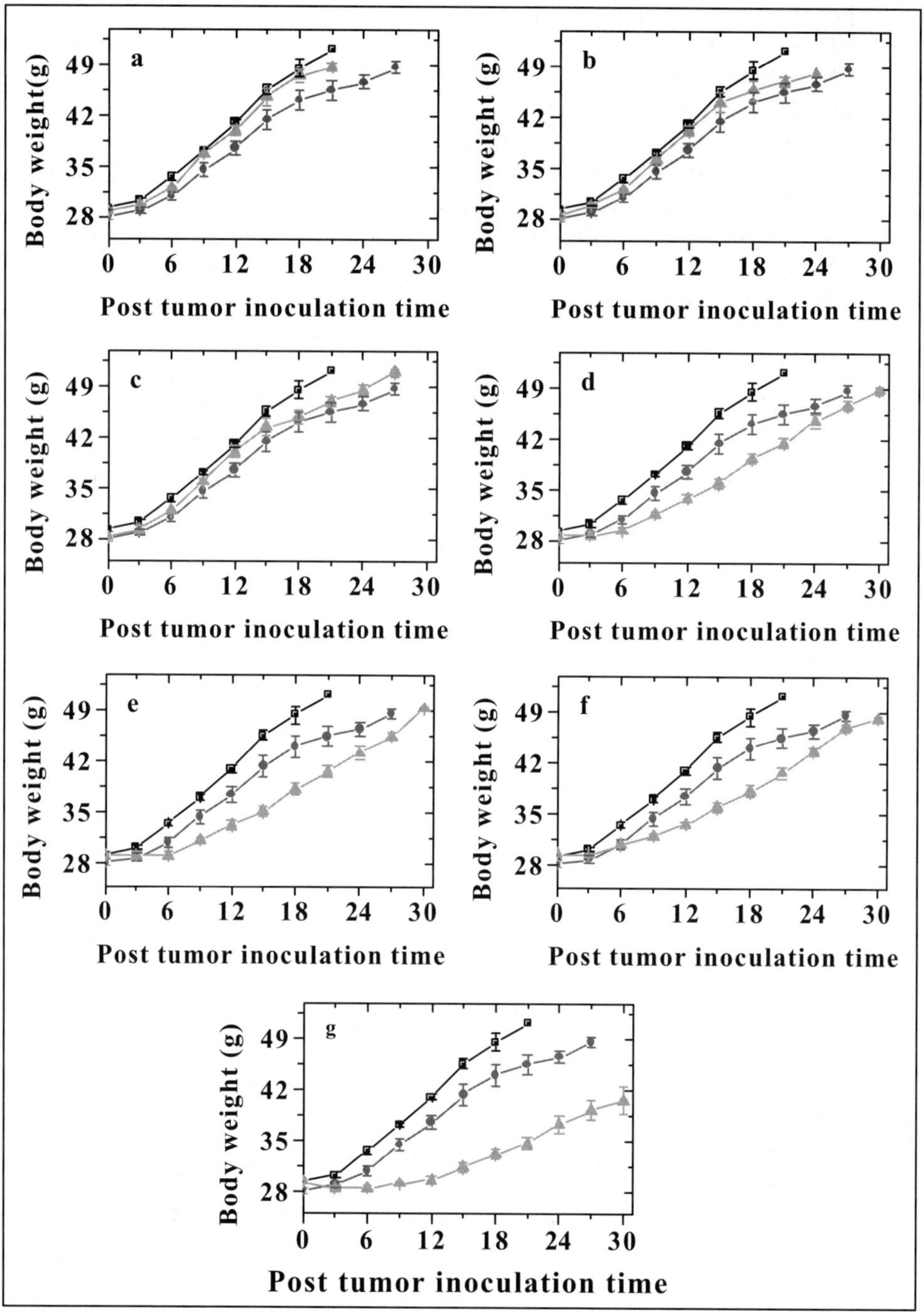

Figure 10.6. Alterations in the body weights of mice injected with EAC cells after treatment with different doses of ASE *in vitro*. Squares: SPS, circles: ECL, triangles: ASE. a: 24, b: 30, c:36, d: 42, e: 48, f: 54, g: 60 µg/ml ASE.

The *in vitro* treatment of EAC cells to 24, 30, 36, 42, 48, 54 and 60 µg/ml of ASE for 6 h *in vitro* and then transplantation into mice resulted in a dose dependent increase in the MST and AST. The exposure of 24 and 30 µg/ml of ASE did not significantly alter the MST and AST (20 and 19.8 days, respectively) when compared with the SPS treated group, whereas a further increase in the ASE doses elevated the MST and AST. The MST was found to be 21.5, 23.5, 27, 30, 32 and 39 days, while AST increased up to 21.3, 25, 27.7, 29.8, 32 and 40.3 days for 24, 30, 36, 42, 48, 54 or 60 µg/ml ASE, respectively. This was accompanied by an increase in the IMLS up to 2.6, 10.2, 20.5, 38.5, 53.8, 64.1 and 100 per cent respectively for 24, 30, 36, 42, 48, 54 and 60 µg/ml of ASE. The IALS also elevated and was found to be 7.6, 15.8, 35.9, 50.5, 61.9, 73.9 and 119 per cent for 24, 30, 36, 42, 48, 54 and 60 µg/ml ASE, respectively (Table 10.1). The ASE treatment increased the MST by 1.2 (48 µg), 1.3 (54 µg) and 1.6 (60 µg) folds and the AST by 1.2 (48 µg), 1.3 (54 µg) and 1.6 (60 µg) folds when compared with the ECL group (Table 10.1).

Biochemical Estimations

Glutathione (GSH)

Treatment of mice with 240 and 420 mg/kg ASE resulted in a time dependent decline in the GSH contents in the EAC cells and a nadir reached at 6 h post treatment. Thereafter, GSH contents elevated steadily and reached to almost normal level by 24 h post-treatment in the tumor bearing mice receiving 240 mg/kg ASE or CPA, however, no such effect was observed for 420 mg/kg ASE (Figure 10.7a). The CPA treatment also caused a decline in the GSH contents and a maximum decline was observed at 9 h post-treatment (Table 10.3).

Lipid Peroxidation (LOO)

Treatment of mice with 240, 420 ASE and 25 mg/kg of CPA resulted in the enhancement of lipid peroxidation with time (Table 10.3). The peak lipid peroxidation was observed for 420 mg/kg ASE followed by 25 mg/kg CPA or 240 mg/kg ASE. The greatest elevation was observed at 9 h post treatment for ASE, whereas 12 h for CPA treatment (Figure 10.7b).

Discussion

Chemotherapy has been the mainstay of cancer treatment for the past 50 years and will continue to be one of the important treatment regimens in the near future. It is a major treatment modality used for the control of advanced stages of malignancies and also as a prophylactic against possible metastases in combination with radiotherapy. The goal of cancer therapy is to completely eradicate the neoplastic cells without causing any appreciable damage to the normal tissues of the host. However, most of the modern clinically used chemotherapeutic drugs exhibit severe normal toxicity, resulting in undesirable side effects. Moreover, many of the potent drugs not only exhibit systemic toxicity, but are mutagenic, carcinogenic, and teratogenic and produce second malignancies, which ultimately prove fatal to the patients. Therefore, a need is felt to find alternative drugs, which may be highly effective at non-toxic doses, inexpensive and accessible to the common man. Plants have

Table 10.3. Alteration in the GSH concentration and lipid peroxidation by hydroalcoholic extract of *Alstonia scholaris* in the EAC mice at various post-treatment time periods.

Time (h)	*Glutathione*				*Lipid Peroxidation*			
	SPS	*ASE 240*	*ASE 480*	*CPA 25*	*SPS*	*ASE 240*	*ASE 480*	*CPA 25*
0	2.63±0.04	2.63±0.03	2.64±0.02	2.62±0.01	4.09±0.03	4.10±0.03	4.10±0.02	4.11±0.02
1.5	2.62±0.03	2.58±0.02	2.53±0.02[a]	2.60±0.02	4.10±0.02	4.17±0.03	4.21±0.03	4.12±0.02
3	2.63±0.04	2.54±0.02[a]	2.46±0.01[b]	2.56±0.01[a]	4.08±0.04	4.21±0.03	4.30±0.03[b]	4.14±0.02
6	2.62±0.03	2.50±0.04[a]	2.41±0.02[c]	2.53±0.01[a]	4.08±0.02	4.32±0.04[b]	4.42±0.02[c]	4.24±0.03[b]
9	2.61±0.04	2.53±0.02[a]	2.44±0.01[b]	2.49±0.02[b]	4.09±0.04	4.41±0.05[c]	4.58±0.04[c]	4.35±0.02[b]
12	2.62±0.03	2.56±0.02[a]	2.48±0.03[b]	2.54±0.02[a]	4.09±0.03	4.37±0.02[b]	4.52±0.02[c]	4.45±0.02[c]
18	2.63±0.04	2.59±0.02	2.51±0.03[a]	2.57±0.02	4.08±0.04	4.24±0.06[b]	4.33±0.04[b]	4.29±0.02[b]
24	2.64±0.04	2.62±0.03	2.54±0.01	2.60±0.03	4.09±0.02	4.11±0.03	4.18±0.03	4.13±0.03

p = a < 0.05; b < 0.01, < 0.001 (compared with SPS).

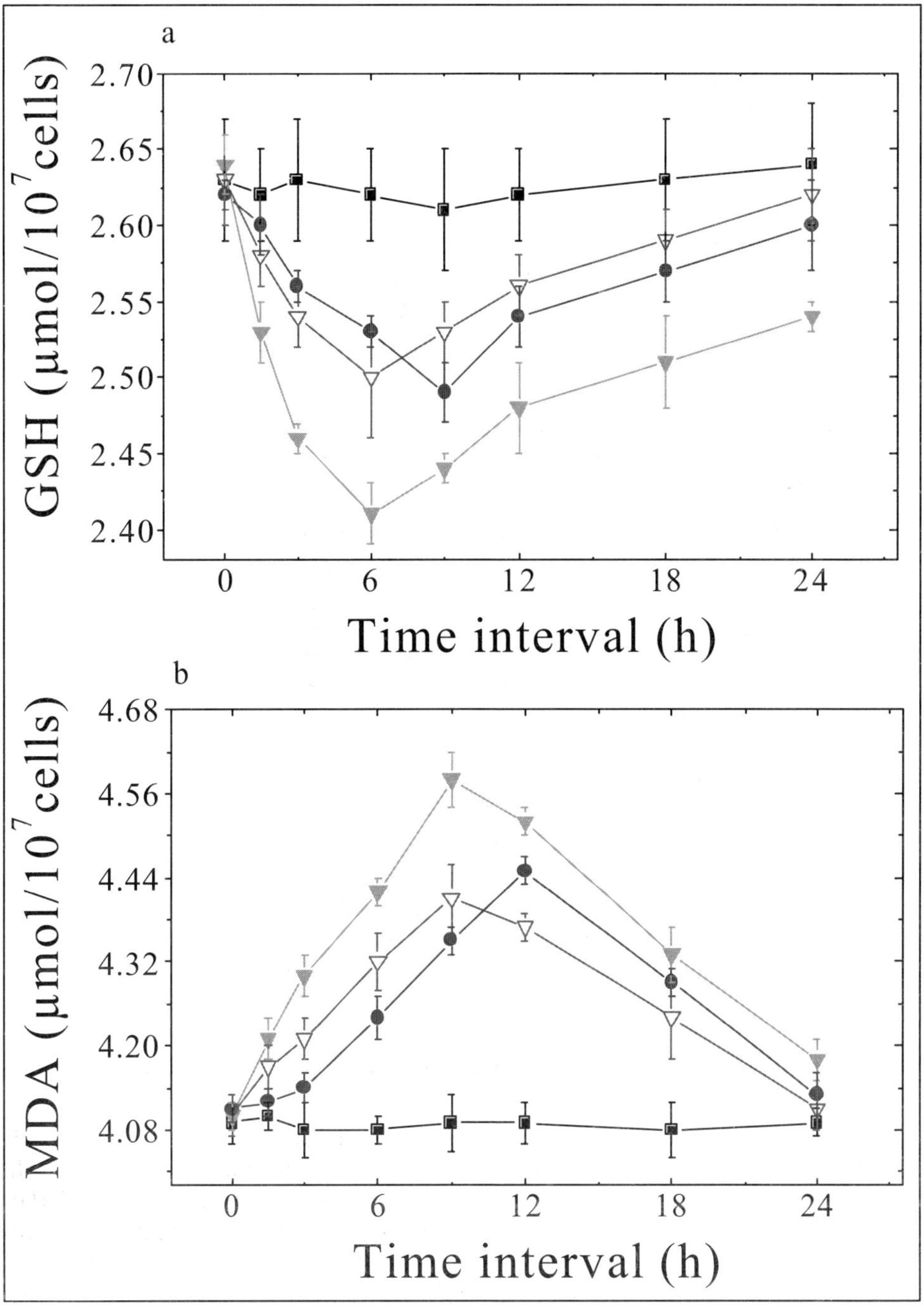

Figure 10.7. Effect of 240 or 480 mg/kg ASE and 25 mg/kg CPA treatment on GSH concentration and lipid peroxidation in the EAC in mice. SPS (squares), 240 mg/kg ASE (open triangles), 480 mg/kg ASE (closed triangles) and 25 mg/kg CPA (circles). a: GSH, b: Lipid Peroxidation. (95 per cent confidence limits).

growth and increase in the life span. The administration of ASE was able to enhance the IMLS by 3.13, 3.73, 4.6 and 5.6 folds for I, II, III, IV, V and VI stages, respectively. Similarly, the IALS was also elevated by 3.7, 2.7, 3.7, 3.7, 5.7 and 6.35 folds for stage I, II, III, IV, V and VI, respectively, when compared with the concurrent CPA group. Treatment of tumor bearing mice with ASE at stage I and III increased the survival by 41.66 and 16.66 per cent respectively at the end of 120 days post tumor inoculation, for stage I and III, no survivors has been reported for the CPA group. The studies of the anticancer activity of plants at different stages of tumor development are scanty, however, withaferin A from *Withania somnifera* and plumbagin, from *Plumbago rosea* have been reported to inhibit EAC growth when administered in mid stages (3 and 5 days after tumor cell inoculation) (Sharda *et al.*, 1996; Devi *et al.*, 1999). The information on the treatment in advanced stages of tumor development is lacking. The stage specific evaluation of ASE has shown that ASE is capable of inhibiting the tumor development even at late stages. This is an interesting finding with respect to clinical application, where the patients turn up late for cancer treatment.

The mechanism of action of herbal drugs and their extract preparations differ in many respects from that of the synthetic drugs or single substances (Wagner, 1999). It can be characterized as a polyvalent action and interpreted as additive or in some cases, potentiating. It is observed that the desired activity of an active compound is rarely present in adequate quantity and when present may contain unwanted activities. Further, it has also been observed that in plants, certain other compounds may be of help in enhancing the potency of the active compounds resulting in an additive or synergistic positive effect and at the same time reducing the toxic implications for the treatment, which in its final total gives immense benefit (Kulkarni, 1997).

The exact mechanism of cell killing effect of ASE is not known. However, operation of following mechanisms for the tumoricidal effect of ASE in the present study cannot be ruled out:

The ASE treatment caused a significant elevation in the LOO and subsequent decline in GSH levels in the EAC cells, which may be responsible for inflicting the damage to tumor cells and arresting the further growth of the tumor. ASE may inflict damage to the cell DNA, which may inhibit further division of tumor cells and finally leading to the cell killing and subsequent shrinkage of the tumor. This is supported by increased lipid peroxidation, which has been reported to cause damage to the DNA (Park *et al.*, 2002). The ASE may have stimulated apoptosis in the tumor cells resulting in the continuous remission of the tumor, thereby eradicating the disease. The ASE treatment may have inhibited the DNA synthesis or mitosis of cells leading to arrest of cell proliferation and further tumor development. Echitamine chloride, one of the constituent of ASE has been reported to inhibit DNA synthesis (Kamarajan *et al.*, 1995; Saraswathi *et al.*, 1997). It may also have killed tumor cells by inhibiting serine proteases, since protease inhibitors have also been reported to inhibit tumor invasion, metastasis and angiogenesis (Dimitroff *et al.*, 1998). The triterpenoids (lupeol linoleate, lupeol palmitate and alpha-amyrin linoleate), present in Alstonia have been reported to inhibit serine proteases and PKA (Rajic *et al.*, 2000). ASE may have also caused immune modulation resulting in the tumor cell kill and shrinkage. *Alstonia scholaris* has been reported to possess immunostimulatory effect in BALB/c mouse and also to enhance the phagocytic activity in normal as well as immunosuppressed mice. It has also prevented the prednisone-induced decline in immune modulation and increased the lytic activity of peritoneal exudate cells against *Escherichia coli* (Iwo *et al.*, 2000).

Conclusions

From present study it is clear that ASE, inhibited the growth of EAC cells and the optimum non-toxic dose of 420 mg/kg was nearly 1/3rd of the LD_{50} (1200 mg/kg) dose. The non-toxic nature of this drug may lie in its composite nature. The exact mechanism of action of ASE is not known, however, the anticancer effect of ASE may be due to multiple actions on the tumor cells, which would have helped to kill the tumor cells effectively resulting in the complete regression of tumors in the survivors. Alternatively, ASE may also increase the immune surveillance and antimetastatic ability. The anticancer activity of Alstonia on EAC tumor may be due to the presence of several alkaloids that have been found to kill tumor cells and inhibition of serine protein kinase or immunomodulatory action. Further studies are required to investigate the active principle/s and their mode of action in tumors of different originin *in vitro* as well as *in vivo*.

Acknowledgements

The financial assistance from The Indian Council of Medical Research (ICMR), Government of India, New Delhi, India is thankfully acknowledged.

References

Adwankar, M.K., and Chitnis, M.P. (1982). *In vivo* anti-cancer activity of RC-18: a plant isolate from *Rubia cordifolia*, Linn. against a spectrum of experimental tumour models. *Chemotherapy*, **28(4):** 291-303.

Beuege, J.A., and Aust, S. D. (1978). Microsomal lipid peroxidation. *Methods in Enzymology*, **30:** 302-310.

Beljanski, M., and Beljanski, M.S. (1986) Three alkaloids as selective destroyers of cancer cells in mice. Synergy with classic anticancer drugs. *Oncology*, **43:** 198-203.

Cassileth, B.R., and Chapman, C.C. (1996). Alternative and complementary cancer therapies. *Cancer*, **77 (6):** 1026-1034.

CHEMEXCIL (1992). Selected medicinal plants of India. Basic Chemicals, Pharmaceutical and Cosmetic Export Promotion Council, Bombay 400 039, India, pp. 205-207.

Chitnis, M.P., Bhatia, K.G., and Phatak M.K. (1979). Anti-tumour activity of the methanol extract *Ervatamia heyneana* (NSC B668619). *Indian Journal of Experimental Biology*, **17 (2):** 212.

Chitnis, M.P., Khandalekar, D.D., Adwankar M.K. and Sahasrabudhe, M.B. (1972). Anti-cancer activity of the extracts of stem and leaf of *Tylophora indica*. *Indian Journal of Medical Research*, **60(3):** 359-362.

Chitnis, M.P., Khandalekar, D.D., Adwankar MK., and Sahasrabudhe, M.B. (1971). Anticancer activity of the extracts of root, stem and leaf of *Ervatamia heyneana*. *Indian Journal of Experimental Biology*, **9(2):** 268-270.

Devi, P.U., Solomon, F.E., and Sharada, A.C. (1999). Plumbagin, A Plant Naphthoquinone with Antitumor and Radiomodifying Properties. *Pharmaceutical Biology*, **37:** 231-236.

Dimitroff, C.J., Sharma, A., and Bernacki, R.J. (1998). Cancer metastasis: a search for therapeutic inhibition. *Cancer Investigation*, **16(4):** 279-290.

Duflos, A., Kruczynski, A., and Barret, J.M. (2002). Novel aspects of natural and modified vinca alkaloids. *Current Medicinal Chemistry and Anticancer Agents*, **2(1):** 55-70.

Erba, E., Ubezio P., Colombo, T., Broggini, M., Torti, L., Vaghi, M., D'Incalci, M., and Morasca, L. (1983). Flow-cytometric analysis of DNA distribution after VP16-213 treatment of Lewis lung carcinoma. *Cancer Chemotherapy and Pharmacology*, **10(3):** 208-211.

Farnsworth, N.R., and Soejarto, D.D. (1985). Potential consequences of plant extinction in the united states on the current and future availability of prescription on drugs. *Economic Botany*, **39:** 231.

Farnsworth, N.R., and Soejarto, D.D. (1991). Global importance of medicinal plant. In: Conservation of medicinal plant, Akerele,O., Heywood. V., and Synge, H. (eds), Cambridge, Cambridge University Press, pp. 25.

Ferlay, J., Shin, H.R., Bray, F., Forman D., Mathers, C., and Parkin, D.M. (2010) Estimates of worldwide burden of cancer in 2008: GLOBOCAN 2008. *International Journal of Cancer*, (in press)

Gandhi,M., and Vinayak, V.K. (1990). Preliminary evaluation of extracts of Alstonia scholaris bark for in vivo antimalarial activity in mice. *Journal of Ethnopharmacology*, **29:** 51-57.

Geran, R.I., Greenberg, N.H., Macdonald, M.M., Schumacher, A,M., and Abbott, B.J. (1972). Protocols for screening chemical agents and natural products against animal tumors and other biological systems. *Cancer Chemotherapy Reports*, **2:** 1-85.

Ghosh, M.N. (1984) Toxicity studies. In: M.N. Ghosh (Ed.), Fundamentals of Experimental Pharmacology, Scientific Book Agency, Calcutta, India, pp.153-158.

Goel, H.C., Prasad, J., Sharma, A., and Singh, B. (1998). Antitumour and radioprotective action of *Podophyllum hexandrum*. *Indian Journal of Experimental Biology*, **36(6):** 583-587.

Iizuka, N., Miyamoto, K., Okita, K., Tangoku, A., Hayashi, H., Yosino, S., Abe, T., Morioka, T., Hazama, S., and Oka, M. (2000). Inhibitory effect of *Coptidis Rhizoma* and berberine on the proliferation of human esophageal cancer cell lines. *Cancer Letters*, **148:** 19-25.

Iwo, M.I., Soemardji, A.A., Retnoningrum, D.S., Sukrasno, and U. UM. (2000). Immunostimulating effect of pule (*Alstonia scholaris* L. R.Br., Apocynaceae) bark extracts. *Clinical Hemorheology and Microcirculation,* **23(2-4):** 177-183.

Jagetia, G.C. (2008) Radiosensitizing activity of guduchi (*Tinospora Cordifolia* Miers Ex h\Hook f & Thonns) in tumor bearing mice. In the Herbal Modulators in Medicine, Homeland Defence and Space. Edited by Rajesh Arora CABI, Oxfordshire, UK, pp 287-304.

Jagetia, G.C., and Baliga M. S. (2005). The effect of seasonal variation on the antineoplastic activity of *Alstonia scholaris* R. Br. in HeLa cells. *Journal of Ethnopharmacology,* **96(1-2):** 37-42.

Jagetia, G.C., and Baliga M. S. (2006). Evaluation of anticancer activity of the alkaloid fraction of *Alstonia scholaris* (Sapthaparna) *in vitro* and *in vivo. Phytotherapy Research,* **20(2):** 103-109.

Jagetia, G.C., and Rao S. K. (2006). Evaluation of the antineoplastic activity of guduchi (*Tinospora cordifolia*) in Ehrlich ascites carcinoma bearing mice. *Biological and Pharmaceutical Bulletin,* **29 (3):** 460-466.

Jagetia, G.C., Nayak, V., and Vidyasagar, M. (1998). Evaluation of the antineoplastic activity of guduchi (*Tinospora cordifolia*) in cultured HeLa cells. *Cancer Letters,* **127:** 71–82.

Jordan, M.A. (2002). Mechanism of action of antitumor drugs that interact with microtubules and tubulin. *Current Medicinal Chemistry and Anticancer Agents,* **2(1):** 1-17.

Kamarajan, P., Ramamurthy, N., and Govindasamy, S. (1995). *In vitro* evaluation of the anti-cancer effects of echitamine chloride on fibrosarcoma cells. *Journal of Clinical Biochemistry and Nutrition,* **18:** 65-71.

Kapoor, L.D. (1990). CRC Hand book of Ayurvedic Medicinal Plants. Baca Raton, FL, CRC.

Keawpradub, N., Eno-Amooquaye, E., Burke, P.J., and Houghton, P.J. (1999) Cytotoxic activity of indole alkaloids from *Alstonia macrophylla. Planta Medica,* **65:** 311-315.

Keawpradub, N., Houghton, P.J., Eno-Amooquaye, E., and Burke, P.J. (1997). Activity of extracts and alkaloids of thai Alstonia species against human lung cancer cell lines. *Planta Medica,* **63:** 97-101.

Krishnaswamy, M., and Purushothaman, K.K. (1983). Anticancer activity of echitamine chloride. *Journal of Research in Ayurveda and Siddha,* **4:** 111-114.

Kulkarni, R.D. (1997). Principles of Pharmacology in Ayurveda. Ram Sangam Graphics, Mumbai, India.

Lin, S.C., Lin, C.C., Lin, Y.H., Supriyatna, S., and Pan, S.L. (1996). The protective effect of *Alstonia scholaris* R. Br. on hepatotoxin-induced acute liver damage. *American Journal of Chinenese Medicine,* **24:** 153-164.

Mazumdar, U.K., Gupta, M., Maiti, S., and Mukherjee D. (1997). Antitumor activity of *Hygrophila spinosa* on Ehrlich ascites carcinoma and sarcoma-180 induced mice. *Indian Journal of Experimental Biology,* **35:** 473-477.

Moron, M.S., Depierre, J.W, and Mannervik, B. (1979). Levels of glutathione, glutathione reductase and glutathione-s-transferase activities in rat lung and liver. *Biochimca Biophysica Acta*., **582:** 67-78.

Nadkarni, A. K. (1976). Indian Materia Medica, 3rd edition, Popular Press Ltd. Mumbai, India. pp 1308-1315.

Newman D.J., Cragg, G.M. and Snader, K.M. (2003). Natural products as sources of new drugs over the period 1981-2002. *Journal of Natural Products,* **66(7)**: 1022-1037.

Nias, A.H.W. (1990). Radiation Biology. In: Sikora K, Halnan KE (Eds) Treatment of cancer. London. Chapman and Hall Medical, pp 53-75.

O'Dwyer, P.J., Leyland-Jones, B., Alonso, M.T., Marsoni, S., and Wittes, R.E. (1985). Etoposide (VP16-213): Current status of an active anticancer drug. *New England Journal of Medicine,* **312:** 692–700.

Omoregbe, R.E., Ikuebe, O.M., and Ihimire, I.G. (1996). Antimicrobial activity of some medicinal plants extracts on *Escherichia coli, Salmonella paratyphi* and *Shigella dysenteriae. African Journal of Medical Sciences,* **25(4):** 373-375.

Park, J.E., Yang, J.H., Yoon, S.J., Lee, J.H., Yang, E.S., and Park, J.W. (2002). Lipid peroxidation-mediated cytotoxicity and DNA damage in U937 cells. *Biochimie,* **84(12):** 1198-1204.

Prieur, D.J., Young, D.M., Davis, R.D., Cooney, D.A., Homan, E.R., Dixon, R.L., and Guarino, A.M. (1973). Procedures for preclinical toxicologic evaluation of cancer chemotherapeutic agents, protocols of the laboratory of toxicology. *Cancer Chemotherapy Reports,* **4:** 1-28.

Rajic, A., Kweifio-Okai, G., Macrides, T., Sandeman, R.M., Chandler, D.S. and Polya, G.M. (2000). Inhibition of serine proteases by anti-inflammatory triterpenoids. *Planta Medica,* **66(3):** 206-210.

Rowinsky, E.K. (1997). Paclitaxel pharmacology and other tumor types. *Seminars in Oncology,* **24(6 Suppl 19):** S19-1-S19-12.

Saraswathi, V., Ramamurthy, N., Subramaniam, S., Mathuram, V., and Govindasamy, S. (1997). Enhancement of the cytotoxic effects of echitamine chloride by vitamin A: an in vitro study on Ehrlich ascites carcinoma cell culture. *Indian Journal of Pharmacology,* **29:** 244-249.

Satyavati, G.V., Gupta, A.K., and Tandon, N. (1987). Medicinal plants of India. *Indian Council of Medical Research, New Delhi, India,* **Vol. 2:** 230-239.

Sharada, A.C., Solomon, F.E., Devi. P.U., Udupa, N., and Srinivasan, K.K. (1996). Antitumor and radiosensitizing effects of withaferin A on mouse Ehrlich ascites carcinoma *in vivo*. *Acta Oncologica,* **35:** 95-100.

Wagner, H. (1999).Phytomedicine research in Germany. *Environmental Health Perspectives*, **107:** 779-781.

Warrier, P. K. Nambiar, V. P. K., and Ramankutty, C. (1996). Indian medicinal plants. Orient Longman Ltd Hyderabad, India, **Vol. 1:** 75-80.

WHO (1999). Hand book for reporting results of cancer treatment, WHO offset publication No. 48.

Medicinal Plants: Phytochemistry, Pharmacology and Therapeutics Vol. 2 (2012) *Pages* **183–194**
Editor-in-Chief: **V.K. Gupta**
Published by: **DAYA PUBLISHING HOUSE, NEW DELHI**

11

Preliminary Study on Adaptogenic Activity of *Plantago erosa* ex Roxb

C.C. Barua[1*], J.D. Roy[1], B. Buragohain[2], A. Talukdar[1], S.A. Begum[1], A.G. Barua[2] and P. Borah[3]

ABSTRACT

The present investigation was undertaken to study the effect of hydroethanol extract of Plantago erosa ex Roxb (PEHE) locally known as "Singapat" on adaptogenic activity in animal models. PEHE was administered by single oral dose (100, 200 and 300 mg/kg) to adult male Wistar rats and adult male Swiss albino mice for evaluation of adaptogenic activity by forced swimming test (rat and mice), tail suspension test (mice) and anoxic stress tolerance test (mice). In forced swimming and tail suspension test, the immobility time was measured during the last 4 min of the total 6 min test period by observer blind to the treatment condition. In anoxic stress tolerance, the time taken for first convulsion was noted. In all the models, Zeetress (14 mg/kg p.o.) was used as the standard drug.

PEHE significantly increased the immobility time in the forced swimming test in rats and mice in a dose dependent manner. Similarly, there was increase in the immobility time in tail suspension test in the treated group. In anoxic stress tolerance model, the time taken for first convulsion increased in dose dependent manner. The effect was comparable with the

1 Department of Pharmacology and Toxicology, College of Veterinary Science, Assam Agricultural University, Khanapara, Guwahati – 781 022, Assam

2 Department of Public Health, College of Veterinary Science, Assam Agricultural University, Khanapara, Guwahati – 781 022, Assam

3 Department of Microbiology, College of Veterinary Science, Assam Agricultural University, Khanapara, Guwahati – 781 022, Assam

* *Corresponding author*: E-mail: chanacin@satyam.net.in; chanacin@gmail.com; Tel: 91-361-2361485 (R); Fax: 91-361-2337700; Cell: 098640-13231

standard drug (i.e. Zeetress). Increase in both immobility time and in the time taken for first convulsion, indicates the adaptogenic activity.

From the above study, it can be concluded that PEHE have potential adaptogenic activity. The presence of diterpenes, triterpenes, tannins and steroids might help in producing the adaptogenic activity.

Keywords: Adaptogenic activity, Anoxic stress tolerance, Forced swimming test, Hydroethanol extract, *Plantago erosa* ex Roxb, Tail suspension test.

Introduction

Stress can be described as the sum total of all the reactions of the body, which disturb the normal physiological condition and result in a state of threatened homeostasis. Stress is an internationally recognized phenomenon fortified by advancement of industrialization in a demanding civilization (Selye,1998). Since the introduction of adaptogens, several plants have been investigated, which were once used as tonics due to their adaptogenic and rejuvenating properties in traditional medicine (Rege *et al.*,1999). The drugs of plant origin are gaining increasing popularity and are being investigated for remedies of a number of disorders including anti stress (adaptogenic) activity (Edzard, 1998).

Plantago erosa ex Roxb locally known as "Singapat" is traditionally used as astringent, antitoxic, antimicrobial, anti-inflammatory as well as demulcent, expectorant and diuretic. The aqueous extract of *Plantago erosa* has been evaluated for analgesic and anti-inflammatory activities (Nunz *et al.*, 1997). It has also been evaluated for anti-diarrhoeal activity on castor oil induced diarrhoel gastrointestinal movements in rats (Atta and Mouneir, 2005). *In vitro,* cytotoxic, anti viral and immunomodulatory effects of *Plantago erosa* and *P. asiatica* have also been reported (Chiang *et al.,* 2003). A composition containing the herbs *Plantago major* and *Piper methysticum* has been patented for its use in producing a diminished desire for tobacco (*i.e.* nicotine) without the use of nicotine itself and advantageously provides anti-depressive and anti-anxiety effects without sedative or hypnotic effects (Cody, 2000). In our earlier studies, the methanolic extracts have shown analgesic and anti-inflammatory activity. The hydroethanolic extract have also shown anti-convulsion and anxiolytic activity (unpublished reports).

Even though, *Plantago erosa* is widely used traditionally in various diseases and stress condition, no scientific investigation have been carried out so far to study the adaptogenic activity of the plant. This has prompted us to study the adaptogenic activity.

Materials and Methods

Collection of Plant Material

The leaves of *Plantago erosa* ex Roxb were collected during the month of July-Sept, 2008 from the medicinal garden of the Department of Pharmacology and Toxicology, C.V.Sc. Khanapara, Guwahati and was identified by Botanical Survey of

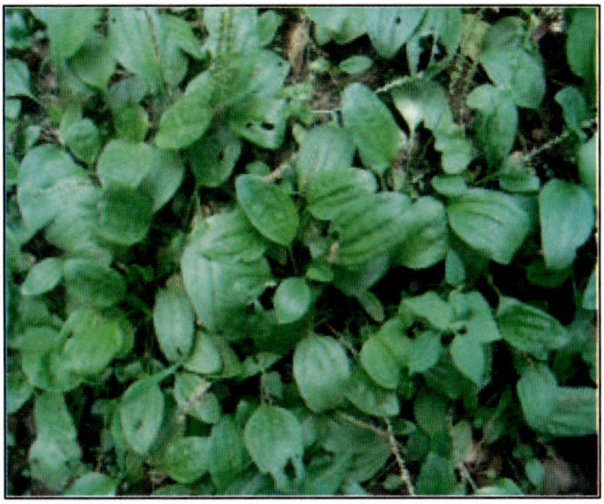

Figure 11.1: The leaves of *Plantago erosa* ex Roxb.

India, Shillong, Meghalaya. A voucher specimen (No. AAU/CVSC/PHT/07-08/03) has also been deposited in the Herbarium of Botanical Survey of India.

Preparation of Extract of Plantago erosa

Fresh leaves of *Plantago erosa* were cleaned and dried under shade in clean dust free environment and grinded and stored in air-tight container. They were (250 g) soaked in 1000 ml of hydroethanol (50:50) for 72 h in separate beakers. The plant materials was stirred every 18 h using a sterile glass rod. The solvent was filtered every 3rd day using muslin cloth and Whatman's filter paper No 1. The filtrate obtained was concentrated in Rotary Evaporator (Equitron, Roteva) at 50°-60°C under reduced pressure leaving a dark brown residue. The *Plantago erosa* hydroethanolic extract (PEHE), thus obtained was transferred to a Petri dish and kept over water bath (50°C) until the solvent gets completely evaporated. It was stored at 4°C for future use. Recovery was 28.62 per cent (w/w).

Animals and Treatment Regimes

Adult male albino Swiss mice and adult Wistar rats weighing around 20-30g and 120-130g, respectively were used for the study. The animals had free access to food and water. The animals were fasted overnight before the experiment They were housed in animal room, with alternating light-dark cycle of 12 h each. The animals were acclimatized to the laboratory conditions for at least five days prior to the behavioral experiments. All experiments were conducted between 0900h – 1800h. The research was conducted in accordance with the ethical rules on animal experimentation, approved by Institutional Animal Ethics Committee, (770/03/ac/CPCSEA/FVSc, AAU/IAEC/06/22).

The animals were divided into five groups, containing six mice in each group and given treatment as follows: Group I-vehicle treated animal as control, Group II-animals received the standard drug- Zeetress (14 mg/kg p.o) as positive control, Group III, IV, and V were fed orally with PEHE at doses 100, 200 and 300 mg/kg respectively.

Drugs and Chemicals

The drugs and chemicals used in this study were obtained from various sources: Zeetress was procured from Indian Herbs Research and Supply Co, Ltd. Darra Shivpuri, Saharanpur, ethanol was purchased from Merck (India). Distilled water was used as vehicle. All the chemicals and solvents were of analytical grade.

Phytochemical Study

Preliminary phytochemical study was done by standard methods for qualitative identification of the phytoconstiteunts (Harborne, 1991).

Acute Toxicity Studies

The LD_{50} of PEHE was estimated by the employment of up-and-down stair case method in mice (Bruce, 1985). Doses were adjusted by a constant multiplicative factor *viz.*, 4, for this experiment. The dose for each successive animal was adjusted up and down depending on the previous outcome. The acute toxicity and gross effect of PEHE was studied in albino mice by using 1/2 LD_{50} dose. A total of six numbers of male albino mice were selected for the experiment. Animals were observed hourly for six hours and again after 24 h. The parameters for motor activity and gross effect were determined after administration of PEHE orally at a dose of 1/2 $LD_{50.}$

Laboratory Models Employed for Testing Adaptogenic Activity

Forced-Swimming Test in Rat

The rats were placed individually in glass cylinders (40 cm in height × 18 cm in diameter) containing water (28°C) in 22 cm depth. The procedure consisted of a pre – swimming and swimming test separated by 24 h. During the pre – swimming test rats were placed in the cylinder for 15 min. They were removed from the cylinder, dried with a towel and warmed them with the electric heater before they were placed back to their home cage (Porsolt *et al.*, 1977). The following day, animals of Group I were treated with vehicle, Group II with Zeetress (14 mg/kg p.o) and Group III, IV and V with PEHE 100, 200, 300 mg/kg p.o. respectively, 1h prior to the swimming test and were placed in the cylinder again. Immobility time was measured during the last 4 min of the total 6 min by observer blind to the treatment condition. Rats were considered to be immobile when floating motionless or making only those movements necessary to keep its head above water surface.

Forced-Swimming Test in Mice

Forced swimming test in mice is a behavioral despair test (Porsolt, 1978). The animals of Group I were treated with vehicle, Group II with Zeetress (14 mg/kg p.o) and Group III, IV and V with PEHE 100, 200 and 300 mg/kg p.o. respectively, 1 h prior to the forced swimming test. The mice were placed individually in glass cylinders (20 cm in height × 10 cm in diameter) containing water (25°C) of 10 cm depth for 6

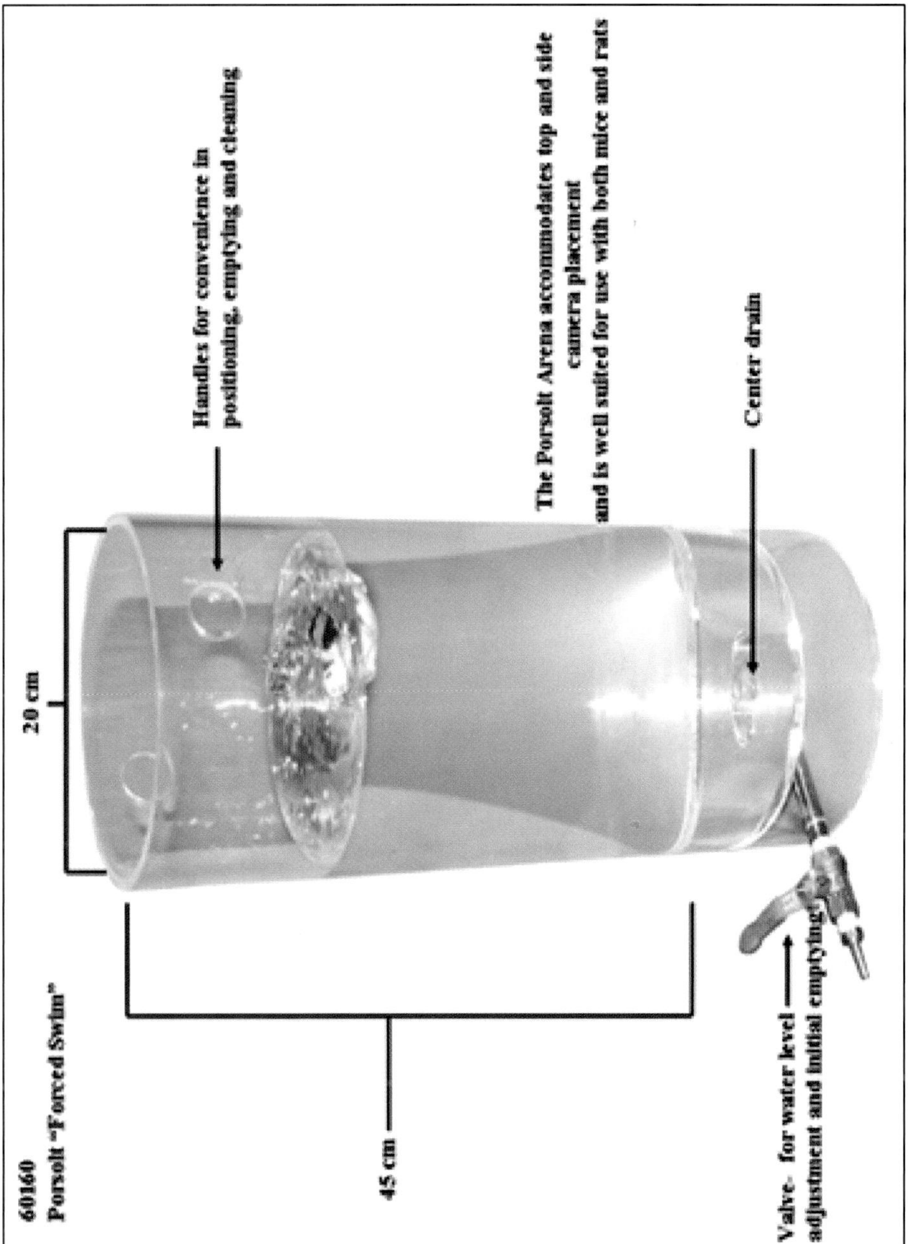
60160
Porsolt "Forced Swim"
20 cm
45 cm
Handles for convenience in positioning, emptying and cleaning
The Porsolt Arena accommodates top and side camera placement
and is well suited for use with both mice and rats
Center drain
Valve- for water level adjustment and initial emptying

Figure 11.2

min. The duration of immobility was measured during the last 4 min of the 6 min period blind to the treatment conditions. Mice were considered to be immobile when floating motion less or making those movements necessary to keep its head above water.

Tail Suspension Test in Mice

Mice were individually suspended 7.5 cm above the surface of the table with an adhesive tape placed 1 cm away from the tip of the tail (Steru, 1985). Mice in Group I were administered with vehicle, Group II with Zeetress (14 mg/kg p.o.) and Group III, IV and V with PEHE 100, 200, 300 mg/kg p.o. respectively, 1 h prior to test and hung to record immobility time during the last 4 min of the total 6 min by observer blind to the treatment condition. They were considered immobile only when hung passively and were completely motionless.

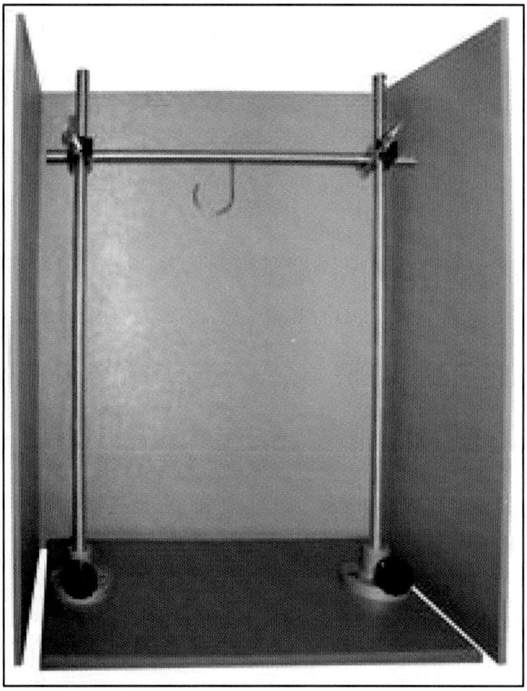

Figure 11.3

Anoxic Stress Tolerance Test

Conical flasks of 250 ml capacity were used for the study. The flasks were made airtight using rubber cork, before the start of the experiment (Kannur *et al.,* 2006). Group I animals were treated with vehicle, Group II with Zeetress (14 mg/kg p.o.) and Group III, IV and V with PEHE 100, 200, 300 mg/kg p.o. respectively, for 14 days. Each animal was then kept in the airtight vessel and the time taken for the first convulsion was noted. The animals were removed immediately from the vessel and resuscitated if necessary.

Statistical Analysis

The statistical analysis of data was done using one-way analysis of variance by using the SPSS software (version 11.5). A probability less than 0.01 was considered to be statistically significant.

Results

Phytochemical Screening

The phytochemical screening of PEHE showed the presence of tannins by ferric chloride and gelatin test, diterpenes, triterpenes by Salkowski's test and Liberman Buchardt's test and steroids by Salkowski's test and Liberman Buchardt's test.

Acute Toxicity Studies

The plant extract was found to be safe up to 5 g/kg body weight p.o. No acute toxicity was observed at 2 g/kg body weight.

Adaptogenic Studies

Forced Swimming Test in Rat

Administration of PEHE significantly (P<0.01) increased the immobility time in dose dependent manner as compared to control group in forced swimming test in rat. The immobility time increased from 121.83 seconds to 133.33 seconds from 100 to 300 mg/kg p.o. respectively. The effect is comparable to the standard drug-Zeetress (14 mg/kg p.o.) which showed the duration of immobility of 141.33 seconds (Figure 10.4).

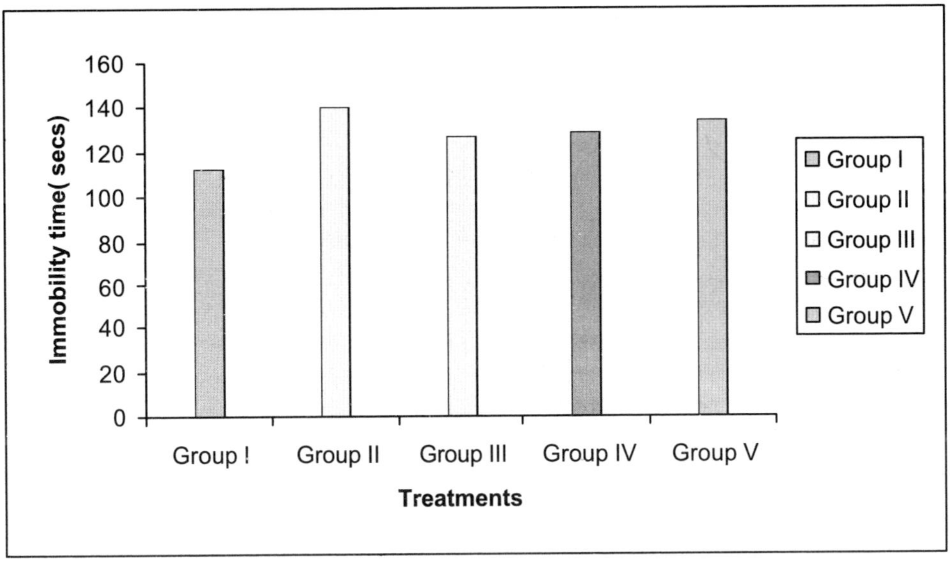

N=6; P<0.01, P< 0.01 vs vehicle (one way ANOVA)

Figure 10.4. Effect of PEHE and zeetress in forced swimming test in rat.

Group I-vehicle treated animal as control, Group II- animals received the standard drug- Zeetress (14 mg/kg p.o) as positive control, Group III, IV, and V were fed orally with PEHE at doses 100, 200 and 300 mg/kg respectively.

Forced Swimming Test in Mice

Similarly, administration of PEHE increased significantly (P<0.01) the duration of immobility time in the forced swimming test in mice in dose dependent manner from 126.16 to 142.00 seconds at 100 (Group III) to 300 (Group IV) mg/kg p.o. respectively, in comparison to the Group II (treated with standard drug-zeetress 14 mg/kg p.o.) which showed the duration of immobility of 182.16 seconds (Figure 10.5).

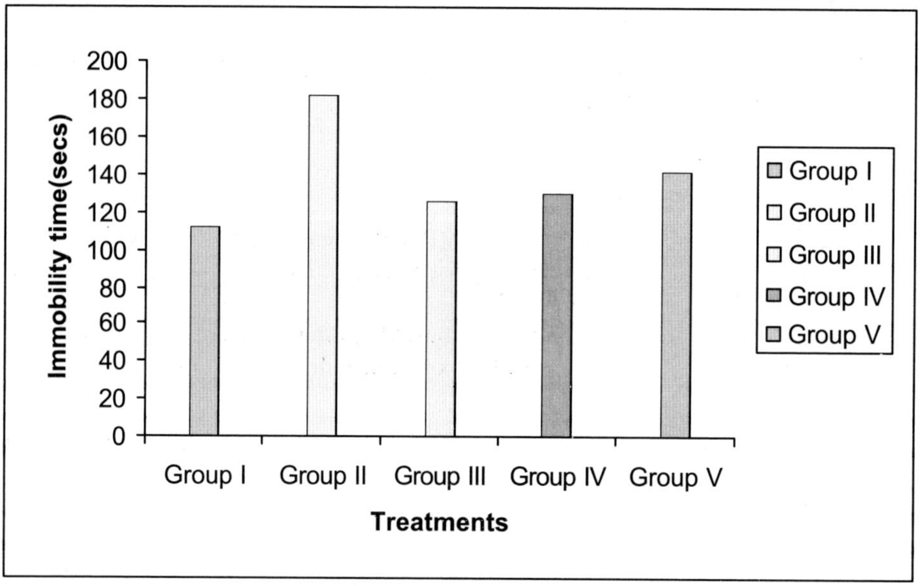

N=6; P<0.01, P< 0.01 vs vehicle (one way ANOVA)

Figure 10.5. Effect of PEHE and zeetress in forced swimming test in mice.

Tail Suspension Test in Mice

The extract also significantly (P<0.01) increased the duration of the immobility time in the tail suspension test in mice in a dose dependent manner from 127.33 to 133.66 seconds with 100 (Group III) to 300 (Group V) mg/kg p.o. dose, respectively. Duration of immobility of standard drug-Zeetress (14 mg/kg p.o.) in tail suspension test was 140.16 seconds (Figure 10.3).

Anoxic Stress Tolerance in Mice

In anoxic stress tolerance, the latency of convulsion increased significantly (P<0.01) in dose dependent manner from 33.56 to 34.82 min with 100 (Group III) to 300 (Group IV) mg/kg p.o. respectively. The effect of PEHE is comparable to Zeetress,

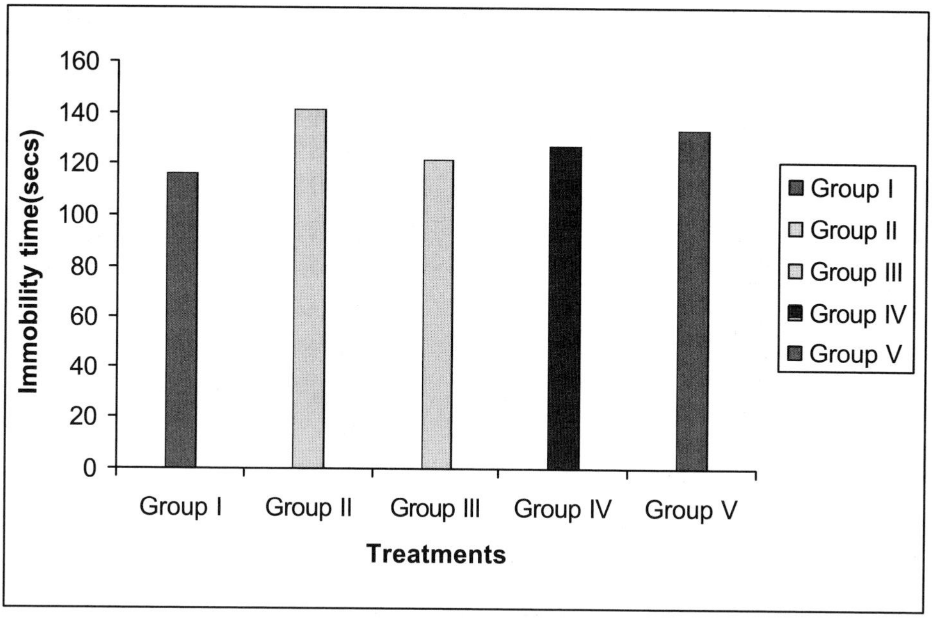

N=6; P<0.01, P< 0.01 vs vehicle (one way ANOVA)

Figure 10.6. Effect of PEHE and zeetress in tail suspension test in mice.

which showed latency of convulsion of 34.42 (Group II) min (Figure 10.7). In all the parameters the standard drug Zeetress showed better activity than the test compound.

Group I-vehicle treated animal as control, Group II- animals received the standard drug- Zeetress (14 mg/kg p.o) as positive control, Group III, IV, and V were fed orally with PEHE at doses 100, 200 and 300 mg/kg respectively.

Discussion

The ability to adapt to a given habitat is a distinctive feature of all living organisms. As adjuvant to other specific treatments, adaptogens can also help in altering the course of the disease. It is non- toxic and is not habit forming, while it exerts a normalizing influence on the body with a wide range of therapeutic benefits, which cause no disturbance to the normal functioning of the body.

One of the best models of stress in rats/mice is forced immobilization. It is most widely used pharmacological model for assessing anti-depressant activity (Cryan *et al.*, 2002). Many psychotropic drugs have been screened with FST (Connor *et al.*, 1998). The development of immobility when the rodents are placed in an inescapable cylinder of water reflects the cessation of persistent escape – directed behavior (Lucki, 1997). The increase in the immobility time signifies the ability of PEHE to tolerate stress induced by the forced swim model.

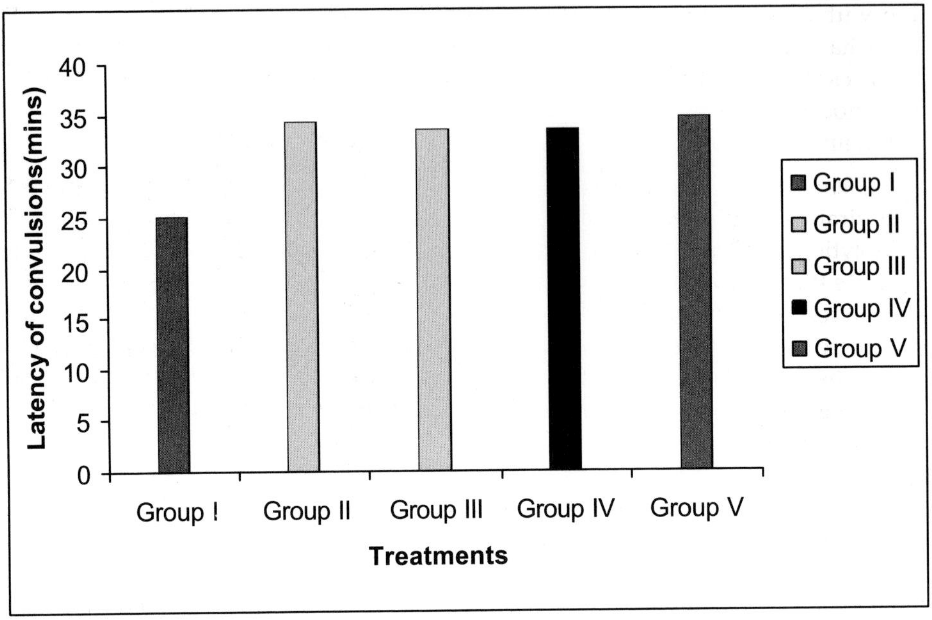

N=6; P<0.01, P< 0.01 vs vehicle (one way ANOVA)

Figure 10.7. Effect of PEHE and Zeetress in anoxic stress tolerance in mice.

Since the introduction of tail suspension test almost 20 years ago, the tail suspension test has become one of the most widely used models for assessing antidepressant-like and adaptogenic activity in mice (Thierry, 1986). The test is based on the fact that animals subjected to the short-term, inescapable stress of being suspended by their tail, will develop an immobile posture. PEHE is able to induce immobility in dose dependant manner as compared to the control group.

The anoxic stress tolerance model shows that administration of PEHE significantly increased the duration of first convulsion in a dose dependent manner in the treated group. Anoxia of the CNS cells plays major role in the development of CNS disorders (Gwyuton, 1981). These disorders may result due to spasm/ arteriosclerosis of CNS blood vessels either due to natural aging process or other causes like thrombosis, cerebral hemorrhage, cellular necrosis and biochemical damage to the cells. PEHE improves anoxic stress tolerance, which might allow cellular functions of CNS at low oxygen supply, thus appears to decrease O_2 demand during anoxia. The increase in anoxia tolerance time by PEHE *per se* is a good indicator for its usefulness in various brain disorders, thus indicating that PEHE not only helps the animal body to adapt to physical stress as well as mental and emotional stress.

Many synthetic drugs in market are available to reduce stress but are also with numerous side effects. Any compound of plant origin with exceptional adaptogenic and with other additional activities is in high demand at present. The Ayurvedic herbs have immense potential in fighting stress, but only a few have been studied so far. These herbs are known to reduce the level of corticosteroids and biogenic amines and modulating the various biochemical parameters, which ultimately help in maintaining homeostasis. The present study is an attempt in this direction.

Plantago erosa have been studied for immunomodulatory, *in vitro* cytotoxic and anti viral property (Chiang *et al.,* 2003). The hydroethanolic extract have shown anxiolytic as well as anti-depressant-like activity (unpublished report). These studies indicate that the plant extract does have effect on CNS. PEHE increased immobility time in forced swim test in both rat and mice and tail suspension test in mice. There was increase in the duration of onset of convulsion in anoxic test model in mice. The phytochemical screening of PEHE showed the presence of tannins, diterpenes, triterpenes and steroids as described above. These phytochemical constituents *viz.,* steroids, tannins, diterpenes and triterpenes might act as mediators (inhibitors/ enhancers) in the various biochemical pathways responsible for reducing stress. However the mechanism by which it can reduce stress is yet to be studied at biochemical and physiological level.

In conclusion, it can be stated that the hydroethanolic extract of *Plantago erosa* showed potential adaptagenic activity in the present investigation. This has opened another hitherto unknown area to study the mechanism of action and further in-depth study of a new adaptagenic plant - *Plantago erosa* ex Roxb.

Acknowledgements

The authors are grateful to National Medicinal Plant Board, Govt. of India, New Delhi for providing financial assistance to carry out this work. Physical facility provided by the Director of Research (Vety) C.V.Sc is also gratefully acknowledged.

References

Atta, A.H., and Mouneir, S.M. (2005). Evaluation of some medicinal plants for anti diarrhoeal activity. *Phytother Res.,* **19:** 481-485.

Bruce, R.D. (1985). An up-and-down procedure for acute toxicity testing. *Fundam Appl Toxicol.,* **5:** 151-177.

Chiang, L.C., Chiang, W., Chang, M.Y., and Lin, C.C. (2003). *In vitro* cytotoxic, antiviral and immunomodulatory effects of *Plantago erosa* and *Plantago asiatica. Chin Med.,* **31:** 225-234.

Cody, Mary E. (2000). *Plantago major* and *Piper methysticum* compound for use in treating a tobacco or nicotine habit: US patent 6,303,647. Mar 14.

Connor T.J., Kelly, J.P., and Leonard, B.E. (1998). Forced swim test induced endocrine and immune changes in the rat: effect of sub-acute desipramine treatments. *Pharmacol Biochem Behav.,* **59**: 171-177.

Cryan, J.F., Markou, A., and Lucki, I. (2002). Assessing anti-depressant activity in rodents: recent development and future need. *Tips., 23:* 238-245.

Edzard, E. (1998). Harmless herbs? A review of the recent literature. *Am J Med.*, 104: 170-178.

Gwyuton, A.C. (1991). Textbook of Medical Physiology. 8th ed. Philadelphia: WB Saunders. p. 459.

Harborne, J.B. (1991). Phytochemical Screening: Guide to modern techniques of plant analysis. 2nd ed. New York: Chapman and Hall. p. 653.

Kannur, D.M., Hukkeri, V.I., and Akki, K.S. (2006). Adaptogenic activity of *Caesalpinia bonducella* seed extract in rats. *J Ethnopharmacol.*, **108**: 327-331.

Lucki, I. 1997).The forced swimming test as a model for core and component behavioral effects of anti-depressant drugs. *Behav Pharmacol.*, **8:** 523-532.

Nunz Guillen, M.E., Silva, D., Emim, J.A., Souccar, C., and Lapa, A.J. (1997). Analgesic and anti- inflammatory activities of the aqueous extract of *Plantago erosa. Int J Pharmacog.*, **35**: 99-104.

Porsolt, R.D., Bertin, A., Blavet, N., and Jalfre, M. (1978). Behavioural despair in rats and mice: strain differences and the effects of imipramine. *Eur J Pharmacol.*, **51**: 291-294.

Porsolt, R.D., LePichon, M., and Jalfre, M. (1977). Depression: A new animal model sensitive to anti- depressant treatments. *Nature,* **266**: 730-732.

Rege, N.N., Thatte, U.M. and Dahanukar, S.A. (1999). Adaptogenic properties of six rasayana herbs used in Ayurvedic medicine. *Phytother Res.*, **13:** 275-291.

Selye, H. (1998). Syndrome produced by diverse nocuous agents. *J Neuropsychr Clin Neurosci.*, 230-231.

Steru, I., Chermat, R., and Thierry Simon, P. (1985). The tail suspension test: new method for screening antidepressants in mice. *Psychopharmacol.*, **85**: 367-370.

Thierry, B., Steru, L., Simon, P., and Porsolt, R.D. (1986). The tails suspension test: Ethical considerations. *Psychopharmacol.*, **90:** 284-285.

Medicinal Plants: Phytochemistry, Pharmacology and Therapeutics Vol. 2 (2012) *Pages* **195–205**
Editor-in-Chief: **V.K. Gupta**
Published by: **DAYA PUBLISHING HOUSE, NEW DELHI**

12

Investigation on the Effects of *Hypericum scabrum* Plant Extract on Signs of Morphine Withdrawal Syndrome in Rats

Khairollah Asadollahi[1*], Koroush Saki[1], Nasser Abassi[1], Amir Faili[1] and Parisa Asadollahi[2]

ABSTRACT

Due to low side effect and expenditure in addition to body's proper physiological adaptations, there is a global trend in using herbal medications. The current study was triggered to investigate the effects of Hypericum scabrum (H.S) plant extract on signs of morphine withdrawal syndrome in rats. For this purpose, 56 healthy Wistar rats (weights 180-200g) were selected and divided into 7 equal groups. Five groups were addicted via the injection of cumulative morphine dosages. Among the five groups being addicted, three groups were injected with different dosages of H. scabrum plant extract (20mg/kg, 40mg/kg and 80 mg/kg), after which naloxan (5mg/kg) was used. For the 2 remained groups one was injected only with 5mg/kg naloxan and the other was treated with 2mg/kg clonidine and 5mg/kg naloxan. Among the two groups not being addicted, one was treated only by normal saline and the other was not injected at all. Morphine withdrawal signs including jumping, standing on feet and gnashing were then measured for all the groups.

Hypericum scabrum plant extract, prevented the occurrence of most signs of morphine withdrawal syndrome in rats. The number of jumpings, standing on feet and gnashings were reduced considerably. Increasing the dosages of H.S plant extract resulted in a more reduction of the signs of morphine withdrawal syndrome. Compared to H.S plant extract (dosages

---

1 Faculty of Medicine, Ilam University of Medical Sciences, Ilam, Iran.

2 Faculty of Science, Chamran University, Ahvaz, Iran.

* *Corresponding author*: E-mail: masoud_1241@yahoo.co.uk,
Tel: 08412227126; Fax. 08412227120

20mg/kg, 40mg/kg), the use of clonidine did not show any significant difference in the occurrence of signs. H.S plant extract in the dosage of 80mg/kg reduced morphine withdrawal signs more than clonidine (p<0.001) but it reduced the lifespan of rats.

As a result, Hypericum scabrum plant extract reduced all signs of morphine withdrawal syndrome in rats. The effect of H.S plant extract can also be investigated solely or synergistically in human along with other chemical drugs.

Keywords: Clonidine, *Hypericum scabrum*, Morphine withdrawal syndrome, Naloxan.

List of Abbreviations

H.S.: *Hypericum scabrum*

H.S.P.E.: *Hypericum scabrum* plant extract

Ip: Intraperitoneal

Introduction

A lot of health problems are currently treated by plant based medications. These medications could also be found in the content of many body care products. Depending on the region where people live, different kinds of plants are used for different purposes. Drug resistance of human pathogens is developing frequently and search for new antimicrobial substances from different sources is of a high priority. Plants have been used traditionally for treating acute and chronic infectious diseases (Martinez *et al.*, 1996; Taylor *et al.*, 1996; Catalano *et al.*, 1998).

Hypericum is a genus of about 400 species of flowering plants in the family of Clusiaceae, subfamily of Hypericoideae. The genus has a nearly world-wide distribution, missing only the tropical lowlands, deserts and Polar Regions. All members of the genus may be referred to as St. John's-worts, though they are also commonly called hypericums, and some are known as tutsans. Among *Hypericum* genus, *Hypericum perforatum* has been more investigated. This plant has been used as an antimigraine (Asian Network for Scientific Information, 2007), antidepressant (Linde *et al.*, 2008: Webpage, 2009), antiretroviral (Lavie, 1990; Abrams, 1990; Ivan, 1979; Moraleda *et al.*, 1993), antimicrobial (Catalano *et al.*, 1998; Dall'Agnol *et al.*, 2003; Kizil *et al.*, 2004; Cecchini *et al.*, 2007; Webpage, 2009), anti-inflammatory (Kakunaga *et al.*, 1966; Webpage, 2009) anti-spasmodic (Asian Network for Scientific Information, 2007) and a painkiller product (Kakunaga *et al.*, 1966). This drug also, inhibits virus replication and therefore it has been used for hepatitis B in ducks (Moraleda *et al.*, 1993). GABA derivations have also been seen in this plant (Lapke, 1995). A review analysis, including 29 clinical trials with more than 5000 patients, showed that the rate of side effects by extracts of St. John's wort was twice as much lower as the newer antidepressants and five times lower than the older tricyclic antidepressants (Linde *et al.*, 2008; Webpage, 2009).

Hypericum scabrum (*Guttiferae*) is a genus of about 370 species of annuals, perennials and deciduous, semi-evergreen and evergreen subshrubs and shrubs, found mainly in temperate regions (Erdoazrol *et al.*, 2004).

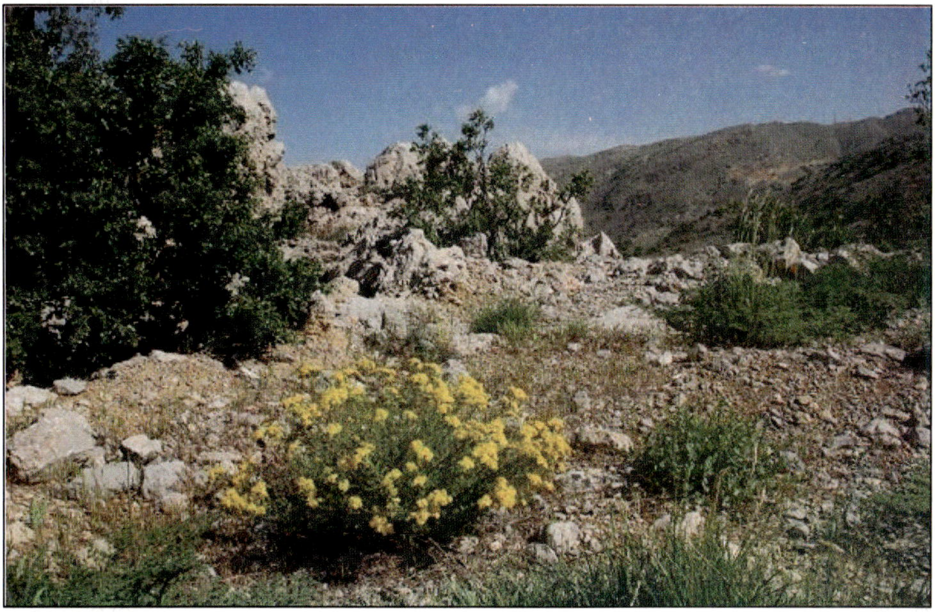

Figure 12.1. *Hypericum scabrum* plant.

Some kinds of *Hypericum* genus have been used as antidepressants and painkillers, which are the signs related to morphine withdrawal syndrome (Linde *et al.*, 2008).

Dependency upon opioid materials can be a physical or mental phenomenon or both (Benjamin and Virginia, 2003). Chronic application of opioid products causes significant mental and behavioural disorder. It starts with joy and well feeling but will change to ill-humour and carelessness gradually. Different signs and symptoms related to opium consumption and opium withdrawal syndrome are listed in Table 12.1.

Some signs of withdrawal syndrome such as depression, irritability, insomnias may extend for more than 6 months (Malekoti, 2002). Withdrawal signs for methadone are started 1-3 days after privation and are gradually settled off in 10-14 days time (Ghaleabandi, 2001).

Opium toxicity is a medical emergency and different drugs have been used for its detoxification, some of which are listed in Table 12.2.

Although opioid withdrawal signs are unpleasant; however, they are not life threatening for healthy people. The main objective for treatment of signs related to opioid withdrawal syndrome is to reduce patients' discomfort and also to disrupt the application of opioid products in 3 weeks time for which three kinds of drugs are currently used. Methadone is a synthetic opioid with a long half life, which is used for treatment of withdrawal syndrome. Opponents of methadone application believe that this drug is expensive and has its effects on a very long period of time or sometimes

Table 12.1. Signs and symptoms related to opium application and opium withdrawal syndrome (Ghaleabandi, 2001).

Overdose use		Hypothermia	Hypotension	Respiratory disorder	Bradycardia	Bradyponea	Coma		
Chronic use		Psychomotor hyperactivity	Psychomotor slow activity	Ill-humour	Carelessness	Judgment disorder	Social and occupational disorder	Pupil narrowness	Dizziness
Withdrawal syndrome	After 12-36 hours	Perspiration	Yawning	Insomnias	Pupil wideness	Lack of appetite	Tremor	Muscle cramp	Mouth dryness
	After 48-72 hours	Abdominal cramp	Diarrhoea, Vomiting	Hypertension	Tachycardia	Fever	Rhinorrhea	Convulsion	

without any effect (Ruiz *et al.*, 1996; Song Xiao-ge, 2005). The second synthetic drug currently used for this purpose is clonidine. Almost 75 per cent of all signs of withdrawal syndrome are treated by clonidine. It doesn't have any effects on insomnias, musculoskeletal pain and opioid eagerness (Katz, 1986; Chen *et al.*, 2007). Naloxan and naltrexone are other long acting drugs which are used for morphine withdrawal syndrome. These drugs are useful in those with high trend to abandon the opioid application and those with a high social support (Mushlin and Cochin, 1976; Malekoti, 2002). The current study aims to investigate the effect of an herbal medication (*Hypericum scabrum*) on signs of morphine withdrawal syndrome in rats and to compare its effect with the current medications used for this purpose.

Table 12.2. Characteristics of drugs used for opium detoxification (Midwest, 2009).

Name of Drug	*Mechanism of Effect*	*Half Life/ Hours*	*Method of Use*	*Daily Amount of Use/mg*	*Drug's Form*
Methadone	Pure agonist of receptors	30	Oral	20-100	Tablet (5mg)
Bupronorphine	Relative agonist of receptors	48-72	Oral/injectional	8-24	Tablet (0.2mg) Ampoule (0.3mg)
Clonidine	Alpha 2 agonist	6-24	Oral/injectional	1.2-2	Tablet (0.2mg) Ampoule (0.3mg)
Naloxane	Pure antagonist	1-2	Injectional	10-40	Ampoule (0.4mg)
Naltrexone	Pure antagonist	4	Oral	50	Tablet (25mg) Capsule (50mg)

Methodology

The sample of collected *Hypericum* plants was confirmed by the Pharmacy Faculty of Mashhad. All parts of the collected plants were dried and then powderised. For each gram of powderised plant 10 ml distilled water was added and the mixture was boiled for 15 minutes. The boiled mixture was filtered by no.1 of Whatman filtering paper. The filtered solution was transferred to the relevant apparatus for removing the surplus water up to 80 per cent. Then the ultimate solution was put in the bath of warm water (30°).

56 healthy male Wistar rats (weights 180-200g) were divided into 7 equal groups. One group was not injected any thing at all and another group was treated only by normal saline. Rats in the remained 5 groups were addicted via the injection of cumulative dosages of morphine subcutaneously 2 times per day until 5 days as follow:

- First day: 15 mg/kg at 8-9 am and 20 mg/kg at 16-17 pm
- Second day: 25mg/kg at 8-9 am and 30 mg/kg at 16-17 pm
- Third day: 35mg/kg at 8-9 am and 40 mg/kg at 16-17 pm
- Fourth day: 45mg/kg at 8-9 am and 50 mg/kg at 16-17 pm
- Fifth day: Only one dosage of 55mg/kg at 8-9 am.

One hour after the last morphine dosage, groups 1, 2 and 3 of the addicted rats were treated by 20mg/kg, 40mg/kg, and 80 mg/kg of H.S. plant extract respectively. For one of the 2 remained addicted groups (control 2), clonidine (0.2 mg/kg ip) was used one hour after last morphine injection and control 1 was remained without any injection at this period. In the last step (30 minutes after H.S or clonidine injection), all addicted rats were injected with 5mg/kg naloxan (Table 12.3). After these stages, morphine withdrawal signs, including jumping, gnashing and standing on feet, were measured for all the groups during a period of 30 minutes.

Using SPSS version 12.0, ANOVA was applied to compare the mean frequency of different signs of morphine withdrawal syndrome between control groups and those injected by H.S.P.E and a P- value smaller than 0.05 was considered significant.

This research was conducted in accordance with the Principles of Laboratory Animal Care (NIH publication, revised in 1985) and was approved prospectively by Ilam Medical Sciences University's Ethics Committee.

Results

Number of jumping, standing on feet and gnashing, which are considered as indications of morphine withdrawal syndrome in rats (Nouri, 1999), were measured in all the study groups. Rats in the group 4 (injected with normal saline) and group 5 (without any injections) did not show any reactions. The mean number of jumpings, standing on feet and gnashings among all study groups are demonstrated in Table 12.4.

Compared to rats in group control 1, there was a lower mean number of jumping, standing on feet and gnashing in the group 1 (20mg/kg H.S) with a significant difference ($p<0.001$) (Figure 12.2). There was also a significant difference between the mean number of signs in the group 2 (40mg/kg H.S) and those in the control group 1 ($p<0.001$). The mean number of signs in the group 3 (80mg/kg H.S.) was considerably lower than those in the group 1, 2 and control 1. The difference between these groups was statistically significant ($p<0.001$).

The mean number of signs in the group control 2 (clonidine 0.2 mg/kg) was significantly lower than those in the group 1 (20mg/kg H.S). There was not a significant difference between the mean number of signs in the group control 2 and that in the group 2 (40mg/kg H.S). The mean number of signs in the group 3 (80mg/kg H.S) was significantly lower than that in the control group 2 (clonidine) ($p<0.001$). However, the mortality rate among the rats in group 3 increased.

Discussion

The results of this study showed that using different dosages of H.S. plant extract (20mg/kg, 40mg/kg, 80mg/kg), one hour before using naloxan, inhibited most of signs of morphine withdrawal syndrome. Therefore, the number of jumpings, standing on feet and gnashings, which have been considered as morphine withdrawal syndrome in rats by previous studies (Nouri, 1999), were all reduced. Also, comparing clonidine and H.S. plant extract in the dosages of 20mg/kg and 40mg/kg did not show any

Table 12.3. Methodology of using morphine, *Hypericum scabrum* and naloxan/clonidine for study groups.

Study Groups		*Group 1*	*Group 2*	*Group 3*	*Group 4*	*Group 5*	*Control 1*	*Control 2*
Morphine injection	First day	15 mg/am 20 mg/pm	15 mg/am 20 mg/pm	15 mg/am 20 mg/pm	Normal saline	Without injection	15 mg/am 20 mg/pm	15 mg/am 20 mg/pm
subcutaneously 2 times/day	2nd day	25 mg/am 30 mg/pm	25 mg/am 30 mg/pm	25 mg/am 30 mg/pm	Normal saline	Without injection	25 mg/am 30 mg/pm	25 mg/am 30 mg/pm
	3rd day	35 mg/am 40 mg/pm	35 mg/am 40 mg/pm	35 mg/am 40 mg/pm	Normal saline	Without injection	35 mg/am 40 mg/pm	35 mg/am 40 mg/pm
	4th day	45 mg/am 50 mg/pm	45 mg/am 50 mg/pm	45 mg/am 50 mg/pm	Normal saline	Without injection	45 mg/am 50 mg/pm	45 mg/am 50 mg/pm
	5th day	55 mg/am	55 mg/am	55 mg/am	Normal saline	Without injection	55 mg/am	55 mg/am
Hypericum scabrum	One hour after last injection	20 mg/kg	40 mg/kg	80 mg/kg	Normal saline	Without injection	–	Clonidine 0.2 mg/kg
Naloxan	30 minute after H.S. injection	5 mg/kg	5 mg/kg	5 mg/kg	Normal saline	Without injection	5 mg/kg	5 mg/kg

difference in reducing the occurrence of signs of morphine withdrawal syndrome. However, the dosage of 80mg/kg, worked significantly better than clonidine ($p<0.001$).

Table 12.4. The mean number of different signs of morphine withdrawal syndrome in different groups of rats 30 minutes after naloxan injection.

Rat's groups	*Jumping (mean± SD)*	*Gnashing (mean ±SD)*	*Standing on Feet (mean ± SD)*	*Sum of Signs (mean ± SD)*
Control 1	21 ± 2.3	55.5 ±1	35.7 ±1.8	37.4±1.7
Group 1	12.2 ±1.5	36.7 ±1.9	22.8 ±1	23.9±1.5
Group 2	8.2 ±1.2	32 ±1.9	18.8 ±1.2	19.7±1.3
Group 3	4.2 ±1.2	23.3 ±1.5	16.2 ±1.2	14.6±1.3
Control 2	5.8 ±1.2	30.7±1	18.7±1.2	18.4±1.1
Group 4	–	–	–	–
Group 5	–	–	–	–

Control 1: morphine addicted rats + naloxan; Group 1: morphine addicted rats + 20mg/kg H.S + naloxan' Group 2: morphine addicted rats + 40mg/kg H.S + naloxan; Group 3: morphine addicted rats + 80mg/kg H.S + naloxan; Control 2: morphine addicted rats + 0.2mg/kg clonidine + naloxan; Group 4: normal saline injected rats; Group 5: rats without any injection.

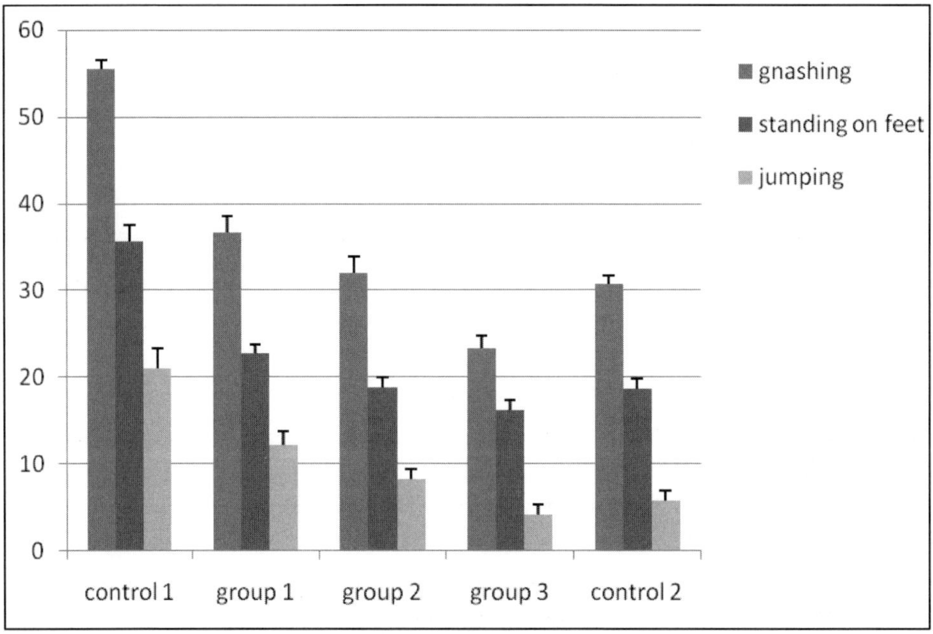

Figure 12.2. Comparing the mean number of morphine withdrawal signs in different groups of rats.

T-sign: standard deviation from the mean; **Control 1**: morphine addicted rats + naloxan; **Group 1** : morphine addicted rats + 20mg/kg H.S + naloxan; **Group 2**: morphine addicted rats + 40mg/kg H.S + naloxan; **Group 3**: morphine addicted rats + 80mg/kg H.S + naloxan; **Control 2**: morphine addicted rats + 0.2mg/kg clonidine + naloxan.

Using key words *Hypericum scabrum* and/or morphine withdrawal syndrome, search engines of Google, ISI web of knowledge, Ovid and Athens were interrogated and there were no published papers to evaluate the effect of H.S on morphine withdrawal syndrome.

A previous study has investigated different dosages of Ca^{++} (10mg, 40mg, 60mg) for treatment of morphine withdrawal syndrome in rat and has reported a high reduction in number of jumping, standing on feet and gnashing (Nouri, 1999). This result was in accordance to the results of the current study. The same study has also evaluated the effect of vitamin D_3 on morphine withdrawal syndrome and has reported a significant reduction of signs in rats (Nouri, 1999). Comparing the effect of Ca^{++} and vitamin D_3 on morphine withdrawal syndrome, they have reported a higher effect of Ca^{++} for this purpose. They have also showed a considerably higher effect of Ca^{++} in the dosage of 80mg/kg than clonidine as a routine chemical drug for treatment of morphine withdrawal syndrome (Nouri, 1999).

Another study has investigated the effect of ascorbic acid on morphine withdrawal syndrome in rats and has reported that using ascorbic acid (5mg/kg, Ip) has prevented most of morphine withdrawal syndrome considerably (Alaei *et al.*, 2005).

According to the results of the current study H.S, which significantly reduced the signs of morphine withdrawal syndrome in rats, can be investigated as morphine withdrawal syndrome inhibitor in human. Also, plants are widely found in the nature and in case of a considerable effect on human as morphine withdrawal syndrome inhibitor, there will be a rich source of natural medications with lower side effects for treatment of morphine withdrawal syndrome.

References

Abrams, D.I. (1990). Alternative therapies in HIV infection. *AIDS*, **4**(12): 1179-87.

Alaei, H., Esmaeili, M., *et al.* (2005). Ascorbic acid decreases morphine self-administration and withdrawal symptoms in rats. *Pathophysiology*, **12(2)**: 103-7.

Asian Network for Scientific Information. (2007). *Pakistan journal of applied sciences.*

Benjamin, S., and Virginia, S. (2003). A summary of psychology, 9 th ed Tehran Arjmand publisher.

Catalano, S., Cioni, P.L., *et al.* (1998). Antimicrobial activity of extracts of *Mutisia acuminata* var. *acuminata*. *J Ethnopharmacol.*, **59(3)**: 207-9.

Cecchini, C., Cresci, A., *et al.* (2007). Antimicrobial activity of seven *Hypericum* entities from central Italy. *Planta Med.*, **73(6)**: 564-6.

Chen, S.Q., Zhai, H.F., *et al.* (2007). Clonidine attenuates morphine withdrawal and subsequent drug sensitization in rhesus monkeys. *Acta Pharmacol Sin.*, **28(4)**: 473-83.

Dallagnol, R., Ferraz, A., *et al.* (2003). Antimicrobial activity of some *Hypericum* species. *Phytomedicine*, **10(6-7)**: 511-6.

Erdoazrol, Ã., Azirak, S., *et al.* (2004). Antimicrobial Activities of *Hypericum scabrum* L. extract. *KSU Journal of Science and Engineering*,**7**: 2.

Ghaleabandi, M. (2001). Clinical psychiatric, first ed. Tehran, Farhangsazan publisher.

Ivan, H. (1979). Preliminary investigations on the application of *Hypericum perforatum* in herpes therapy. *Gyogyszereszet*, **23**: 217-218.

Johnston, P.A., Chahl, L. A. (1992). Chronic treatment with ascorbic acid inhibits the morphine withdrawal response in guinea-pigs. *Neurosci Lett.*, **135(1)**: 23-7.

Kakunaga, T., Kaneto, H., *et al.* (1966). Pharmacologic studies on analgesics. VII. Significance of the calcium ion in morphine analgesia. *J Pharmacol Exp Ther.*, **153(1)**: 134-41.

Katz, J.L. (1986). Effects of clonidine and morphine on opioid withdrawal in rhesus monkeys. *Psychopharmacology (Berl)*, **88(3)**: 392-7.

Kizil, G., Toker, Z., *et al.* (2004). The antimicrobial activity of essential oils of *Hypericum scabrum, Hypericum scabroides* and *Hypericum triquetrifolium*. *Phytother Res.*, **18(4)**: 339-41.

Lapke, C. (1995). GABA in *Hypericum perforatom* L and in other herbal drugs. *Amino Acids*, **(9)**: 55-56.

Lavie, G.M.Y., Lavie, D., *et al.* (1990). Hypericin as an antiretroviral agent; mode of action and related analogues. *Annals of the New York Academy of Sciences*, **616**: 556-562.

Linde, K., Berner, M.M. *et al.* (2008). St John's wort for major depression. *Cochrane Database Syst Rev*. **(4)**: CD000448.

Malekoti, S. (2002). A practical guide for treatment of addiction, First ed. Tehran, Pourshokoh publisher.

Martinez, M.J., Betancourt, J., *et al.* (1996). Screening of some Cuban medicinal plants for antimicrobial activity. *J Ethnopharmacol.*, **52(3)**: 171-4.

Midwest, D.S. (2009). Opiate Drugs, Narcotics, and other related Medications and Drugs. from http: / /www.mrods.com.

Moraleda, G., Wu, T.T., *et al.* (1993). Inhibition of duck hepatitis B virus replication by hypericin. *Antiviral Res.*, **20(3)**: 235-47.

Mushlin, B.E., and Cochin, J. (1976). Tolerance to morphine in the rat: its prevention by naloxone. *Life Sci.*, **18(8)**: 797-801.

Nouri, G. (1999). Investigation of the effect of calcium and vitamin D on morphine withdrawal symptoms in rats. *Isfahan University of medical sciences publication*, 61-72.

Ruiz, F., Fournie-Zaluski, M.C., *et al.* (1996). Similar decrease in spontaneous morphine abstinence by methadone and RB 101, an inhibitor of enkephalin catabolism. *Br J Pharmacol.*, **119(1)**: 174-82.

Song, Xiao-ge., Wang Zhen-hua, Z.H., *et al*. (2005). Clinical observation on improvement of heroin withdrawal syndrome by acupuncture plus methadone. *Journal of Acupuncture and Tuina Science,* **3**: 6-8.

Taylor, R.S., Manandhar, *et al*. (1996). Antiviral activities of Nepalese medicinal plants. *J Ethnopharmacol*., **52(3)**: 157-63.

Webpage. (2009). St John's wort, 2009, from <http: //en.wikipedia.org/wiki/ Hypericum_perforatum>.

Medicinal Plants: Phytochemistry, Pharmacology and Therapeutics Vol. 2 (2012) *Pages* **207–214**
Editor-in-Chief: **V.K. Gupta**
Published by: **DAYA PUBLISHING HOUSE, NEW DELHI**

13

The Role of Herbal Medicine Use in HIV/AIDS Treatment

R.O. Orisatoki[1] and O.O. Oguntibeju[2*]

ABSTRACT

Herbal medicine use is becoming very popular in many countries especially in the western world, where public health safety has become a concern especially its concomitant use with orthodox medicine. The devastating impact of HIV/AIDS pandemic coupled with the severe shortage of health personnel has compelled patients to develop coping mechanisms by adopting alternative sources of primary health care, one of which has been the use of herbal therapies. In the treating and management HIV/AIDS, the medication should be capable of controlling diarrhea, increasing absorption activities in the gastrointestinal tract and improving immunity. It is known that acquired immunity from drug prophylaxis is not a long-term effective solution especially if such drugs demonstrate severe side-effects. It has been shown that remedies derived from plants are common to many cultures and a number of advanced pharmaceutical drugs were derived from plants. It has been also shown that not just herbalists but naturopaths, homeopathic, ayurvedic, Chinese and Native American medical practitioners use herbs as one component in an overall system of medicine and traditional medicine is reported common among individuals with moderate and advanced HIV disease. This review

1 Department of Medical Physiology, School of Medicine, Spartan Health Sciences University, Vieux Fort, Saint Lucia, West Indies.

2 Department of Biomedical Sciences, Faculty of Health and Wellness Sciences, Cape Peninsula University of Technology, Bellville, South Africa.

* *Corresponding author*: E-mail: oguntibejuo@cput.ac.za; bejufemi@yahoo.co, Tel: +27219538495, Fax: +27219538490.

briefly examines the role of herbal medicine in HIV/AIDS treatment and management. It is hoped that this review will provide important and relevant information that will help policy makers to put in place control measures against the abuse of herbal therapy.

Keywords: Herbal medicine, HIV/AIDS, Developed countries, Developing countries, Supplement, Orthodox medicine.

Introduction

The use of herbal medicine is increasingly becoming more popular in many countries (Bannerman, 1993; Kisangau *et al.*, 2007). This practice has continued to be a main source of health care in the rural communities especially in developing countries since modern medicine has not been able to reach the majority of the populace. Also, herbal medicines are still being commonly sold by practitioner and their agents without any restriction with most of the health care providers receiving little or no formal training in this area. This lack of proper training may be associated with the inability of herbal practitioners or their agents to answer questions patients have about its efficacy either as a supplement to orthodox medicine or as a therapy to treat or prevent disease. Their inability to answer questions may partly be linked to the fact that herbal medicine involves a sophisticated theory or system, with the knowledge that is often passed on, verbally or otherwise, from generation to generation (David, 1997; Zhang, 2000; Stephen *et al.*, 2003). Notwithstanding, there have been a remarkable increase in the popularity of herbal preparations especially in developed countries which has stimulated considerable public health concern among physicians who are sometimes uncertain about the safety of herbs especially when used concomitantly with regular orthodox medications (UNAIDS, 2007).

HIV/AIDS pandemic is currently the most socio-economic challenge that is facing the world at large as it affects mostly the young and economically productive population (Kisangau *et al.*, 2007; UNAIDS, 2007). A study has shown that majority of people living with HIV/AIDS are susceptible to fungal and bacterial opportunistic infections that result from immunosuppression and treatment of such infections is therefore one of the areas that traditional health services for the control of the disease is prevalent (Kisangau *et al.*, 2007). The World Health Organization (WHO) estimates that 4 billion people (80 per cent of the World's population) use herbal medicines for some aspect of primary healthcare (WHO, 2002). Treatment of diseases using traditional remedies is an age old art which has been confined into the backstage due to access to western biomedicine, adequate education, employment opportunities and economic growth (Liu *et al.*, 2005).

Regional Use of Herbal Medicine

Herbal Medicine in the Caribbean

Afro-Caribbean pharmacopoeia is that body of knowledge and practices around medicinal plants with its origins in the cultures of African slaves brought to the Caribbean (Lagurrre, 1987). Herbal baths are common in Haitian culture for both spiritual and medicinal practices and represent the second most important category of administration after ingestion in the region (Volpato *et al.*, 2009) There is a significant use of herbal remedies in the Caribbean and recent studies in Trinidad show relatively high prevalence of use for symptomatic relief in asthma and therapeutic management in diabetes mellitus and other chronic diseases (Mahabir and Gilliford, 1997; Clement *et al.*, 2005).

Herbal Use in North America

The increasingly diverse US immigrant populations have led to the growing use of medicinal herbs. A survey conducted by the National Center for Complementary and Alternative Medicine in 2004 revealed that the use of herbal therapy or of other natural products was most common of the complementary and alternative medicines and the commonest reason for use of herbal medicines by Americans was that they believed they would improve health when used in combination with conventional medical treatments (National Center for Health Statistics, 2004).

Herbal Use in Africa

Herbs has a long history in African traditional medicine, however there has been increasing attention and interest in its use in recent times (David, 1997). Traditional herbal medicine has continued to be a main source of health care in the rural communities and heavy reliance on it by the majority of the sub-Saharan African population has led to the generally accepted conclusion that it is most preferred form of treatment of HIV-related symptoms (Bamidele *et al.*, 2009).

Herbal Use in Asia

Medicinal herbs are a major component of Traditional Chinese Medicine. It is estimated that over 600 different herbs have been used to treat various human diseases including those caused by viral infection, accounting for approximately one-fifth of the entire Chinese pharmaceutical market and are regarded as the state cultural treasure by the Chinese government (Li, 2009). Studies on the anti-HIV activities and mechanisms of TCMs are very limited but are expected to accelerate. Herbs native to Japan were classified in the first pharmacopoeia of Japanese traditional medicine in the ninth century (Saitoh, 2000). Ayurveda is a herbal medical system primarily practiced in India. It includes diet and herbal remedies, while emphasizing the body, mind and spirit, in disease prevention and treatment (Morgan, 2009).

Herbal Use in Europe

Complementary or unconventional treatments are used by many doctors and other therapists throughout Europe. The major forms are acupuncture, homoeopathy, manual therapy or manipulation, and phytotherapy or herbal medicine. The relative popularity of therapies differs between countries, but public demand is strong and growing. Regulation of practitioners varies widely: in most countries, only registered health professionals may practice, but in the United Kingdom practice is virtually unregulated. Germany and some Scandinavian countries have intermediate systems. Legal reforms are in progress in the Netherlands and the United Kingdom. European institutions are starting to influence the development of complementary medicine (Fisher and Ward, 1994).

In Germany, herbal medications are dispensed by pharmacists, subjected to same criteria for efficacy, safety and quality as are other drug products. Despite the progress in orthodox medicine, interest in alternative medicine, including herbal medicine is on the increase. A great variety of plants are used for medicinal treatments, either the dried plant or a specific part of it (root, leaves, fruit, flowers, seeds), is formulated into suitable preparations-compressed as tablets or made into pills, used to make infusions (teas), extracts, tinctures or mixed with excipients to make lotions, ointments, creams (Zudek, 1994; Tapsell, 2006).

Herbal Medicine in the Treatment of HIV/AIDS

Traditional herbal use has been reported to be common among individuals with moderate and advanced HIV disease (Langlois-klassen *et al.*, 2007). In Africa, traditional herbal medicines are often used as primary treatment for HIV/AIDS and for HIV-related problems including dermatological disorders, nausea, depression, insomnia and weakness (Hodgson and Rachanis, 2002). The use of traditional herbal medicine by AIDS patients after HIV diagnosis was noted in a study in Uganda (Langlois-Klassen *et al.*, 2007).

Despite a paucity of evidence on effectiveness and the possibility of serious side effects, some African ministries of health currently promote traditional medicines for the treatment of HIV and associated-symptoms. In the case of South Africa, the Ministry of Health is actively promoting the use of traditional medicines with antiretroviral treatments (Manfred and Chiodo, 2000). Two principal African herbal compounds used for HIV/AIDS treatment in sub-Saharan Africa include *hypoxis hemerocallidea* (African potato-an immunostimulant) and *Sutherlandia*. These two herbal remedies are currently recommended by the South African Ministry of Health for HIV/AIDS management (SADC, 2002).

We believe that medical practitioners and researchers ought to be informed about the use of herbal medicine for both HIV-related illnesses and other co-morbid conditions as part of their history taking and clinical assessments. Failure to do so may cause health-care workers to inadvertently overlook the full spectrum of potential herb-drug interactions that may be experienced by an AIDS patient. For instance, a study in Canada found that more than 53 per cent of HIV outpatients taken traditional herbs did not report its use to their treating physician (Furler *et al.*, 2003). Also, antiretroviral therapy recipients have been reported to use herbs to alleviate some of the negative side effects of antiretroviral (ARV) drugs such as nausea and diarrhea (Langlois-Klassen *et al.*, 2007).

In North America, commonly used herbal dietary supplements have been found to impede on ARV drug effectiveness. Specifically, garlic supplements (*Allium sativum*) and St John's Wort (*Hypericum perforatum*) have been shown to have detrimental effects on the plasma concentrations of *saquinavir* and *indinavir* (Piscitelli *et al.*, 2000). The most common reasons patients gave for using herbs include general wellbeing, relaxation, pain, stress, spiritualism and healing. It was reported of outpatients that 9 per cent believed that it was possible to treat HIV solely with the use of herbs, while others use it to improve energy level, to supplement dietary intake and to enhance response. However, in a US study, the most common treated conditions using herbal medicine in relation to AIDS include anxiety/fear, depression, pain and neuropathy (Furler *et al.*, 2003; Dhalla *et al.*, 2006). Fogarty *et al.* (2007) also found that 44.3 per cent of an Australian HIV patient sample reported mixed use of marijuana for therapeutic and recreational purposes.

Although modern medicine may exists side-by-side with such traditional practice, herbal medicines have often maintained their popularity for historical and cultural reasons, so such people see traditional medicine as a complementary health care not alternative to modern medicine (Langlois-Klassen *et al.*, 2007). However, there are some challenges to collaboration between traditional herbal medicine and orthodox medicine especially in the developing countries mainly due to shortage of mutual trust and appreciation between the two health system, limited availability of training in basic preventive medicine, palliative care for traditional herbal healer, lack of meaningful referral between conventional health providers and traditional herbal healers, exclusion of traditional healing methods from the training curricula of doctors and traditional healers fear of losing their treatments secrets to scientists and researchers (Bamidele *et al.*, 2009). A patient's level of knowledge about HIV disease, a belief that ART is effective and prolongs life and recognition that poor adherence may result in viral resistance and treatment failure all impact negatively upon a patient's ability to adhere. Beliefs about the medications (including traditional) themselves also play a role in adherence. Patients who report low confidence in the efficacy of the medications and perceive minimal benefits resulting from ART are less likely to be adherent. It is estimated from other studies that at least 30 per cent of patients on ART will use any form of traditional complementary and alternative medicine (Liu *et al.*, 2005; Peltzer *et al.*, 2008;).

Because the exact level of risk and/or benefits resulting from traditional herbal medicine-antiretroviral- drug co-therapy amongst AIDS patients is largely unknown, the concerns raised about herb-ARV drug interactions, communication between patients and physicians about herbal medicine is valuable in enabling physicians to address issues of potential herb-drug interactions and ensuring appropriate medical care (Astin, 1998). The range of care for patients encompassed a broad range of treatment options. South Africans living with HIV/AIDS are now encouraged to make their own informed choices about the types of treatment they wish to seek including antiretroviral (ART), exercise, nutrition as well as traditional and complementary medicines (Drew and Myers, 1997). The devastating impact of HIV/AIDS pandemic in the region (Southern Africa) coupled with the severe shortage of health personnel might have forced the inhabitants to develop coping mechanisms by adopting alternative sources of primary health care, one of which has been the use of herbal therapies (Hollenburg *et al.*, 2008).

Conclusions

The inclusion of traditional herbal healers in the health care system especially in primary healthcare team in developing countries could improve quality of life and safety standards and their use as a complimentary therapy could play a role in the palliative care of people living with HIV/AIDS.

While many years of herbal use in traditional settings can be used as a testimony that a particular herbal ingredient is effective or safe, several problems need to be addressed. It is now known that ingredients that form part of herbal preparations are incorporated into modern practice and are now used in developed countries as part of health promotion or disease prevention strategies. One of the most difficult issues to contend with in translating traditional herbal practices into conventional western medicine is the individualization of prescription containing multiple herbal and other ingredients.

Whether backed by medical science or simply by years of use, traditional treatments remain popular and as more research is carried out, some may play a complementary role in modern medicine.

There is an urgent need for educational intervention with regard to herbal medicine in the training of our physicians. We propose that an integration of herbal medicine into the current medical curriculum so that future physicians would be better prepared to communicate with their patients on this healthcare modality. Continuing education programme are also recommended so that practicing physicians would have the opportunity to upgrade their knowledge in this rapidly expanding area of significant public health concern.

References

Astin, J A (1998). Why patients use alternative medicine: results of a national study. *J Am Med Assoc.*, **279**: 1548-1553.

Bamidele, J.O., Adebimpee, W.O., and Oladele, E.A. (2009). Knowledge, attitude and use of alternative medical therapy amongst urban residents of Osun state, SouthWestern, Nigeria. *Afri J Trad, Compl and Alternat Med.*, **6 (3):** 281-288.

Bannerman, R.H.(1993). Traditional medicine and healthcare. Geneva. World Health Organization.

Clement, Y.N., Williams, A.F., Aranda, D., Chase, R., Watson, N., Mohammed, R., Stubbs, O., and Williamson, D. (2005). Medicinal herbal use among asthmatic patients attending a specialty care facility in Trinidad. *BMC Compl and Altern Med.*, **5:** 3-6.

David, M.E. (1997). Advising patients who seek alternative medical therapies. *Annals Int Med.*, **27(1):** 61-69.

Dhalla, S., Chan, K.J., Montaner, J.S., and Hogg, R.S. (2006). Complementary and alternative medicine use in British Columbia- a survey of HIV positive people on antiretroviral therapy. *Complement Therapeutic Clin Pract.*, **12(4):** 242-248.

Drew, A.K., and Myers, S.P. (1997). Safety issues in herbal medicine: implications for the health professions. *Med. J. Aust.*, **166**: 538-541.

Fisher, P., and Ward, A. (1994). Complementary medicine in Europe. *Brit Med J.*, **9:** 107-111.

Forgarty, A., Rawstorne, P., Prestage, G.,Crawford, J., Grierson, J., and Kippax, S. (2007). Marijuana as therapy for people living with HIV/AIDS: social and health aspects. *AIDS Care*, **19 (2):** 295-301.

Furler, M.D., Einarson, T.R., Walmsley, S., Millson, M., and Bendayan, R. (2003). Use of complementary and alternative medicine by HIV-infected outpatients in Ontario, Canada. *AIDS Patient Care STDs.*, **17(4):** 155-168.

Hodgson, T. and Rachanis, C. (2002). Oral fungal and bacterial infections in HIV-infected individuals: an overview in Africa. *J Oral Dis.*, **8:** 80-87.

Hollenburg, D., Zakus, D., Cook, T., and Xu, X.W. (2008). Re-positioning the role of traditional, complementary and alternative medicine as essential health knowledge in global health: do they still have a role to play? *World Health Population,* **10 (4):** 62-75.

Kisangau, D.P., Lyaruu, H.V.M., Hosea, K.M., and Joseph, C.C.(2007). Use of traditional medicines in the management of HIV / AIDS opportunistic infections in Tanzania: a case in the Bukoba rural district. *J Ethnobiol and Ethnomed.*, **3:** 29-33.

Laguerre, M. (1987). Afro-Caribbean folk medicine. South Hadley, MA: Bergin and Garvey Publishers.

Langlois-Klassen, D., Kipp, W., Jhangari, G.S., and Rubaale, T. (2007). Use of traditional herbal medicine by AIDS patients in Kabarole District, Western Uganda. *Am J Trop Med and Hyg.*, **77(4):** 757-763.

Li, L. (2000). Opportunity and challenge of traditional Chinese medicine in the face of the entrance to World Trade Organization. *Chin. Inform.Trad.Chin.Med.*, **7**: 7-8.

Liu, J.P., Manheimer, E., Yang, M. (2005). Herbal Medicines for treating HIV infection and AIDS. *Cochrane Database Syst Rev.*, **20(3):** CD003937.

Mahabir, D., and Gilliford, M.C. (1997). Use of medicinal plants for diabetes in Trinidad and Tobago. *Rev Panam Salud Publica.*, **1(3):** 174-179.

Manfred, R., and Chiodo, F. (2000). The effects of alternative treatments for HIV disease on recommended pharmacological regimens, *Int J Antimicrobial Agents*, **13:** 281-285.

Morgan, K. (2009).Medicine of the gods: Basic principles of Ayurvedic medicine. http: / /www.compulink.co.uk/~mandrake/ayurveda.htm (accessed on the 20 April 2010).

National Center for Health Statistics (2004). Complementary and alternative medicine use among adults.

Peltzer, K., Preez, N.F., Ramlagan, S., and Fomundam, H. (2008). Use of traditional complementary and alternative medicine for HIV patients in KwaZulu-Natal, South Africa. *BMC Public Health*, **8:** 255-259.

Piscitelli, S.C., Burstein, A.H., Welden, N., Gallicano, K.D., Falloon, J. (2000). Indinavir concentrations and St. John's wort. *Lancet*, **255**: 547-548.

SADC (2002). Southern African development community (SADC) ministerial consultative meeting on Nutrition and HIV / AIDS. Johannesburg.

Saito, H. (2000). Regulation of herbal medicines in Japan. *Pharmacol. Regul.*, **41:** 515-519.

Stephen, M.L., Margaret, L.W.L., and Robert, M.M. (2003). Complementary and alternative medical practices: training, experiences, and attitudes of a primary care medical school faculty. *J Am Board Fam Pract.,* **16**: 318-326.

Tapsell, L.C. (2006). Health benefits of herbs and spices: the past, the present, the future. *Med J Austr.,***185 (4 Suppl):** S4-S24.

UNAIDS (2007). AIDS epidemic update Geneva.

Volpato, G., Godinez, D., Beyra, A., and Barreto, A. (2009). Use of medicinal plants by Haitian immigrants and their descendants in the Province of Camaguey, Cuba. *J Ethnobiol and Ethnomed.,* **5**: 16-22.

WHO (2002). Traditional medicine; growing needs and potential. WHO policy perspectives on medicines. *World Health Organization, Geneva,* 1-6.

Zhang, X. (2000). Integration of traditional and complimentary medicine into national health care systems. *J Manipulative and Physiol Therap.,* **23**: 139-140.

Zudek, E.M. (1994). Traditional native healing: alternative or adjunct to modern medicine? *Can Fam Physician.,* **40:** 1923-1931.

Medicinal Plants: Phytochemistry, Pharmacology and Therapeutics Vol. 2 (2012) *Pages* **215–225**
Editor-in-Chief: **V.K. Gupta**
Published by: **DAYA PUBLISHING HOUSE, NEW DELHI**

14

Effect of *Alternanthera brasiliana* (L.) Kuntze on Modified Forced Swimming Test in Rats

C.C. Baruah[1]*, S.A. Begum[1], A. Talukdar[1], B. Buragohain[1], J.D. Roy[1], A.G. Barua[2], P. Borah[3] and M. Lahkar[3]

ABSTRACT

Alternanthera brasiliana (L.) Kuntze (Amaranthaceae) is a herbaceous plant commonly known in Brazil as Penicillin. The present study was designed to investigate the antidepressant-like effect of the plant by using modified forced swimming test (MFST). The methanol extract of A. brasiliana (MEAB) leaves were used to investigate the putative psychotherapeutic effects of this plant as antidepressant. The animals were randomly allocated into six groups of six animals each. Group I served as vehicle control, group II, III, IV received MEAB p.o. at the dose rate of 100, 300 and 600 mg/kg body wt. and group V received Desipramine hydrochloride (DMI) @ 30 mg/kg and group VI, Citalopram (CIT) @ 15 mg/kg body wt. i.p. as standard drug. Following administration, the immobility time in MFST in rats were decreased significantly ($P<0.01$) in MEAB treated group as compared to the control group. There was significant ($P<0.01$) increase in the climbing behavior in the treated groups as well as in the DMI treated group compared to the control group in a dose dependant manner without much

1 Department of Pharmacology and Toxicology, College of Veterinary Science, Assam Agricultural University, Khanapara, Guwahati – 781 022, India

2 Department of Public Health, College of Veterinary Science, Assam Agricultural University, Khanapara, Guwahati – 781 022, India

3 Department of Microbiology, College of Veterinary Science, Assam Agricultural University, Khanapara, Guwahati – 781 022, India

* *Corresponding author*: E-mail: chanacin@gmail.com; chanacin@satyam.net.in, Tel: 098640-13231, Fax: 02364941 (O)

effect on the swimming component. The study revealed antidepressant-like activity of MEAB. The pattern of effects observed in the MFST suggests involvement of the noradrenergic neurotransmitter system.

Keywords: *Alternanthera brasiliana,* Antidepressant, Citalopram, Desipramine hydrochloride, Modified forced swimming test.

Introduction

At present, depression is one of the most frequent psychiatric conditions commonly encountered, but till date the efficacy of antidepressant drugs are very limited due to their side effects. Hence, need for newer, better tolerated and more efficacious treatment is remaining high. The plant extracts being more efficacious, free from undesirable side effects compared to their pure active principle revalidated the therapeutic benefits of herbs due to totality of constituents rather than the single molecule. In spite of phenomenal development of the synthetic drug industry and antibiotics, medicinal plants still constitute an important part of pharmacopoeias in both the developed and developing countries. These plants are important elements of traditional medicine in virtually all cultures. Therefore, herbal therapies could be considered as alternative/complementary medicines.

The search for novel pharmacotherapy from medicinal plants for psychiatric illness has progressed significantly in the past decade (Zhang, 2004). This is reflected in large number of herbal medicines whose psychotherapeutic potential has been assessed in a variety of animal models. The forced swimming test (FST), described originally (Porsolt *et al.,* 1977) is widely used as an animal model to assess the antidepressant action (Cryan *et al.,* 2002). The test is relatively simple to perform and has the ability to measure behavioral effects common to antidepressant treatments that have diverse pharmacological and physiological effects. The test can also distinguish drugs that are not antidepressant. Nonetheless, almost all members of an important group of antidepressants–the selective serotonin reuptake inhibitors (SSRIs) - had been found not to be active in classic Porsolt's test in rats (Cryan *et al.,* 2002). Therefore, certain procedural modifications had to be introduced in order to measure the behavioral effects of those drugs (Cryan *et al.,* 2005; Lucki, 1997).

The MFST, besides allowing to observe the effects of SSRIs in rats was found to be very useful in distinguishing that group of compounds from those drugs acting via the inhibition of noradrenalin reuptake. The latter drugs, as for example reboxetine or desipramine, increases rather climbing, while SSRIs increases swimming behavior (Kusmider *et al.,* 2007). Thus, SSRIs such as Fluoxetine, paroxetine or sertraline decrease immobility and increase swimming (Cryan and Lucki, 2000; Page *et al.,* 1999), while the selective noradrenergic and dopaminergic reuptake inhibitors, like DMI, maprotiline and bupropion decrease immobility accompanied by an increase in climbing behavior (Hemby *et al.,* 1997).

Alternanthera brasiliana Kuntz (Amaranthaceae), a herbaceous plant commonly known in Brazil as Penicillin or Brazilian Joy Weed is a neotropical native species, which grows easily on poor and deforested soil. The plant is used against inflammation, cough and diarrhea in Brazilian popular medicine (Macedo *et al.*, 1999). The extracts of *A. brasiliana* exhibited antinociceptive effects in mice (Bivattti *et al.*, 2003), antimicrobial effect (Lagrota *et al.*, 1994) and also anti-herpes simplex virus activity (Brochadoa *et al.*, 2003). Aqueous or ethanolic extracts of *A. brasiliana* are able to block human mitogen induced lymphocyte proliferation without any toxic effect (Wagner *et al.*, 1984).

In our previous study, methanol extract of leaves of *A. brasiliana* showed wound healing activity in both *in vivo* (excision and incision wound model) as well as *in vitro* (Chorioallantoic membrane) model (Barua *et al.*, 2009). In another study, *A. brasiliana* showed antinociceptive activity in both peripheral and non-narcotic models like acetic acid induced writhing syndrome test and narcotic analgesic models like tail flick and hot plate test (Barua *et al.*, 2009a). The methanol extract was found to possess antidepressant-like activity in forced swimming test in rat and mice as well as tail suspension test in mice which was comparable with DMI, a noradrenalin reuptake inhibitor, used as antidepressant drug. As MFST differentiates swimming behavior (which is sensitive to SSRIs, 5-HT receptor agonists) from climbing behavior (which is sensitive to tricyclic antidepressants and drugs with selective effects on catecholamine transmission like DMI) (Lucki, 1997), hence, to elucidate the mechanism of antidepressant-like action of *A. brasiliana* at neurotransmitter level, the present study was undertaken.

Materials and Methods

Plant Material

The leaves of the plants were collected during the month of Feb - June, 2009 from the medicinal garden of the Department of Pharmacology and Toxicology, College of Veterinary Science, Khanapara, Guwahati and were identified by Taxonomist of NEIST, Jorhat, Assam; a voucher specimen (No AAU/CVSC/PHT/02) was deposited.

Preparation of Methanol Extract of Alternanthera brasiliana

Fresh leaves of *A. brasiliana* were cleaned and washed thoroughly with water and rewashed with distilled water. Washed fresh leaves were dried under shade in clean and dust free environment and grinded and stored in air tight container. About 250 g of powdered leaves were soaked in 1000 ml methanol for 72 hours in beaker. The mixture was stirred every 18 hours using a sterile glass rod. The solvent was filtered every 3rd day using muslin cloth and Whatman filter paper no 1. The filtrate obtained was concentrated in Rotary Evaporator (Equitron, Roteva) at 50- 60°C under reduced pressure leaving a dark brown residue. *A. brasiliana* extract thus obtained was transferred to a Petri dish and kept over water bath (50°C) until the solvent gets completely evaporated. It was stored in air tight container at 40°C for further use. Recovery was 6.12 per cent (w/w).

Phytochemical Screening

The freshly prepared methanol extract of *A. brasiliana* (MEAB) was subjected to standard screening tests for various phytoconstituents (Harborne, 1991).

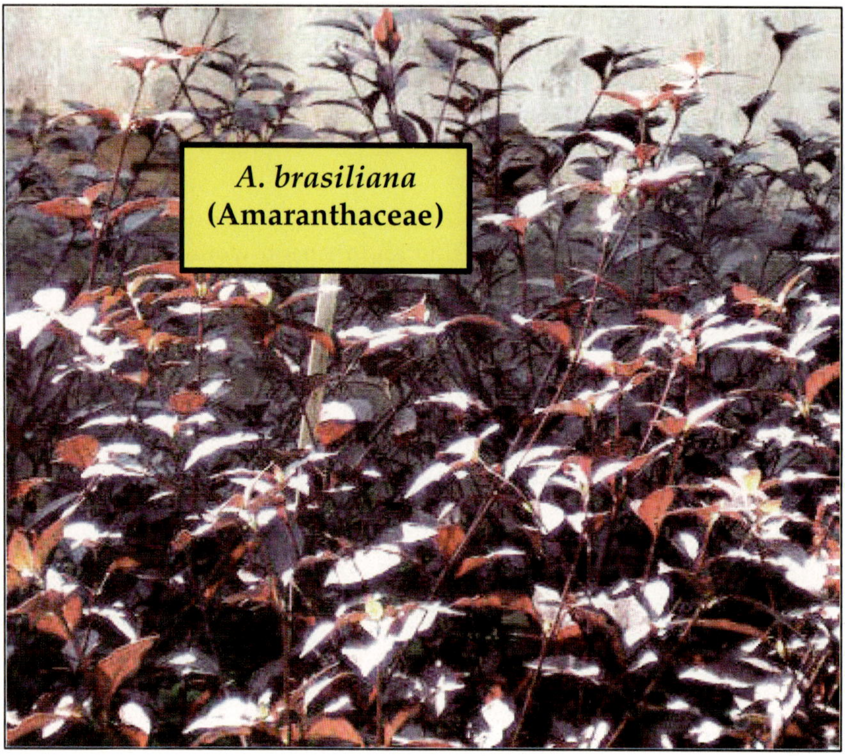

Figure 14.1.

Determination of LD_{50}

The LD_{50} of MEAB was estimated by the employment of up-and-down stair case method in mice. Doses were adjusted by a constant multiplicative factor *viz.*, 4, for this experiment. The dose for each successive animal was adjusted up and down depending on the previous outcome. The acute toxicity and gross effect of MEAB was studied in albino mice by using 1/2 LD_{50} dose. A total of six numbers of male albino mice were selected for the experiment. Animals were observed hourly for six hours and again after 24 hours. The parameters for motor activity and gross effect were determined after administration of MEAB orally at half LD_{50} dose.

Animals

Healthy Sprague Dawley rats of either sex, approximately of same age (6-8 weeks), weighing between 150-220 g were used for the study. They were housed under controlled conditions of temperature (25±30°C), relative humidity (50±5 per cent), 12:12 hour light-dark cycle and free access to food and water. Animals were housed individually in polypropylene cages containing sterile paddy husk bedding. The animals were randomly allocated into six groups of six animals each. Group I served as vehicle control, group II, III, IV received MEAB p.o. at the dose rate of 100, 300 and 600 mg/kg body wt. and group V received the standard drug DMI @ 30 mg/

kg and Group VI, Citalopram @ 15 mg/kg body wt. p.o. The study was conducted after obtaining the approval of the Institutional Animal Ethics Committee (770/03/ac/CPCSEA/FVSc, AAU/IAEC/06/21). The animals were fasted for 14 hours before tests to achieve better drug absorption through gastrointestinal tract.

Drugs

Desipramine hydrochloride (DMI) obtained from Sigma–Aldrich Inc. (St. Louis MO.USA) and Citalopram (CIT) from Lundbeck were used in the study. Both were dissolved in distilled water and administered i.p.

Modified Forced Swimming Test

In order to asses the antidepressant activity of plant extract, the modified forced swimming test (MFST) as suggested by Porsolt (1977) was conducted. An important group of antidepressants, the selective serotonin reuptake inhibitors (SSRIs) had been found not to be active in classic Porsolt's test in rats (Cryan *et al.,* 2002). Hence, certain procedural modifications had to be introduced to measure the behavioral effects of those drugs (Cryan *et al.,* 2005; Lucki, 1997). The modification that have been introduced, concerned the water depth - in the modified procedure, it was increased from 15-18 cm to 30 cm resulting in worse support of floating animals and not only the immobility time has been measured, but also the mode of active behavior (climbing, swimming, diving or head shaking) (Detke *et al.,* 1995). In the first trial, the

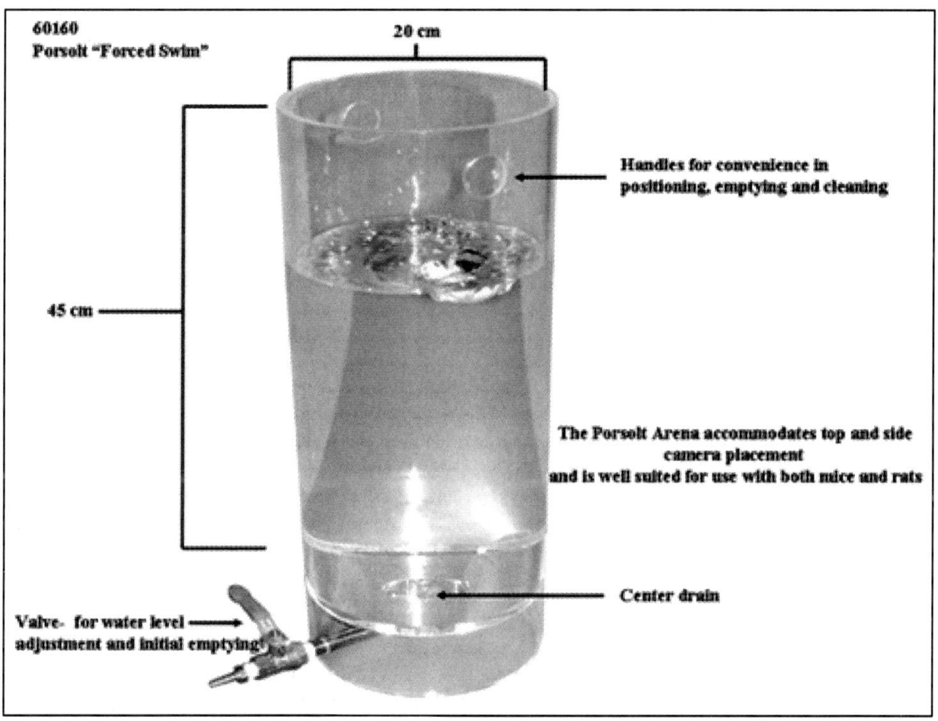

Figure 14.2.

untreated rats were forced to swim for 15 min in a glass cylinder (21cm in diameter) filled with water (23-25°C) to 30 cm depth. The next day, animals received different doses of the plant extracts (100 to 600 mg/kg p.o.). One hour after feeding, the animals were again placed inside the cylinders filled in the same way as during the pre-test and observed for 5 min. Upon removal from water the animals were towel dried before placing them to the respective cage.

Behavioral Scoring

A time sampling technique was employed to score three different behaviors (Detke *et al.*, 1995). During the test session, the following behaviors in rats were recorded by observers blind to the treatment conditions. (1) immobility - floating in the water without struggling, and doing only those movements necessary to keep the head above the water; (2) swimming - showing moderate active motions around in the cylinder, more than necessary to merely keep the head above water; and (3) climbing - presenting active vigorous movements with forepaws in and out of the water, usually directed against the walls. Upon removal from the water, rats were towel-dried and finally returned to their home cage.

Statistical Analysis

The results were subjected to statistical analysis as per standard method (Snedecor and Cochran, 1994).

Results

Qualitative phytochemical screening of the MEAB revealed the presence of alkaloid, steroid and triterpenes by various tests. In acute toxicity study, there was no change of motor activity and gross behavior during 24 hours of observation and the plant extract was found to be safe up to 2g/kg body wt. p.o. The low toxicity of the plant extract suggests that MEAB is relatively safe and devoid of acute toxicity.

In MFST three criteria were measured for antidepressant activity *viz* climbing, immobility and swimming (Table 14.1). The MEAB when administered orally at dose of 100, 300 and 600 mg/kg significantly ($P<0.01$) increased duration of climbing behavior (65.16, 91.58 and 124.95 sec respectively) in a dose dependent manner; for DMI and CIT, it was 142.91 and 63.83 sec, respectively (Figure 14.3).

Significant reduction in duration of immobility time in MEAB treated group at the above dose (133.96, 86.84 and 65.28 sec) was recorded in a dose dependent manner (Figure 14.4). Duration of swimming in MEAB treated group was 100.88, 121.58 and 109.77 sec; in case of DMI and CIT it was 81.16 and 158.97 sec., respectively (Figure 14.5).

Discussion

The present study characterized the antidepressant- like effect of the MEAB using MFST. The behaviors selected for scoring were climbing, swimming as well as immobility as per modified forced swimming method, which was slightly different from the classical Porsolt's model. The results demonstrated that administration of MEAB significantly ($P<0.01$) decreased the duration of the immobility time in MFST

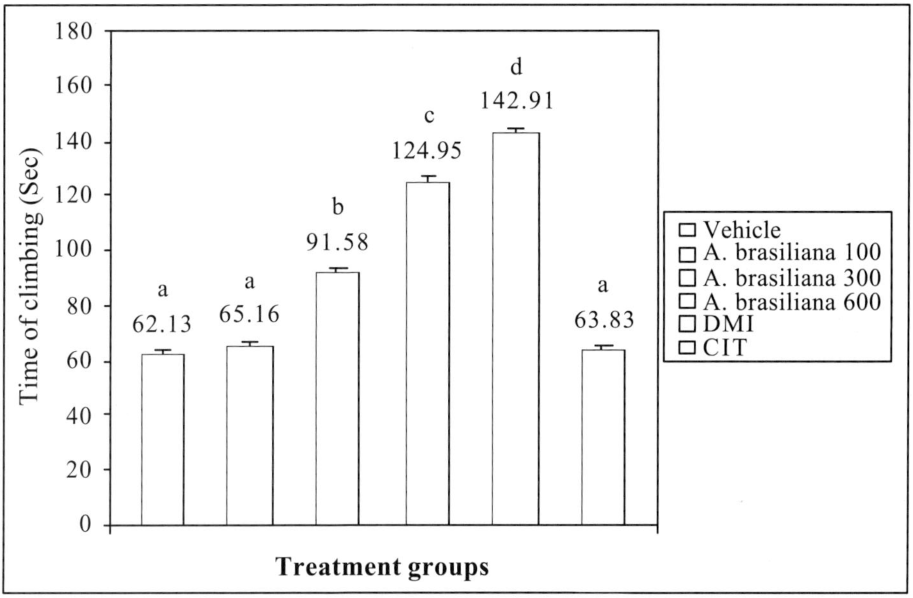

Figure 14.3. Effect of MEAB on climbing behavior in modified forced swimming test in rats.

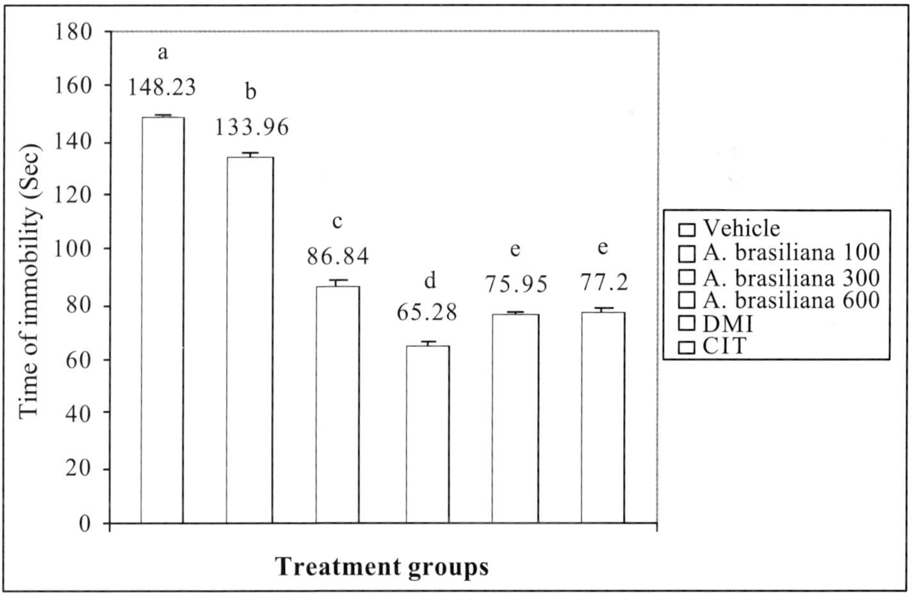

Figure 14.4. Effect of MEAB on immobility time in modified forced swimming test in rats.

in rat in a dose dependant manner as compared to the control group, indicating the antidepressant activity of MEAB. The extract was able to reduce immobility time and simultaneously enhance active behaviors like climbing.

Table 14.1. Effect of MEAB in modified forced swimming test in rats.

Sl.No.	*Treatment Groups*	*Dose (mg/kg, po)*	*Climbing (Sec)*	*Swimming (Sec)*	*Immobility (Sec)*
Group I	Control	10	62.13^{a}±1.28	89.64^{a}±1.04	148.23^{a}±1.13
Group II	*A. brasiliana*	100	65.16^{a}±1.65	100.88^{b}±2.09	133.96^{b}±1.26
Group III	*A. brasiliana*	300	91.58^{b}±1.55	121.58^{c}±3.36	86.84^{c}±1.96
Group IV	*A. brasiliana*	600	124.95^{c}±1.89	109.77^{d}±3.20	65.28^{d}±1.53
Group V	DMI	30 (ip)	142.91^{d}±1.70	81.16^{e}±1.16	75.95^{e}±1.34
Group VI	CIT	15 (i.p.)	63.83^{a}±1.05	158.97^{f}±1.79	77.20^{e}±1.64

(n = 6, mean ± SE)

Means bearing same superscript in a column don't differ significantly (P< 0.01).

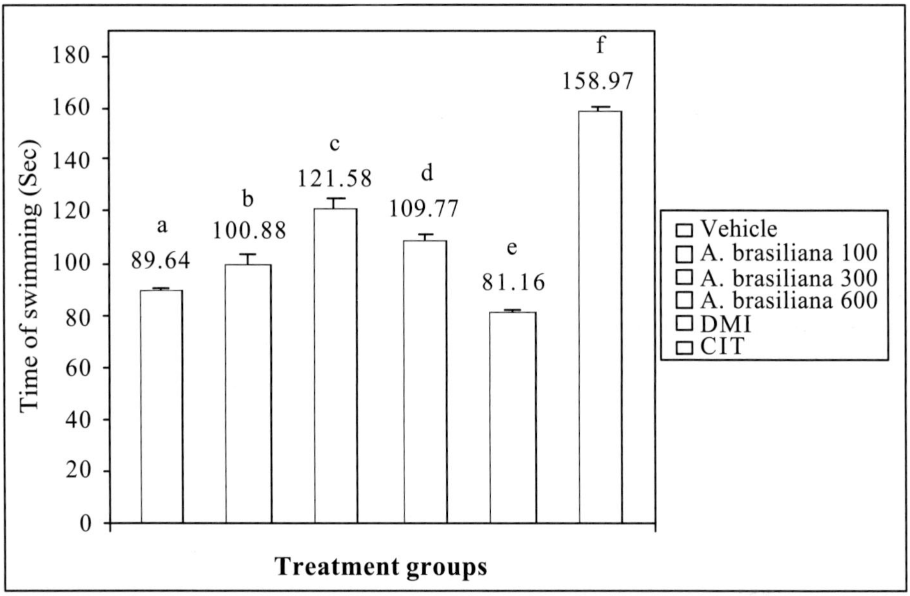

Figure 14.5. Effect of MEAB on swimming behavior in modified forced swimming test in rats.

Acute administration of most of the antidepressant decreases immobility (Cryan *et al.,* 2005). The immobile behavior is thought to reflect either a failure to persist in escape-directed behavior after persistent stress or the development of passive behavior that disengages the animal from active forms of coping with stressful stimuli (Cryan *et al.,* 2005). A broad spectrum of antidepressant drugs selectively prevents the development of behavioral immobility in the FST (Borsini and Meli, 1988). In a study, the hydroethanolic extract of the Brazilian medicinal plant *Trichilia catigua* produced antidepressant-like effects in the forced swimming model in both mice and rats suggesting the antidepressant-like effect of the plant (Campos *et al.,* 2005).

In our study, reduction of immobility time in case of treatment groups were comparable to that observed after i.p. administration of the reference antidepressant drug DMI without any effect on the swimming component. Similar results were reported by other workers (Kusmider *et al.,* 2007) that DMI, the noradrenaline reuptake inhibitor significantly augmented the climbing behavior without any effect on the swimming component. The finding is also in agreement with the report by another author (24) who indicated that drugs affecting noradrenergic system modify rather climbing behavior without any significant change in the swimming in MFST. Another study (Estrada-Camarena *et al.,* 2003) conducted to evaluate the possible antidepressant action of natural estrogen 17β-estradiol ethynyl estradiol and diethyl-stilbesterol also confirms the antidepressant-like effect of fluoxetine (FLX) and DMI. The reduction in immobility induced by FLX was accompanied by increased swimming, while in case of DMI, an increase in climbing behavior is observed. In another report (Kusmider *et al.,* 2007), CIT which belongs to SSRIs was found to increase swimming behaviour at the cost of climbing and immobility in the MFST in rats while comparing with the effect of DMI at the same dose. Likewise, in our study also CIT increased swimming behaviour at the cost of climbing.

Therefore, the present study revealed that MEAB possess significant antidepressant-like activity which is similar to DMI, a noradrenaline reuptake inhibitor. Presence of monoterpenoid compounds like carvone and thujone in the essential oil of *Aloysia polystachya* are responsible for their anxiolytic and antidepressant like effects (Mora *et al.,* 2005). As triterpenes is one of the phytoconstituents of MEAB, it may be possible that its antidepressant-like effect might be due to its triterpenes content. The pattern of effects of *Alternanthera brasiliana* observed in the MFST suggests the involvement of the noradrenergic neurotransmitters system on its antidepressants like effect. However the precise mechanism underlying this change still requires further investigation to confirm and extend these results before the application in human.

Acknowledgements

The authors are grateful to Defence Research Development Organization (DRDO), Govt. of India, New Delhi for financial help and the Director of Research (Vety), FVSc, Khanapara for providing necessary facilities to carry out the research work.

References

Barua, C.C., Talukdar, A., Begum, S. A., Sarm, D. K., Pathak, D.C., and Borah P. (2009a). Antinociceptive activity of methanolic extract of leaves of *Alternanthera brasiliana* Kuntz. in animal models of nociception. *Pharmacologyonline,* **3:**49-55.

Barua, C.C., Talukdar, A., Begum, S.A., Sarma, D.K., Pathak, D.C., Barua, A.G., and Bora, R.S. (2009). Wound healing activity of methanolic extract of leaves of *Alternanthera brasiliana* Kuntz using *in vivo* and *in vitro* model. *Indian J Exp Biol.,* **47**: 1001-1005.

Bivattti, M.W., Bellever, M.H., Valpato, L., Costa, C., and Bellaver, C. (2003). Preliminary studies of alternative feed additives for broilers: *Alternanthera brasiliana* extract, propolis extract and linseed oil. *Rev Bras Cienc Avic Campinas*, **5:** 1516-1635.

Borsini, F., and Meli, A. (1988). Is the forced swimming test a suitable model for revealing antidepressant activity? *Psychopharmacol.*, **94:** 147-160.

Brochadoa, C.O., Almeidaa, A.P., Barretoa, B.P., *et al.* (2003). Flavonol Robinobiosides and Rutinosides from *Alternanthera brasiliana* (Amaranthaceae) and their effects on lymphocyte proliferation *in vitro*. *J Braz Chem Soc.*, **14:** 451.

Bruce, R.D. (1985). An up-and-down procedure for acute toxicity testing. *Fundam Appl Toxicol.*, **5**: 151-157.

Campos, M.M., Fernandes, E.S., and Ferreira, J. (2005). Antidepressant-like effects of *Trichilia catigua* (Catuaba) extract: evidence for dopaminergic-mediated mechanisms. *Psychopharmacol.*, **182**: 45-53.

Cryan, J.F., and Lucki, I. (2000). Antidepressant-like behavioral effects mediated by 5-Hydroxytryptamine 2c receptors. *J Pharmacol Exp Ther.*, **295**: 1120-1126.

Cryan, J.F., Markou, A., and Lucki, I. (2002). Assessing antidepressant activity in rodents: recent developments and future needs. *Trends Pharmacol Sci.*, **2:** 238-245.

Cryan, J.F., Mombereau, C., and Vassout, A. (2005). The tail suspension test as a model for assessing antidepressant activity: review of pharmacological and genetic studies in mice. *Neurosci Biobehav Rev.*, **29**: 571- 625.

Cryan, J.F., Valentino, R.J., and Lucki, I. (2005). Assessing substrates underlying the behavioral effects of antidepressants using the modified rat forced swimming test. *Neurosci Biobehav Rev.*, **29:** 547-569.

Detke, M.J., Rickels, M., and Lucki, I. (1995). Active behaviors in the rat forced swimming test differently produced by serotonergic and noradrenergic antidepressants. *Psychopharmacol.*, **121**: 66-72.

Estrada-Camarena, E., Fernandez-Guasti, A., and Lopez-Rubalcava C. (2003). Antidepressant like effect of Different estrogenic Compounds in the Forced Swimming Test. *Neuropsychopharmacol.*, **28**: 830-838.

Harborne, J.B. (1991). Phytochemical methods-Guide to modern techniques of plant analysis, 2nd ed. Chapman and Hall India, 653.

Hemby, S.E., Lucki, I., Gatto, G., *et al.* (1997). Potential antidepressant effects of tropane compounds, selective for serotonine or dopamine transporters. *J Pharmacol Exp Ther.*, **282**: 727-733.

Kusmider, M., Solich, J., Palach, P., *et al.* (2007). Effect of citalopram in the modified forced swim test in rats. *Pharmacological reports,* **59**: 785-788.

Lagrota, M.H., Wigg, M.D., Santos, M.M.G., *et al.* (1994). Inhibitory activity of extracts of *Alternanthera brasiliana* (Amaranthaceae) against the herpes simplex virus. *Phytother Res.*, **8**: 361.

Lopez-Rubalcava, C., and Lucki, I. (2000). Strain differences in the behavioral effects of antidepressent drugs in the rat forced swimming test. *Neuropsychopharmacol.*, **22:** 191-199.

Lucki, I. (1997). The forced swimming test as a model for core and component behavioral effects of antidepressant drugs. *Behav Pharmacol.*, **8:** 523-532.

Macedo, A.F., Barbosa, N.C., Esquibel, M.A., Souza, M.M., and Cechinel-Filho, V. (1999). Pharmacological and phytochemical studies of callus culture extracts from *Alternanthera brasiliana*. *Pharma Zic.*, **54** : 771.

Mora, S., Diaz-veliz, G., Millan, R., *et al.* (2005). Anxiolytic and antidepressant like effect of the hydroehanolic extract from *Aloysia polystachya* in rats. *Pharmacol Biochem Behav.*, **82**: 373-378.

Page, M., Detke, M., Dalvi, A., *et al.* (1999). Serotonergic mediation of the effects of fluoxetine, but not desipramine, in the rat forced swimming test. *Psychopharmacol*, **147**: 62-67.

Porsolt, R.D., LePichon, M., and Jalfre, M. (1977). Depression: a new animal model sensitive to antidepressant treatments. *Nature*, **266**: 730-732.

Snedecor, G.W., and Cochran, W.G. (1994). Statistical methods, 8th ed. Oxford and IBH Publishing Co New Delhi.

Wagner, H., Bladt, S., and Zgainski, E.M. (1984). Plant Drug Analysis. Springer-Verlag: Berlin: 334.

Zhang ZJ. (2004). Therapeutic effects of herbal extracts and constituents in animal models of psychiatric disorders. *Life Sci.*, **75**: 1659-1699.

Medicinal Plants: Phytochemistry, Pharmacology and Therapeutics Vol. 2 (2012) *Pages* **227–235**
Editor-in-Chief: **V.K. Gupta**
Published by: **DAYA PUBLISHING HOUSE, NEW DELHI**

15

Growth Characteristics, Phytochemicals and Mineral Composition of *Ocimum gratissimum* Applied with Albit® Biosubstance

S.T. Anjorin[1]* and N.H. Ugwu[2]

ABSTRACT

Ocimum gratissimum (basil) was seed-dressed and foliar sprayed with Albit® bioregulator/biopesticide and assessed for its growth characteristics, phytochemicals and mineral composition. Those applied with Albit® had increased number of leaves (two/plant), increased shoot height (2cm/plant) at 28 days after sowing (DAS), increased shoot weight (7.4g/plant) and roots weight (3g/plant) at 182 DAS than the control without Albit® application. Albit® application induced flowering 15 days earlier than those in the control plots. Steroid phytochemical were present in the leaves and roots of basil applied with Albit® while alkaloid was absent in basil leaves applied with the biosubstance. The potassium, magnesium, zinc and calcium contents in the basil leaves applied with Albit® were significantly higher (P≤0.05) than from the basil in the control. Albit® has proven to be a promising alternative input for producing lamiaceous culinary plants with enhanced growth characteristics and mineral composition.

Keywords: Albit® biosubstance, Growth characteristics, Minerals, Phytochemicals, *Ocimum gratissimum.*

1 Department of Crop Science, Faculty of Agriculture, University of Abuja, Abuja, Nigeria.

2 Department of Biological Sciences, University of Abuja, Abuja, Nigeria.

* *Corresponding author*: E-mail: oyindamola35@yahoo.com

Introduction

Ocimum gratissimum L. (Family Lamiaceae) commonly called basil, is a culinary herb with pungent sweet smell. Propagation of basil is through seeds and also reliably from cuttings. (Calixto, 2000; Ehiagbonare, 2004). The foliage is commonly used fresh in cooked recipes or added at the last moment, as cooking quickly destroys the flavour (Giami *et al.*, 2005). Studies have established that compounds in basil oil have potent antioxidant, anticancer, antiviral and antimicrobial properties (Essawi and Srour, 2000; Rabelo *et al.*, 2003 Adebolu and Salau, 2005). Basil has also been used from time immemorial both prophylactically and curatively (Gills, 1992; Chen *et al.*, 1994; George, 1994 and El-said *et al.*, 2001).

Albit®-a plant growth regulator and biofungiscide is reported to have improved germinability and seedling vigour, improve vegetative growth, accelerates maturity and yield of cereals and vegetables (Albit Biotechnology LLC, 2008). Albit® TPS is composed of hydrolysate of microorganisms (*Bacillus megaterium H. Pseudomonas aurefaciens*); microelements, growth substances (poly-β-hydroxybutyrate (6.2g PHB L^{-1}) and terpenes, extracted from plant shoots (Zlotnikov, 2006). Albit® is formulated as an alternative farm input to synthetic fertilizer and fungicide which are less environment-friendly. There is a dearth of information on the performance of Lamiaceous crops applied with Albit®. This study was carried out to assess the effect of Albit® seed dressing and foliar spraying on the germination, growth characteristics, biomass, phytochemicals and mineral composition of the shoot and root of *O. gratissimum*.

Materials and Methods

Loamy soil was collected from the Biological Science Experimental garden, University of Abuja, Abuja. Each of the 30cm-diameter polythene pots was filled with two kilograms (2 kg) of the soil.

Collection of Seeds, Albit® and Sowing of Treated Seeds

O. gratissimum seeds were collected from farmers in Kwali, Abuja. The matured brown fruits were splitted to bring out the small dried black seeds. Seeds were pre-soaked for 4h in Albit® at concentration of 2 ml/L distilled water in a 9cm-diameter Petri-dish. The seeds for the control were not pre-soaked with the Albit®. After the solution was drained off, 10 seeds per polypots were sown at 2cm depth. The seeds treated with Albit® were sown in a total of 24 polypots and the control was sown in 24 polypots. Watering was done every other day and weeding was also done when necessary. First foliar sprayings of the seedlings was carried out at 4-5 leaf stage (3 weeks after sowing-WAS) and the second at 10-12 leaf stage (7 WAS) each at the rate 2 mL Albit® L^1 water evenly sprayed with a hand sprayer.

Growth Parameters Measured

The number of leaves per plant was counted at 28 and 38 DAS respectively. Also the shoot length was obtained at the same periods. Leaf area was obtained by using graph paper. Dry weight of the stem, root and leaf were obtained by the use of electronic balance (Hx-6000, MAX 6100g).

Phytochemical Analysis

The phytochemical screening of the ethanolic leaf extract took place in Natural product chemistry laboratory of Sheda Science and Technology Complex (SHESTCO) Sheda-Abuja. The roots, shoots and leaves of the basil were dried in the oven at 70°C for 24h before being grounded into powder with a 240v Warring blender (3 M 821 Thomas scientific, Swedesborn, U.K). One gram (1g) each of the respective leaf powder was soaked in 100ml of ethanol for 48h. They were later filtered with cheese cloth and the liquid filterate concentrated with rotary vacuum evaporator. The extracts were analysed for the presence of glycosides, flavonoid, tannins, terpenoids, alkaioid, steroids, balsam and saponin derivatives in line with the procedures described by Sofowora (1993).

Determination of Mineral Composition

Preparation of Samples

The dried basil leaves, stems and roots were separately pulverized to fine powder using the Warring blender. One gram (1g) of each samples were digested with nitric acid (HNO_3), filtered and make to 100ml mark in a volumetric flask. The resulting solution was concentrated in rotary vacuum evaporator (RE 300B, Bar Loworld Scientific Ltd OSA, U. K).

Reagents and Apparatus

All the reagents and chemicals used were of analytical grade obtained from BDH and syma-Aldrich. The standards used were prepared in the laboratory, Chemistry Advanced Laboratory (CAL, SHESTCO), Sheda, Abuja. Distilled water and acid washed glass wares were used throughout the analysis.

Wet Digestion Method

One (1g) of each of the samples was weighed into separate beakers and treated with 10 ml of concentrated HNO_3, heated to reflux on an electric hot plate at 90?C until digestion is complete. Side by side 10 ml of nitric acid was also added to empty beakers which served as blank. The content of the beaker was allowed to cool, filtered through Whatman No. 42 filter paper into volumetric flasks and make up to volume of 100ml with distilled water. The flasks were then covered.

Determination of Minerals

The mineral contents of basil were determined in six samples namely; the leaf with Albit®, leaf without Albit®, stem with Albit®, stem without Albit®, root with Albit® and root without Albit®. Working standard solutions of Magnesium (Mg), Zinc (Zn), Calcium (Ca), Iron (Fe), Manganese (Mn), Potassium (K), Phosphorous (P) were prepared from stock standard solution (1000ppm) and absorbance were noted for standard solutions of each elements and samples using Atomic Absorption Spectrometer (AAS) 969 UNICAM (Sahito *et al.*, 2002). While (K) was analysed using flame photometer. A blank reading was also taken and necessary correction was made during the calculation of concentration of various elements.

Data collected were subjected to Analysis of Variance (ANOVA) and differences among the mineral components of the plant parts were determined with Duncan Multiple Range Test (DMRT) at 0.05 level of probability, using SAS 9.0 (2002) statistical package. P values ≤ 0.05 were considered statistically significant.

Results

Growth Characteristics of O. gratissimum Applied with Albit® and Without Albit®

As a result of seed treatment and foliar spraying with Albit®, the number of leaves, shoot height, leaf area, number of flower, shoot and root weights were higher than the ones without Albit® (Table 15.1).

At 28 DAS, the mean value of the leaves of basil applied with Albit® had two leaves more than that of the control and shoot height applied with Albit® was 2 cm higher than the ones with no Albit® application. At 38 DAS (*i.e.* 10 days interval), the mean values of the leaves of basil applied with Albit® had two leaves more than that of the control and shoot height applied with Albit® was 3 cm higher than the control. At 42 DAS, the mean leaf area of basil applied with Albit® was 31cm^3 more than that of the control. The mean days of basil without Albit® to flower was 15 days more than that with Albit®. The number of flower on basil applied with Albit® was eight (8) more than those with Albit® application at 182 DAS. Shoot weight of basil with Albit® at 182 DAS was 7.4g heavier than the control. The mean root biomass of basil applied with Albit® at the same time was 3g more than those in the control plots.

Saponin was present in leaves and stems of basil applied with or without Albit® but was absent in their roots (Table 2). Flavonoid was present only in the leaves of basil, applied with and without Albit® but was absent in their stems and roots. Tannin and balsam were present in all the leaves, stems and roots applied with or without Albit®. Glycoside was absent in the leaves of basil applied with and without Albit® and was present in the stems and roots applied with and without Albit®. Terpenoid was absent in all the leaves, stems and roots applied with and without Albit®. Steroid was present in the leaves and roots with Albit® and absent in those without the Albit®. However alkaloid was in the leaves applied with Albit® and present in those without Albit®. Albit® application did not alter the composition of phytochemicals in the stem of basil. Tannin and balsam were present in all the basil parts applied with and without Albit® while terpenoid was absence in all the parts.

Table 3 shows that the highest K content (3.289 mg g-^{1}) was found in the leaves of basil applied with Albit® and was not significantly different($P>0.05$) from the K content in basil root without Albit®. The K content in the root from basil applied with Albit® was significantly lower ($P>0.05$) than all other treatment. The Mg content in basil stem with no Albit® application was significantly higher (P? 0.05) than every other treatment. There was no significant difference ($P>0.05$) between the Mg content in basil leaf applied with Albit® and basil root applied with Albit®. However, the Mg content in the basil root without Albit® was significantly lower (P ? 0.05) than any other treatments.

Table 15.1. Growth characteristics of *O. gratissimum* applied with Albit® and without Albit®.

Treatment	*No. of Leaves at 28 DAS*	*Shoot-height (cm) 28 DAS*	*No. of Leaves at 38 DAS*	*Shoot-height 38 DAS*	*Leaf-Area (cm^2) at 42 DAS*	*Days to 50 per cent Flowering (DAS)*	*No. of Flowers (182 DAS)*	*Shoot Weight (g) (DAS)*	*Root Weight (g) (DAS)*
With Albit®	8	5	12	16	85	148	11	23.6	7
Control (no Albit®)	6	3	10	13	54	163	3	16.2	4

DAS: Days After Sowing. Data is mean of three replicates.

Table 15.2. Phytochemicals in *O. gratissimum* applied with Albit® and without Albit®

Phytochemical	*Leaves with Albit®*	*Leaves Without Albit®*	*Stem with Albit®*	*Stem Without Albit®*	*Root with Albit®*	*Root Without Albit®*
Saponin	+	+	+	+	–	–
Flavonoids	+	+	–	–	–	–
Steroids	+	–	+	+	+	–
Alkaloid	–	+	–	–	–	–
Tannin	+	+	+	+	+	+
Glycoside	–	–	+	+	+	+
Terpenoids	–	–	–	–	–	–
Balsam	+	+	+	+	+	+

Note: +: Present; –: Absent.

Minerals Content in O. gratissimum Parts

Table 15.3 shows the results of mineral contents in the parts of basil applied with and without Albit® biosubstance.

Table 15.3. Mineral Composition of Leaves, Stem and Roots of *O. gratissimum* applied with and without Albit®

Treatment	*mg g⁻¹*						
	K	*Mg*	*Zn*	*Ca*	*Fe*	*P*	*Mn*
Leaf with Albit®	3.289a	8.264b	4.761a	31.175a	3.265b	2.319a	0.657a
Leaf without Albit®	2.194b	6.944c	2.766b	26.611b	4.839a	1.648bc	0.721a
Stem with Albit®	2.116b	6.110d	1.502c	23.6553cd	1.309e	1.136d	0.440bc
Stem without Albit®	1.948b	10.948a	1.132d	25.549bc	1.349e	1.748bc	0.514b
Root with Albit®	1.094c	7.668b	2.768b	21.946de	2.307c	1.914b	0.357c
Root without Albit®	3.108a	5.236e	1.168d	20.676e	1.809d	1.448cd	0.442bc

Means followed by the same letter(s) within each column are not significant at 5 per cent significant level, using DMRT.

The Zn content in basil leaf with Albit® was significantly higher (P?0.05) than any other treatment. There was no significant difference (P>0.05) between the Zn content in basil leaf without Albit® and basil root with Albit®. The Zn content in the basil stem with Albit® was significantly lower (P?0.05) than any other treatments. The highest Ca content (31.175 mg g^{-1}) was found in basil leaf with Albit® and was significantly higher (P?0.05) than any other treatments. There was no significant difference (P>0.05) between the Ca content in basil stem with Albit and basil stem without Albit®.

The Fe content in basil leaf with no Albit® application was significantly higher ($P \leq 0.05$) than any other treatments. Meanwhile, the Fe content in the stem of basil applied with or without Albit® was significantly lower (P≤0.05) than other treatments. The highest P content (2.319 mg g^{-1}) was found in the leaf of basil applied with Albit® was significantly higher (P≤0.05) than other treatments. There was no significant difference (P>0.05) between the P content in basil leaf without Albit® and basil stem without Albit®. The highest Mn content was found in the leaf of basil applied with Albit® and was not significantly different (P > 0.05) from the Mn content in basil leaf without Albit®. There was no significant difference (P > 0.05) between the Mn content in basil stem with Albit® and basil root without Albit®.

The mineral content in the leaf of basil applied with Albit® was in the order of Ca > Mg > Zn > K > Fe > P > Mn while the mineral content in the basil leaf with no Albit® application was in order of Ca > Mg > Fe > Zn > K > P > Mn. This indicated that Albit® application altered the concentration of Zn and K concentration in the leaf. The mineral content in the basil stem applied with Albit® was in the order of Ca > Mg > K > Zn > Fe > P > Mn while the mineral content in the basil stem without Albit applicator was in the order of Ca > Mg > K > P > Fe > Zn > Mn. This indicated that Albit® application alters the concentration of P and Zn concentration in the stem. The mineral content in the root of basil applied with Albit® was in the order of Ca > Mg > Zn > Fe > P > K > Mn while the mineral content in the basil root without Albit® application was in order of Ca > Mg > K > Fe > P > Zn > Mn. This also indicated that Albit® application could alter the concentration of K and Zn concentration in the root.

Discussion

Unsterilized garden soil was used for raising the *O. gratissimum* in order to simulate natural garden soil. *O. gratissimum* applied with Albit® had higher number of leaves, shoot height, leaf area and flower earlier than those without Albit®. These results is similar to that of Yakhtanigova (2009) who reported that Albit® application enhanced the productivity of various corn subspecies in Russian agroecology. Enhanced crop productivity by Albit® might be due to synergism between the plant growth hormone, nutrients and biofungicide it is composed of. This is evident in the result obtained during the foliar application of plant growth regulator (GA3 - 20mgL-1)) and nutrient solution for improvement of lily flowers (*Lilium longifolium*) by Mustafa *et al.* (2009). The mean shoot length of the plants sprayed with both the hormones and nutrients increased by 33 per cent over the control plants and by 6 per cent over the other set of plants, which received the treatment of nutrients alone. Number of nodes per stem was also found to increase in the dually treated plants by 71 per cent and 42 per cent in that order. The plants receiving dual treatment harbored 92 per cent greater number of buds per stem over the control plants whereas nutrients- alone treated lily plant showed only 28 per cent greater number of buds.

The phytochemicals observed in the basil with or without Albit® in this study was in line with the report of Pessoa *et al.* (2002) that basil plant contained terpenoid, eugenol, saponins and alkaloids. It was observed that Albit® application resulted in higher K, Mg and Ca yield than those reported by Giami *et al.* (2005) and El-Adawy and Taha (2001) for basil plant treated with indole butyric acid (IBA). However, the Fe, P and Mn content was similar to those reported by the same researchers under the IBA application. It is indicated from this work, that higher content of K, Mg and Ca could be induced in basil plant by Albit® treatment. This might be due to presence of a balanced set of macro and micro elements and terpenes in Albit® biosubstance (Kudrjavcevs *et al.*, 2005; Zlotnikov, 2006).

This study indicated that seed and foliar treatments of basil with Albit® enhanced the yield and quality of basil through improved growth characteristics and mineral composition. This might be due to the growth promoting and protective potential of the plant by Albit®. Thus it proved to be a recommendable input in the cultivation of culinary plants like basil. Further field research work is imperative in order to confirm the efficacy of Albit® biosubstance on the growth and yield of leafy vegetables on various agroecolological zones in the tropics.

References

Adebolu, T. T., and A. O. Salau (2005). Antimicrobial activity of leaf of *Ocimum gratissimum* on selected diarrhoea causing bacteria in South Western Nigeria. *African Journal of Biotechnology*, **4(7)**: 682-684.

Albit Biotechnology LLC (2008). An innovative biopesticide for organic and traditional farming Prospekt Naoka 5, Pushino,Moscow Oblast. 142290. Russia.

AOAC, (1990). Association of Official Analytical Chemist. *Official Methods of Analysis*, 15th ed. Washington DC.

Chen, M., Theander, T.G., Christensen, S.B., Hviid, L., Zhai L., and Kharazmi, A. (1994). Lincochalcone A, a new antimalarial agent and antifungal properties. Preliminary screening of 35 essential oils. *J. Sci. Ind. Res.*, **28:** 25-34.

Calixto, J.B. (2000). Efficacy, safety, quality control marketing and regulatory guidelines for herbal medicines (phytotherapeutic agents) *Braz. J. Med. Biol. Res.*, **33**: 179-189.

Ehiagbonare, J.E.(2004). A Study of the effect of various depth of sowing on seed germination and seedling emergence on *Ocimum gratissimum* (De wild and Th.Dur) *Nig. J. Appl. Sci.*, **22:** 195-197.

El-Adawy, T. A., and Taha, K.M. (2001). Characteristics and composition of different seed oils and flours. *Food Chem.*, **74**: 47-54.

El-said, F., Sofowora, E. A., Malcom, S.A., and Hofer, A. (2001). An investigation Into the efficacy of *Ocimum gratissimum* as used in Nigeria native Medicine. *Planta medica*, **17**: 195-200

Essawi,T., and Srour, M. (2000). Screening of some Palestinian medicinal plants For antibacterial activity. *J. Ethnopharmacol.*, **70**: 343-349.

George, C. (1994). Development in food science spices; Herb and Edible Fungi 2nd Edition Elsevier publ. Ansterdam London. pp309-327.

Gill, L.S (1992) Ethno medical uses of plants in Nigeria, Uniben press. University of Benin, Edo State, Nig. pp196-177.

Giami, S. Y., Achinewhu, S.C., and Ibaakee, C. (2005). The quality and sensory attributes of cookies supplemented with basil (*Ocimum gratissimum*). *J. Food Sci. Technol.*, **40**: 613-620.

Kudrjavcev, A., Zaiceva, A., Zlotnikov, A., and Zlotnikov, K. (2005). Biopesticide Albit® as a part of flax protection system. *Zemledelie,* p 34-35.

Mustafa, G. S., Mahmoona, K., and Zahoor, A. (2009). Foliar application of plant growth regulator (PGRS) and nutrients for improvement of lily flowers. *Pak. J. Bot.,* **41(1)**: 233-237

Pessoa, L.M., Morais, S.M., Bevilaqua, C., and Luciano, J.H.S. (2002) Anthelmintic activity of essential oil of *Ocimum gratissimum* Linn. and eugenol against *Haemonchus contortus. Vet. Parasitol.,* **109**: 59-63

Rabelo, M., Souza, E.P., Soares, P.M.G., Miranda, A.V., Matos, F.J.A., and Criddle, D.N. (2003). Antinociceptive properties of the essential oil of *Ocimum gratissimum* L. (Labiatae) in mice. *Brazilian Journal of Medical Research,* **36:** 521-524.

Sahito, A.T.G., Kazi, M.A., Jakhrani, G.H., Kazi, G.Q., and Memon, M.A. (2002). Elemental investigation of *Momordica charantia* Linn. and *Syziginm jambolana* Linn. using atomic absorption spectrophotometer. *The Nucleus,* **39:** 49-54.

SAS - Statistical Analysis System (2002). User's guide. Statistics SAS Institute Inc. Cary N.C., USA.

Sofowora, A. (1993). Medicinal plants and traditional medicine. Spectrum Books Ltd. Ibadan, Nigeria. pp. 224-227.

Zlotnikov, A.K. (2006). Biopesticide Albit® for increasing yield and protection of agricultures against diseases. Ed. Prof. A. Melkumova. All-Russia Institute of Plant Protection. Russia.

Yakhtanigova, Z. M. (2009). Effect of growth regulators on productivity of various corn subspecies in the Piedmont zone of Kabardino-Bulkaria. *Russian Agricultural Sciences,* **25**: 2 84-85.

Medicinal Plants: Phytochemistry, Pharmacology and Therapeutics Vol. 2 (2012) *Pages* **237–244**
Editor-in-Chief: **V.K. Gupta**
Published by: **DAYA PUBLISHING HOUSE, NEW DELHI**

16

Effect of Mulberry (*Morus indica* L.) Leaves on Blood Glucose, Glycosylated Hemoglobin and Serum Gluconeogenic Enzymes in NIDDM Patients

B. Andallu[1]*, B.L. Srikanthi[1] and A.V. Vinay Kumar[2]

ABSTRACT

Mulberry leaves, rich in protein, minerals, fibre, and vitamin C, containing trigonelline bases, a glycoprotein Moran A and N-containing sugar-Fagomine have been found to possess antidiabetic effect. Administration of dried mulberry leaf powder at a dose of 3g/day to NIDDM patients for a period of 60 days, decreased significantly blood glucose, glycosylated hemoglobin (HbA_{1c}) and also decreased the activities of serum gluconeogenic enzymes viz., glutamate pyruvate transaminase (GPT), glutamate oxaloacetate transaminase (GOT), glucose-6-phosphatase (G6pase), lactate dehydrogenase (LDH) and acid and alkaline phosphatases indicating control over hyperglycemia in diabetics is by the regulation of the formation of glucose via gluconeogenesis.

Keywords: NIDDM patients, Mulberry, Antidiabetic, Blood glucose, Glycosylated hemoglobin.

1 Department of Home Science, Sri Sathya Sai Institute of Higher Learning, Anantapur – 515 001, India

2 The Institute of Environmental and Human Health (TIEHH), Texas Tech University, Lubbock, Texas 79415, USA

* *Corresponding author*: E-mail: bandallu@gmail.com, Mobile: 09247450990

Introduction

Mulberry (*Morus indica*.L) leaves, the sole feed for silk worm possess many medicinal properties. The leaves were reported to possess hypoglycemic (Bart, 1932; Kelkar *et al.*, 1996), hypotensive (Ramachandran, 1986), antipyretic and anti-inflammatory (Chatterjee *et al.*, 1983) effects. These effects of mulberry leaves have been ascribed to a glycoprotein Moran A (Burman, 1985), trigonelline bases (Watanabe, 1958) and Moranoline (Yoshikuni, 1988). Present chapter deals with a comparative study on the effect of mulberry leaves with that of standard drug-glibenclamide on blood glucose, glycosylated hemoglobin levels and on the activity of gluconeogenic enzymes in NIDDM patients.

Materials and Methods

Fresh young mulberry leaves (*Morus indica* L.) procured in bulk from Regional Seri cultural Research Station, Rapthadu, Anantapur district, Andhra Pradesh, were washed thoroughly under running tap water, shade dried, powdered and loaded in the capsules (500mg/capsules).

Forty male mild NIDDM patients (blood glucose >150mg/dl) in the age group of 40-60 yrs. and with the body weights ranging from 50-60 kg with no other complications were selected from a local diabetic clinic under the guidance of a diabetologist. Out of the selected patients, 20 served as controls and 20 as experimental subjects. To study the effect of mulberry leaves in isolation, the subjects undergoing any treatment before the study period were instructed to terminate the same and were subjected to initial clinical check up. After one week of stabilization period, treatment of experimental subjects with mulberry leaf powder (6 capsules per day, two after every meal accounting to a dose of 3g/day) and treatment of control subjects with glibenclamide (5mg/day) were started and continued for a period of 60 days under the supervision of local diabetologist. Both control and experimental subjects were put on a prescribed diet which was in fact, the same diet consumed by the subjects in day to day life with appropriate changes in it to make the protein, fat and carbohydrate ratio ideal (20:20:60). Each patient was provided with a diet chart, food exchange list and approximate house hold measures for each food. By learning the use of these food exchanges patients could make the diet flexible to match their taste and keep their caloric needs constant.

At the initial stage and at the end of 60 days of experimental period, fasting blood samples of control and experimental subjects were collected and used for the determination of blood glucose (Huggett and Nixon, 1957), glycosylated hemoglobin (Eross *et al.*, 1984), serum enzymes *viz.*, lactate dehydrogenase (Henry *et al.*, 1960), glucose-6-phosphatase (Koide and Oda,1959), glutamate pyruvate transaminase (GPT), glutamate oxaloacetate transaminase (GOT) (Bergmeyer and Bernt,1974), acid and alkaline phosphatases (Gutman and Gutman,1940; King and Armstrong, 1988). All the values were analyzed statistically to obtain mean ± SD and were subjected to Student's't' test (Gupta, 1997) to assess significant differences after treatment.

Results and Discussion

In diabetes, fasting blood glucose, glycosylated hemoglobin (HbA1c) and the activity of gluconeogenic enzymes are elevated. Effect of administration of mulberry leaf powder and glibenclamide on blood glucose and glycosylated hemoglobin levels in NIDDM patients is given in Table 16.1 where as Table 16.2 shows the effect of mulberry treatment on the activities of serum gluconeogenic enzymes *i.e.* lactate dehydrogenase, glucose-6-phosphatase, SGOT and SGPT, Table 16.3 depicts the effect on the activities of acid and alkaline phosphatases.

The fundamental mechanism underlying hyperglycemia in diabetes mellitus involves over production (excessive hepatic glycogenolysis and gluconeogenesis) as well as under utilization of glucose (Latner, 1958). The elevated blood glucose levels in NIDDM patients when treated with mulberry leaves, significantly ($p<0.01$) decreased (27 per cent) whereas in glibenclamide-treated group, the decrease (8 per cent) was comparatively lesser as indicated in Table 16.1. The hypoglycemic response of mulberry could be attributed to trigonelline bases in mulberry similar to that isolated from fenugreek and/or due to the presence of Moran A, which showed a good glycemic control in alloxan induced diabetic mice (Burman, 1985). The observed beneficial effect of mulberry leaves is attributed to be brought about by the activity of various specific principal bioactive constituents present in mulberry leaves *viz.*, deoxynojirimycin-DNJ, galactopyranosyl-DNJ, fagomine, moran A, quercetin, isoquercitrin, phytosterols, etc.(Kimura *et al.*, 1995; Yamzaki *et al.*, 1997; Doi *et al.*, 2001). High fiber content (13.85 per cent) of mulberry leaves also contributed to the effect as reported in curry leaves-treated- type 2 diabetics (Iyer and Mani,1990).

Glycosylated hemoglobin is a good measure to indicate the average blood glucose concentration over the preceding weeks while a single glucose determination gives a value which is true only at the time the blood sample is drawn (Murray *et al.*, 1993). HbA_{IC} is formed progressively and irreversibly over a period of time and is stable till the life of the RBC and is unaffected by diet, insulin or exercise on the day of testing (Bunn, 1981).

Table 16.1 shows a significant ($p<0.01$) decrease (10 per cent) in HbA_{IC} after mulberry treatment, while in glibenclamide-treated group, no much change has been noticed. A higher decrease (27 per cent) in HbA_{IC} was reported in NIDDM subjects treated with insulin for a period of four weeks (Tilvis *et al.*, 1988) and glibenclamide treatment for a period of three months resulted in a decrease of HbA_{IC} by 24 per cent (Baynes *et al.*, 1993). Mulberry was found to be effective in controlling HbA_{IC} levels as insulin and more effective than glibenclamide as the effect was evident within one month. Therefore, on prolonged intake, mulberry may further reduce HbA_{1c} levels and probably help in achieving a good glycemic control.

Activities of Serum Gluconeogenic Enzymes

There is a significant increase in the activity of lactate dehydrogenase (LDH) in diabetics due to excessive accumulation of pyruvate that is converted to lactate for which enzyme LDH is needed and therefore the activity of LDH is increased due to less insulin availability in diabetes (Chang and Schneider, 1972). Mulberry treatment showed a decrease (7 per cent) in the activity of LDH while in glibenclamide-treated group, the decrease (4 per cent) was lesser than that of mulberry-treated group (Table 16.2). The decrease in the activity of LDH following mulberry treatment in the present study could be due to a decrease in pyruvate levels in blood in mulberry-treated group as result of decrease in the conversion of alanine to pyruvate via gluconeogenesis.

Table 16.1. Fasting blood glucose and glycosylated hemoglobin levels in control and experimental diabetics.

Groups	*Diabetic–Glibenclamide*		*Diabetic–Mulberry*	
	Pre-treatment	*Post-treatment*	*Pre-treatment*	*Post-treatment*
Fasting blood glucose (mg/dl)	154.4±17.5 (8)	141.8±10.4** (27)	152.7±13.3	110.5±14.0**
Glycosylated Hemoglobin (per cent)	12.5±2.2	12.4 ±2.1 (1)	10.8±1.9	9.6 ± 1.7** (11)

Values are mean ± SD of 20 subjects.

Figures in parentheses indicate per cent decrease over pre-treatment values **p<0.01.

Table 16.2. Activities of serum gluconeogenic enzymes in control and experimental diabetics.

Groups	*Diabetic–Glibenclamide*		*Diabetic–Mulberry*	
	Pre-treatment	*Post-treatment*	*Pre-treatment*	*Post-treatment*
Lactate dehydrogenase (IU/l)	339.1 ± 3.0	326.7 ± 60.7 (4)	343.6±1.6	320.0 ±4.0** (7)
Glucose–6 phosphatase (units/ml)	21.0 ± 3.7	15.0 ±3.7* (29)	19.4 ±3.3	12.4±2.6** (36)
Glutamate pyruvate transaminase (IU/l)	24.0±1.2	26.0±1.2* (8)	33.0±5.0	23.7±1.5** (28)
Glutamate oxaloacetate transaminase (IU/l)	24.0±1.5	21.0±2.6* (13)	31.3±2.5	26.3±2.5** (16)

Values are mean ± SD of 20 subjects.

Figures in parentheses indicate per cent decrease over Pre-treatment values *p<0.05; **p<0.01.

Raised activity of glucose-6-phophatase was observed in plasma of diabetics due to glucose-6-phosphatase flux from hepatocytes into the blood. Inadequate availability of insulin also allows cortisol to enhance the activity of G-6-pase in diabetes (Montogomery *et al.*, 1973).

It was interesting to find that (Table 16.2) diabetes patients when treated with mulberry, showed a significant (p< 0.05) decrease (36 per cent) in glucose-6-phosphatase activity compared to glibenclamide-treated group which showed a lesser decrease (29 per cent). Controlled blood glucose levels induced by mulberry in diabetics could be attributed to a decrease in the activity of glucose-6-phosphatase following mulberry treatment thereby decreasing the release of glucose from glucose-6-phosphate via gluconeogeniesis.

Accelerated gluconeogenesis, negative nitrogen balance and muscle wasting are among the hallmarks of uncontrolled diabetes (Buse *et al.*, 1972). There is catabolism of branched chain amino acids and alanine release by skeletal muscles (Odessey *et al.*, 1974). Glutamate is an obligate precursor of alanine and glutamine production by muscles. The latter two amino acids comprise more than 50 per cent of all the amino acids released by muscle, alanine being the preferred amino acid precursor of gluconeogenesis in the liver and glutamine in the kidney (Cahill *et al.*, 1972). The activity of GPT significantly ($p<0.01$) decreased (28 per cent) in mulberry-treated group while glibenclamide treatment showed a significant ($p<0.01$) increase (8 per cent) as shown in Table 16.2. Mulberry treatment decreased pyruvate levels thereby making it unavailable for alanine synthesis which is a gluconeogenic amino acid.

Increased activity of GOT was observed in diabetes when compared to that of normal (Unakami *et al.*, 1990).The activity of GOT was found to be significantly ($p<0.01$) decreased (16 per cent) in mulberry-treated as well as in glibenclamide-treated (13 per cent) groups as depicted in Table 16.2. However, the decrease was two fold higher in mulberry-treated group when compared to glibenclamide-treated group. The reduction in the activities of GPT and GOT following mulberry treatment could be attributed to a partly regulated gluconeogenesis which otherwise would be elevated in uncontrolled diabetes.

Table 16.3. Activities of serum acid and alkaline phosphatases in control and experimental diabetics.

Groups	*Diabetic–Glibenclamide*		*Diabetic–Mulberry*	
	Pre-treatment	*Post-treatment*	*Pre-treatment*	*Post-treatment*
Acid phosphatase (K.A. units/dl)	5.7±0.4	5.6±0.5 (2)	12.7±1.6	11.9±1.7** (6)
Alkaline phosphatase (K.A.units/dl)	5.5±1.2	4.7±1.4* (14)	12.9±1.6	10.8±1.6* (16)

Values are mean ± SD of 20 subjects in each group.

Figures in parentheses indicate per cent decrease over Pre-treatment values *$p<0.05$; **$p<0.01$.

During diabetes, an increase in the activity of serum alkaline phosphatase (ALP) has been observed and this has been reported to be the soluble form of intestinal ALP leached from intestine and translocated into the circulation and a decrease in the activity of ALP was observed during insulin treatment (Caspary *et al.*, 1972). In mulberry treatment, the activity of serum ALP was significantly ($p<0.01$) lowered (16 per cent) while in glibenclamide group, it was decreased to a comparatively lesser extent (14 per cent) as indicated in Table 16.3. The high fibre content of mulberry (14 per cent) could have decreased the rate of absorption of the soluble form of ALP thereby its release into the circulation would have been minimized. Activity of acid phosphatase which is elevated in diabetics was found to be significantly ($p<0.05$) decreased (14 per cent) following mulberry treatment, whereas glibenclamide treatment did not show much change (Table 16.3).

Conclusions

In NIDDM patients, mulberry treatment ameliorated some of the metabolic abnormalities. The mechanism by which mulberry leaves improve the metabolic status in the diabetics is probably by way of controlling glucose production via gluconeogenesis as evidenced by remarkably decreased activities of serum gluconeogenic enzymes. The antihyperglycemic effect of mulberry leaves is more potent than that of glibenclamide, as evidenced by fasting plasma glucose and glycosylated hemoglobin levels in the mulberry –treated group compared to the control group who received glibenclamide. The observed beneficial effects of mulberry leaves are postulated to be brought about by the synergistic action of various specific principal bioactive constituents present in mulberry leaves. In addition, its nutrient composition (protein, fiber, vitamins, and minerals) also played a role, as diabetic therapy is indispensably associated with therapeutic nutrition. Further pharmacological and biochemical investigations are in progress to elucidate the mechanism of action of various bioactive compounds of *M. indica* L. leaves.

Acknowledgements

The authors are grateful to the diabetic patients for their co-operation, the diabetologist for his supervision and the Institute for providing the financial assistance and facilities.

References

Bart, C. (1932). Hypoglycemic action of the leaves of Morus alba. Compt. Rend. Soc. Biol., 109, 897–899, In: *Chemical Abstracts* (1932): **26.2**: 3294.

Baynes, C., Elkeles, R.S., Henderson, A.D., Richmond, W., and Johnston, D.G. (1993). The effects of glibenclamide on glucose homeostasis and lipoprotein metabolism in poorly controlled type 2 diabetes. *Hormone Metabolic Research*, **25**: 96-101.

Bergmeyer, H.U., and Bernt, E. (1974). In: *Methods of Enzymatic Analysis*, 2nd edn, ed by Bergmeyer, HU., Verlag-Chemie Weinheim. Academic Press, Inc., New York. **2**: 727-735, 752-753.

Bunn, H.F. (1981).Evaluation of glycosylated hemoglobin in diabetic patients. *Diabetes*, **30**: 613-617.

Burman, T.K.(1985). Isolation and hypoglycemic activity of Glycoprotein moran A from mulberry leaves. *Planta Medica*, **6**: 482-484.

Buse, M.G., Biggers, J.F., and Friderici, K.H. (1972). Oxidation of branched chain amino acids by isolated hearts and diaphragms of the rat. The effect of fatty acids, glucose and pyruvate respiration. *Journal of Biological Chemistry*, **247**: 8085-8096.

Cahill, G.F., Aoki, T.T., and Marless, E.B.(1972). Insulin and muscle protein, In: Handbook of Physiology and Endocrinology, Vol I. Steiner, DF.,and Frienkel, N., Washington. D.C. (eds) *American Physiololgical Society*. pp 563-577.

Caspary, W.F., Rhein, A.M., and Creutzfeldt, W.(1972). Increase of intestinal brush border hydrolases in mucosa of streptozotocin-diabetic rats. *Diabetologia*, **8**: 412-414.

Chang, A.Y., and Schneider, D.I.(1972): Blood glucose and gluconeogenic enzymes. *Biochemica et Biophysica Acta*, **222**: 587-592.

Chatterjee, G.K., Burman, T.K., and Pal, S.P.(1983). Antiinflammatory and antipyretic activities of *Morus indica*. *Planta Medica*, **48**: 116-119.

Doi, K., Kojima, T., Makino, M., Kimura, Y., and Fujimoto, Y. (2001). Studies on the constituents of the leaves of *Morus alba* L. *Chemical Pharmacological Bulletin*, **49**: 151–153.

Eross, J., Kreutzmann, D., Jimenez, M., Keen, R., Roger, S., Colwell, C., Vines, R., and Sinik, M. (1984). Colorimetric measurement of glycosylated protein in whole blood cells, plasma and dried blood. *Annals of Clinical Biochemistry*, **21**: 519-522.

Gupta, S.P. (1997). Statistical methods 28th Ed. New Delhi: Sulthan Chand and Sons, pp E-7.5, E-8.18.

Gutman, A.B., and Gutman, E.B. (1940). Estimation of acid phosphatase activity of blood serum. *Journal of Biological Chemistry*, **136**: 201-209.

Henry, R.J., Chiamori, N.,Golub, O.J., and Berkman,S.(1960). *Am. J. Clin. Pathol.*, **34**: 381. In: *Practical Clinical Biochemistry*. (1988) 4th edn, Ed by Varley, H., CBS publishers and distributors. New Delhi, India. pp. 278-279.

Huggett, A.St.G., and Nixon, D.A.(1957). Use of glucose oxidase, peroxidase and o-dianisidine in the determination of blood and urinary glucose. *Lancet*, **273**: 366-370.

Iyer, U.M., and Mani, U.V.(1990). Studies on the effect of curry leaves supplementation (*Murraya koenigii*) on lipid profile, glycated proteins and amino acids in non-insulin dependant diabetic patients. *Plant Foods for Human Nutrition*, **40**: 275-282.

Kelkar, S.M., Bapat, V.A., Ganapathi, T.R., Kaklij, G.S., Rao, P.S., and Heble, M.R. (1996). Determination of hypoglycemic activity in *Morus indica* L. (mulberry) shoot cultures. *Current Science*, **71(1)**: 71-72.

Kimura, M., Chen, F., Nakashima, N., Kimura, I., Asano, N., and Koya, S. (1995). Antihyperglycemic effects of N-containing sugars derived from mulberry leaves in streptozotocin-induced diabetic mice. *Journal of Traditional Medicine*, **12**: 214–219.

King, E.J., and Armstrong, A.R. (1988). *Canad. Med.Assoc. J.*, **31**. 376. In: *Practical Clinical Biochemistry*, 4th edn.(1988) ed by Varley, H. CBS Publishers and Distributors, New Delhi, India. pp. 461.

Koide, H., and Oda, T. (1959). Pathological occurrence of glucose 6-phosphatase in serum in liver diseases. *Clinica Chimica Acta*, **4**: 554-561.

Latner, A. (1958). Clinical Biochemistry 2nd Ed. W.B. Saunders Co., Philadelphia. pp. 47- 50.

Montogomery, R., Dryer., R.L., Conway, T. W., and Specter, A.A. (1973), In: Biochemistry, A case oriented approach, 2nd edn. The CV Mosby co. St. Louis., Toronto. London, pp. 330.

Murray, R.K., Granner, D.K., Mayes, P.A., and Rodwell, N.W.(1993). Harper's Biochemistry 23rd edn. Prentice Hall of India private limited, New Delhi.pp. 58.

Odessey, R., Khairallah, E., and Goldberg, A.L.(1974). Origin and possible significance of alanine production by skeletal muscle. *Journal of Biological Chemistry*, **249**: 7623- 7629.

Ramachandran, K. (1986).The useful plants of India. Publications and Information Directorate, CSIR. Hill side road, New Delhi, pp.381-382.

Tilvis, R.S., Taskinen, M.R., and Mielliner, T.A. (1988). Effect of insulin treatment on fatty acids of plasma and erythrocyte membrane lipids in type 2 diabetes. *Clinica Chimica Acta*, **171**: 293-304.

Unakami, S., Komoda, T., and Sakagishi, Y. (1990).Translocation of intestinal alkaline phosphatase in streptozotocin-induced diabetic rats. *Journal of Biochemistry*, **22 (11)**: 1325-1331.

Watanabe.(1958). Volatile components of mulberry leaves. *Journal of Sericulural Science Japan*, **20**: 448-452.

Yamzaki, M., Nakamura, N., and Kurioka, A. (1997). Identification of isofucosterol in mulberry leaves (*Morus alba*). *Journal of Seri cultural Science Japan*, **66**: 136–137.

Yoshikuni,Y. (1988).Inhibition of intestinal glucosidase activity and postprandial hyerglycemia by moranoline and its N-Alkyl derivatives. *Agricultural Biological Chemistry*, **52 (1):** 121-128.

Medicinal Plants: Phytochemistry, Pharmacology and Therapeutics Vol. 2 (2012) *Pages* **245–306**
Editor-in-Chief: **V.K. Gupta**
Published by: **DAYA PUBLISHING HOUSE, NEW DELHI**

17

Treating Diabetes Mellitus with Natural Products

Z. Ahmed[1*], A. Bhagat[1], R.K. Johri[1] and M.Z. Chishti[2]

ABSTRACT

Since antiquity, the natural products have been used in treating diabetes mellitus. Recent scientific investigation has confirmed the efficacy of many of these natural preparations and molecules, some of which are remarkably effective. Herbs are very effective in treating patients with Type II diabetes mellitus. When prescribed correctly, they may lower blood glucose level manage common signs and symptoms, and treat the complications of diabetes mellitus. Patients generally respond to herbal treatment within three-to-four weeks, with significant reduction in blood glucose level and little fluctuation throughout the day. However, some patients may require up to six-to-eight weeks. For patients with Type I diabetes mellitus, some herbs are used in conjunction with insulin to manage symptoms and complications. Herbs can also reduce the frequency and dosage of insulin injections. However, it is important to keep in mind that herbs cannot replace insulin, and patients with IDDM will still require insulin injections. Only those herbs that appear most effective, are relatively non-toxic and have substantial documentation of efficacy are covered in this chapter.

Keywords: Diabetes mellitus, Insulin resistance, Homeostasis, Insulin dependent diabetes mellitus, Non-insulin dependent diabetes mellitus, Insulin, Hyperglycemia, Hypoglycemia.

1 Diabetes Pharmacology Division, Indian Institute of Integrative Medicine (IIIM), CSIR, Canal Road, Jammu – 180 001, India

2 PG Department of Zoology, University of Kashmir, Srinagar – 190 006, India

* *Corresponding author*: E-mail:zahmed@iiim.ac.in; zabeerahmed@gmail.com

of weight, there is an accompanying deficiency of the pancreatic β-cells response to glucose. Both the tissue resistance to insulin and the impaired β-cell response to glucose appears to be further aggravated by increased hyperglycemia and both of these defects are ameliorated by the therapeutic maneuvers that reduce hyperglycemia.

Gestational Diabetes (GD) Mellitus

Gestational Diabetes (GD) mellitus refers to the onset or initial recognition of glucose intolerance during pregnancy, usually in the second or third trimester (American Diabetes Association, 2001). It occurs in about 4 per cent of all pregnancies. Patients with GD have a 30 per cent to 50 per cent chance of developing DM.

Other types include genetic defects of the pancreatic *b*-cells or in insulin action pathways (insulin receptor mutations or post-receptor defects) (Raffel *et al.*, 1997) as well as disease of the exocrine pancreas (*e.g.*, Pancreatitis, pancreatic reaction, or cystic fibrosis) are less common causes of diabetes mellitus (DM) (American Diabetes Association, Gestational diabetes mellitus, 2001). Endocrinopathies producing insulin counter regulatory hormones excess (*e.g.*, Cushing's syndrome, acromegaly) may result in DM (Kumar, 2002). Certain drugs like glucocorticoids, pentamidine, niacin and a-interferon may also lead to diabetes mellitus (DM) (Pandit, 1993).

Symptoms

Although the symptoms are similar in both types of diabetes, they vary in their intensity. The presentation is most typical and the symptoms develop most rapidly in patients with type 1 diabetes mellitus (DM). These symptoms include polyuria (increase in urine output) due to osmotic diuresis, polydipsia (increase in thirst) due to depletion of intracellular water triggering osmoreceptor of the thirst center, polyphagia (increased appetite) due to catabolism of protein and fat induce negative energy balance that lead to increase appetite, weight loss, fatigue, cramps, constipation, blurred vision and candidiasis (Kumar, 2002). Long-standing type 1 diabetes mellitus (DM) patients are susceptible to microvascular complications, (nephropathy, neuropathy, retinopathy); and macrovascula disease (coronary artery, heart, and peripheral vascular diseases) (Kannel and McGee, 1979).

Beside these, hyperglycemia (increase in blood glucose concentration), glucosuria (presence of glucose in urine), ketonuria and ketonemia (increased concentration of ketone bodies in the urine and blood respectively) and muscular weakness have also been reported.

Symptoms in patients with type 2 diabetes mellitus (DM) are similar but insidious in their onset. Many cases are diagnosed incidentally or because of the presence of diabetic complications. Type 2 diabetes mellitus (DM) carries a high risk of large vessel atherosclerosis; commonly associated with hypertension, hyperlipidaemia, and obesity. Myocardial infarction is also common and accounts for about 60 per cent of the deaths in diabetic patients. Moreover, human studies have shown that diabetes mellitus can be associated with altered cardiac function (Grossman and Messerli, 1993) and this can occur independently of cardiovascular complications. Enhanced susceptibility to infection of skin, tuberculosis, pneumonia and pyelonephritis found in type 2 diabetic patients.

Pathogenesis of Diabetes

In order to better understand the role of each drug class in the treatment of diabetes, it is important to have a basic understanding of the pathogenesis of diabetes (Figure 17.2) and the interplay between insulin and glucose at different sites. Postprandial elevations in serum glucose levels stimulate insulin synthesis and release from pancreatic β-cells. Insulin secreted into the systemic circulation binds to receptors in target organs (skeletal muscle, adipose tissue and liver). Insulin binding initiates a cascade of intracellular signal transduction pathways that inhibits glucose production in the liver, suppresses lipolysis in adipose tissue and stimulates glucose uptake into target cells (muscle and fat) by mechanisms such as the translocation of vesicles that contain glucose transporters to the plasma membrane

Type 2 diabetes is characterized by 2 major defects: decreased secretion of insulin by the pancreas and resistance to the action of insulin in various tissues (muscle, liver and adipose), which results in impaired glucose uptake (Cheng, 2005). The precise molecular mechanism of insulin resistance is not clearly understood, but

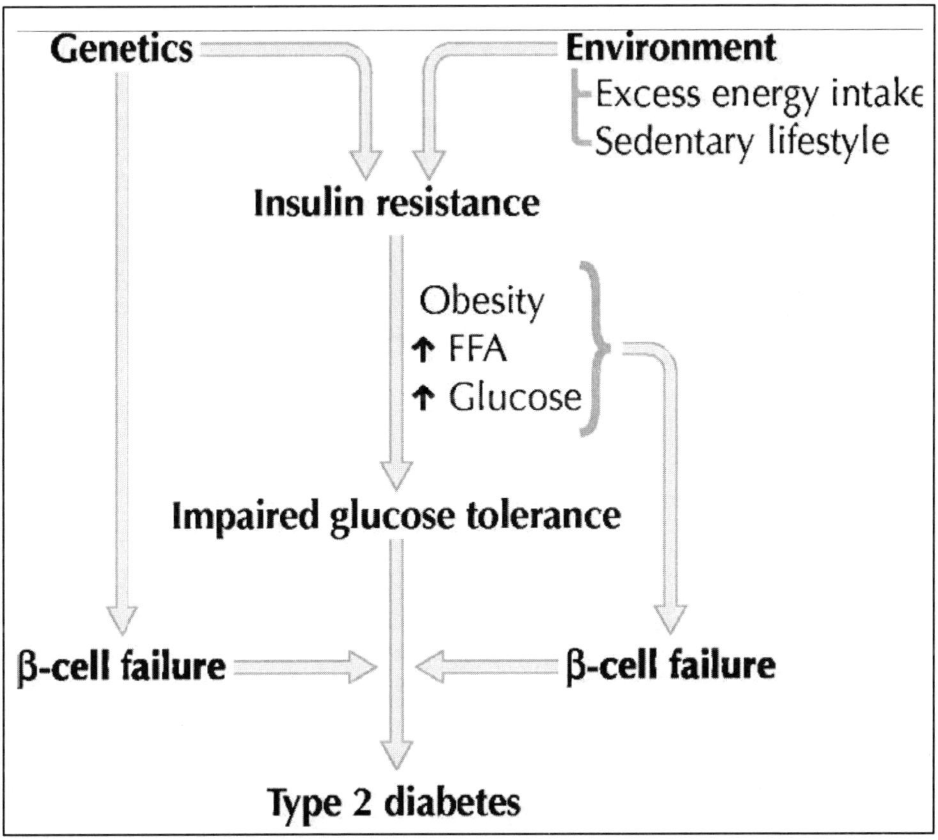

Figure 17.2. Overview of the pathogenesis of type 2 diabetes mellitus. FFA = free fatty acids.

deficits in the post-insulin receptor intracellular signaling pathways are believed to play a role. Insulin resistance, which is usually present before the onset of diabetes, is determined by a number of factors, including genetics, age, obesity and, later in the disease, hyperglycemia itself. Excess visceral adiposity, dyslipidemia and hypertension often accompany insulin resistance (Ramarao and Kaul, 1999). Other findings may include impaired fibrinolysis, increased platelet aggregation, vascular inflammation, endothelial dysfunction and premature atherosclerosis.

The increase in lipolysis by adipose cells that are resistant to insulin and the subsequent increased levels of circulating free fatty acids also contribute to the pathogenesis of diabetes by impairing *b*-cell function, impairing glucose uptake in skeletal muscles and promoting glucose release from the liver. In addition to its role as a source of excess circulating free fatty acids, adipose tissue has emerged in the last decade as an endocrine organ. Adipose tissue is a source of a number of hormones (adipo-cytokines or "adipokines") that appear to regulate insulin sensitivity (*e.g.*, adiponectin, resistin), as well as appetite regulation (*e.g.*, leptin), inflammation (*e.g.*, tumour necrosis factor-α, interleukin-6) and coagulability (*e.g.*, plasminogen activator inhibitor-1) (Devi *et al.*, 2005). Moreover, some studies suggest that reactive oxygen species (including free radical) may also involved in the initiation and development of vascular complication in diabetics (Lapolla *et al.*, 1993). Oxidative stress combined with mitochondria dysfunction leads to the activation of inflammatory signaling pathways, which may damage insulin-producing cells and further aggravate the complication of diabetes (Leonid and Philipson, 2004).

Management of Diabetes Mellitus

Conventional Therapies

The general consensus on treatment of type 2 diabetes mellitus is that lifestyle management is at the forefront of therapy options. In addition to exercise, weight control, medical nutrition therapy, oral glucose-lowering drugs and injections of insulin are the conventional therapies. Pharmacological treatment is indicated when fasting glucose level exceeds 140 mg/dL, the post-prandial glucose level exceeds 160 mg/dL or HbA1c exceeds 8.0 per cent (DeFronzo, 1999).

Insulin was the first, and remains the primary mean of treatment for Type 1 diabetes and is administered by subcutaneous injection. This method is necessary since insulin is destroyed by gastric stomach secretions when it is taken by mouth. During the past several years a large number of different classes of drug therapies for patients with both Type 1 and Type 2 diabetes have been developed. The concept of genetic re-engineering of insulin to produce insulin analogs (synthetic insulin) with improved properties has enhanced the ability to affect glycaemic control with fewer adverse reactions. For Type 2 patients, the number of orally active antidiabetic agents has increased from one class of agents (the sulfonylureas - sulfa drugs) to the current total of four classes of agents. The three new classes include agents of potentially even greater glycaemic efficacy, such as Biguanide 'Metformin'; agents directly improving the underlying insulin resistance of Type 2 diabetes, specifically thiazolidinediones such as 'Troglitazone'; and finally agents that alter the rate of hydrolysis and absorption of oligosaccharides, such as the alpha-glucosidase inhibitor 'Acarbose'. The sulfonylureas as a group have proven to be not very effective. After three months of continual treatment at an adequate dosage, only about sixty percent of Type 2 diabetics are able to control blood sugar levels using these drugs. Furthermore these agents generally lose their effectiveness over time. After an initial period of success they fail to produce a positive effect in about thirty- percent of the cases at best.

Traditionally, lifestyle changes including losing excess weight, eating a healthful diet and engaging in regular exercise are the first-line treatments for type 2 diabetes. When these modifications do not make enough of a dent in the disease, medications can be prescribed. Some medications help the pancreas produce more insulin, while others help the body use the insulin that it does produce more efficiently. If these drugs don't work, a person may need to take insulin. Conventional therapies for diabetes have been geared toward regulating blood glucose with a combination of diet modification, insulin and/or oral pharmacological agents, weight loss when appropriate, and exercise. Although Western medicine and Traditional Chinese medicine (TCM) share the diabetes treatment goals of reducing symptoms and preventing complications, their approaches to conceptualizing, diagnosing, and treating the disease are very different.

Insulin Treatment in Diabetes Mellitus

The introduction of insulin to treat diabetes mellitus has saved an estimated 5 million lives of patients with type 1 diabetes mellitus during the year 2000. Considerable progress has been made, in recent years, in the production, formulation and delivery of insulin preparations, as well as the development of insulin treatment regimens which maintains long-term-normoglycaemia, with a low risk of hypoglycaemia (Bolli, 1997). The importance of the aim of preventing or slowing the progression of chronic microvascular complications has been conclusively proven during the last decade, in both type 1 and type 2 diabetes mellitus (UK Prospective Diabetes Study Group, 1998). Unfortunately, patients treated with insulin have uniformly poorer glycaemic control compared to those treated with other therapies. It is an accepted fact that insulin is the most potent glucose-lowering agent, with hypoglycaemia being the only major dose-limiting factor. Unlike all oral agents that have limited maximum action, insulin has progressively more side effects as the dose is increased. Insulin is a hormone with extensive effects on both metabolism and several other body systems (*e.g.*, vascular compliance). Insulin causes most of the body's cells to take up glucose from the blood (including liver, muscle, and fat tissue cells), storing it as glycogen in the liver and muscle, and stops use of fat as an energy source. When insulin is absent (or low), glucose is not taken up by most body cells and the body begins to use fat as an energy source (*i.e.*, transfer of lipids from adipose tissue to the liver for mobilization as an energy source). As its level is a central metabolic control mechanism, its status is also used as a control signal to other body systems (such as amino acid uptake by body cells). It has several other anabolic effects throughout the body. When control of insulin levels fails, diabetes mellitus results.

Insulin is used medically to treat some forms of diabetes mellitus. Patients with Type 1 diabetes mellitus depend on external insulin (most commonly injected subcutaneously) for their survival because the hormone is no longer produced internally. Patients with Type 2 diabetes mellitus are insulin resistant, have relatively low insulin production, or both; some patients with Type 2 diabetes may eventually require insulin when other medications fail to control blood glucose levels adequately. Insulin is a peptide hormone composed of 51 amino acid residues and has a molecular weight of 5808 Da (Figure 17.3). It is produced in the islets of Langerhans in the pancreas. The name comes from the Latin *insula* for "island". Insulin's structure varies slightly between species of animal. Insulin from animal sources differs somewhat in 'strength' (*i.e.*, in carbohydrate metabolism control effects) in humans because of those variations. Porcine (pig) insulin is especially close to the human version.

Alternative Treatments

The term alternative medicine means the mode of healing by alternative system of medicine having a similar degree of efficacy without the troublesome side effects associated with conventional treatments. Alternative treatments for diabetes have become increasingly popular for the last several years (Sinha *et al.*, 1996), including medicinal herbs, nutritional supplementation, acupuncture and hot tub therapy.

Ayurveda, an ancient Indian system of medicine had mentioned several plants that are useful in the correction of metabolic disorders such as diabetes mellitus. Numerous herbal drugs such as *Momordica charantia, Tinospora cordifolia, Terminalia chebula, Azadirachta indica, Gymnema sylvestris* and *Syzygium cumini* have been used by people of various cultures to treat diabetes (Gupta *et al.*, 2006).

Herbal Treatment for Diabetes

Herbs are very effective in treating patients with Type II diabetes mellitus. When prescribed correctly, they may lower blood glucose levels, manage common signs and symptoms, and treat the complications of diabetes mellitus. Patients generally respond to herbal treatment within three-to-four weeks, with significant reduction in blood glucose levels and little fluctuation throughout the day. However, some patients may require up to six-to-eight weeks. For patients with Type I diabetes mellitus, some herbs are used in conjunction with insulin to manage symptoms and complications. Herbs can also reduce the frequency and dosage of insulin injections. However, it is important to keep in mind that herbs cannot replace insulin, and patients with IDDM will still require insulin injections.

Thus treatment of diabetes mellitus through herbs requires a balance stabilize the parameters and markers of diabetes which is known as Equilibrium. The Equilibrium is the formula of choice for treating diabetes mellitus. From the perspective of Western medicine, Equilibrium contains herbs with excellent hypoglycemic effects, lowering blood glucose levels and reducing synthesis of fatty tissues. In addition, Equilibrium contains herbs that lower blood cholesterol levels and improve blood circulation to the coronary arteries and peripheral parts of the body- thus managing

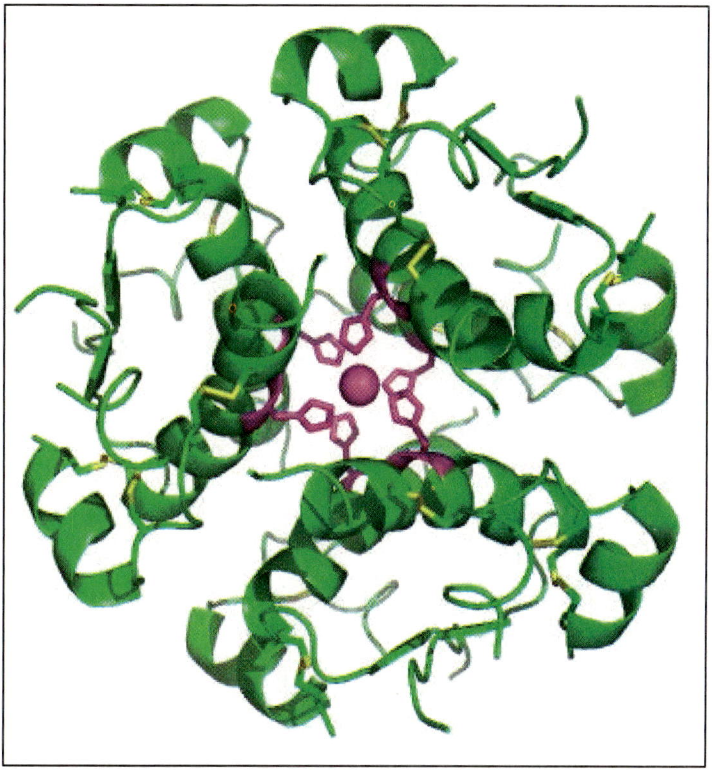

Figure 17.3. Computer-generated image of insulin hexamers highlighting the threefold symmetry, the zinc ions holding it together, and the histidine residues involved in zinc binding (Chang *et al.*, 1997).

common complications of diabetes, such as hyperlipidemia, atherosclerosis, coronary artery disease, peripheral neuropathy, etc.

Thus the herbal medicines effectively work as alternative diabetes treatment. These medicines have been used in treating diabetes for centuries. Herbs regulate the glucose levels in the body. Some of the herbs those are safe and effective as alternative diabetes treatment are discussed briefly herein below:

Acacia arabica (Lam.) Muhl. *ex* Willd. (Family: Mimosaceae)

Acacia arabica is a moderate sized, almost evergreen tree found throughout the drier parts of India, ascending to an altitude of 900 m. The bark of this plant has various traditional uses (Anonymous, 1976). The plant extract acts as an antidiabetic agent by acting as insulin secretagouge. It induces hypoglycemia in control rats but not in alloxanized animals. Powdered seeds of *Acacia arabica* when administered to normal rabbits induced hypoglycemic effect by initiating release of insulin from pancreatic beta cells (Wadood *et al.*, 1989).

Aegle marmelos (L.) Correa ex Roxb. (Family: Rutaceae)

The aqueous extract of *A. marmelos* leaves significantly ($P < 0.05$) increased the plasma insulin level from day 3 onward. It is evident from the results that an aqueous extract of *A. marmelos* leaves exhibited significant hypoglycaemic activity both in normoglycaemic and streptozotocin-diabetic rats. A similar effect of *A. marmelos* leaves has been documented in alloxan diabetic animals (Rao, 1992; Ponnachan *et al.*, 1993) with two different possible mechanisms of hypoglycaemic effect, *i.e.*, reduced absorption of glucose from gut and insulin-like activity, respectively. However, in our experiment an insulin release effect of *A. marmelos* leaves similar to glibenclamide (reference oral hypoglycaemic drug), *i.e.*, stimulation of the surviving β-cells to release more insulin is a possible explanation of the hypoglycaemic effect. It was substantiated by significantly increased levels of plasma insulin.

Allium cepa L. (Family: Liliaceae)

Allium cepa commonly known as onion, is an essential dietary ingredient, cultivated throughout India. Several studies indicated the hypoglycemic activity of this plant along with its hypolipidemic and antioxidant activity (Roman-Ramos *et al.*, 1995; Campos *et al.*, 2003; El-Demerdash *et al.*, 2005). A study with the seedling, seedling parts and callus cultures of onion suggested that the callus cultures exhibited much higher hypoglycemic activity as compared to natural bulbs of onion and the same can be used as an alternative source for the isolation of hypoglycemic compounds (Kelkar *et al.*, 2001). Investigations revealed the presence of a sulfur containing amino acid, S-methyl cysteine sulphoxide, in onion, which shown to impart potent hypoglycemic activity when administered at a dose of 200 mg/kg for 45 days to alloxan induced diabetic rats (Kumari *et al.*, 1995). Another compound S-allyl cysteine sulphoxide was also found to be effective in reducing the blood glucose level of alloxan induced diabetic rats (Sheela *et al.*, 1995). Several clinical studies also strongly substantiated the hypoglycemic claim of *Allium cepa* (Mathew and Augusti, 1975; Sharma *et al.*, 1977; Tjokroprawiro *et al.*, 1983).

Allium sativum L. (Family: Alliaceae)

Allium sativum is more commonly known as garlic, belongs to family Liliaceae and is thought to offer antioxidant properties (Liu *et al.*, 2007; Jain and Vyas, 1975). This is another essential dietary component cultivated throughout India, and familiar worldwide as garlic. The hypoglycemic activity of garlic has been extensively studied and reported. Pioneering works by many researchers proved the potent hypoglycemic activity of *Allium sativum* (Zacharias *et al.*, 1980; Roman-Ramos *et al.*, 1995; Kasuga *et al.*, 1999). Garlic contains S-allyl cysteine sulphoxide, a sulphur containing amino acid, which produced significant blood glucose lowering activity in experimental diabetic animals (Sheela and Augusti, 1992). Allicin (thio-2-propene-1-sulfinic acid S-allyl ester) another sulphur compound isolated from garlic (Figure 17.4, [I]) resulted in pronounced hypoglycemia in mildly diabetic rabbits upon oral administration (0.25 mg/kg) but failed to produce such effect in severe diabetes in the animals at same dose (Mathew and Augusti, 1973)

Aloe vera (L.) Burm.f. (Family: Aloaceae)

An acaulescent herb cultivated through out India. Aloes have long been used all over the world for their various medicinal properties. The extract of aloe gum is effective in enhancing glucose tolerance in normal as well as diabetic rats (Al-Awadi and Gumaa, 1987). Several other works have revealed the hypoglycemic activity of this plant along with possible mode of action.

Areca catechu L. (Family: Arecaceae)

Areca catechu commonly known as betel nut, is a handsome tree cultivated throughout India. The nut contains a large quantity of tannin, gallic acid, fixed oil gum, volatile oil, lignin and alkaloids like arecoline, arecain, guracine, etc. Arecoline (Figure 17.4, [II]) was investigated and reported to have hypoglycemic activity in an animal model of diabetes upon subcutaneous administration (Chempakam, 1993).

Artemisia pallens Wall. ex DC. (Family: Compositae)

It is a shrub used in the treatment of diabetes mellitus in the southern part of India as folk medicine. Oral administration of the methanol extract of the aerial parts of *Artemisia pallens* led to significant blood glucose lowering effect in glucose-fed hyperglycaemic and alloxan-induced diabetic rats. This effect of the extract was dose dependent and significant at 100 mg/kg level in glucose-fed rats. In fasted normal rats, the extract caused a moderate hypoglycaemic effect at a higher dose (1000 mg/kg), whereas water extract (1000 mg/kg) did not show any activity (Subramoniam *et al.*, 1996).

Annona squamosa L. (Family: Annonaceae)

Annona squamosa commonly known as sugar apple is a 10–20 ft long tree found in different parts of India. According to the folklore claim *Annona squamosa* has hypoglycemic properties, which has been further supported by different research findings.

The claim by some tribal populations in parts of Northern India that the young leaves of the custard apple tree, *Annona squamosa* has antidiabetic properties was investigated (Unpublished results). Diabetes mellitus was induced with streptozotocin-nicotinamide and graded doses of the aqueous leaf extracts were then administered in drinking water to normal and experimental diabetic rats for 12 days. Fasting plasma glucose levels, serum insulin levels, serum lipid profiles and changes in body weight were evaluated in normal rats while liver glycogen levels and pancreatic TBARS levels were evaluated additionally in diabetic rats. The diabetic groups treated with the aqueous leaf extract were compared with standard glibenclamide. The findings of the study support the antidiabetic claims of *Annona squamosa* (Shirwaikar *et al.*, 2004).

Andrographis paniculata Nees (Family: Acanthaceae)

It is an erect annual herb commonly known as Kalmegh or 'King of Bitters', found throughout India and cultivated in many states of India. A number of studies have shown that *Andrographis paniculata* extract and the active metabolite andrographolide (Figure 17.4, [III]) can exert potent antihyperglycemic activity.

the clonal pancreatic beta-cell line. The insulin-releasing effect of the aqueous extract of *Eucalyptus globulus* is probably responsible for antihyperglycemic activity (Gray and Flatt, 1998).

Enicostemma littorale Blume (Family: Gentiaceae)

Perennial herb attaining height of 5–20 inches, found throughout India up to height of 1500 ft. The hypoglycemic potential of the plant was studied by several workers, indicating significant blood glucose lowering activity. A clinical study involving 84 patients with Type II Diabetes showed that pills prepared from *Enicostemma littorale* Blume administered for three months reduced blood glucose as well as serum insulin levels and prevented the progression of complications in diabetic patients. It also improved kidney function, lipid profile and blood pressure significantly (Upadhyay and Goyal, 2004).

Eugenia jambolana Lam. (Family: Myrtaceae)

Large evergreen tree of Indian subcontinent, also known as *Syzygium cumini* commonly known as 'jamun'. In India, the decoction of kernels of *Eugenia jambolana* is used as a household remedy for diabetes. The seeds and decoction of dry leaves were found to produce hypoglycemic effect (Mahapatra *et al.*, 1985; Coimbra *et al.*, 1992; Nandkarni, 1992). The protective effect of the alcoholic (100 mg/kg) and the aqueous (5 g/kg) extracts of the seed of this plant against tissue damage in diabetic rat brain was studied and it was observed that both the extract effectively protected the tissues, the alcoholic extract having more pronounced effect than the water extract (Stanely *et al.*, 2003).

Ficus bengalensis L. (Family: Moraceae)

It is a very large tree with spreading branches distributed throughout India. Various active components isolated from the plant including the dimethoxy derivative of leucocyandin 3-*O*-beta-d-galactosyl cellobioside, dimethoxy derivative of perlargonidin 3-*O*-alpha-l rhamnoside, glycoside of leucopelargonidin, leucodelphinidin (Figure 17.4, [V]), isolated from the bark of this plant have been reported for their hypoglycemic activity (Deshmukh *et al.*, 1960; Brahmachari and Augusti, 1964; Kumar and Augusti, 1994).

Ficus carica is well known as a diabetic remedy in Spain and South-western Europe (Serraclara *et al.*, 1998), but its active component is unknown. Some studies on animals suggest that fig-leaf facilitates glucose uptake. The efficacy of the plant is, however, still yet to be validated in the treatment of diabetes.

Gymnema montanum Hook.f. (Family: Asclepiadaceae)

It is an endemic and endangered plant species of India found mainly in Western Ghats. Blood glucose lowering activity of alcoholic leaf extract (200 mg/kg orally) was studied in alloxan diabetic rats along with an increase in plasma insulin level (Ananthan *et al.*, 2003a). The extract also produced significant antioxidant and antiperoxidative activity in alloxanized rats (Ananthan *et al.*, 2003b, 2004; Ramkumar *et al.*, 2004). The leaf extract was also reported to exert potent antihyperlipidemic activity in alloxanized rats (Ananthan *et al.*, 2003c).

Gymnema sylvestre R. Br. (Family: Asclepiadaceae)

Gymnema sylvestre is one of the Asclepiad strains, native to the tropical regions of India and commonly known as the "sugar destroyer" because the leaves effectively block sweet tastes in the mouth when chewed. The plant has been used in the treatment of diabetes mellitus for a long time in India and reported by different workers for its blood glucose lowering activity both *in vitro* and *in vivo* (Shanmugasundaram *et al.*, 1983; Fushiki *et al.*, 1992; Tominaga *et al.*, 1995; Shimizu *et al.*, 1997; Yoshikawa *et al.*, 1997a, b; Chattopadhyay, 1998, 1999; Persaud *et al.*, 1999; Sugihara *et al.*, 2000; Gholap and Kar, 2003).

G. sylvestre is also employed in traditional ayurvedic medicine (Chattopadhyay, 1998; Shanmugasundaram *et al.*, 1990b; Okabayashi, 1990). The plant grows in the tropical forests of southern and central India, and has been linked with significant blood glucose lowering. Anti-hyperglycemic effect of dried leaf powder of *G. sylvestre* was seen in alloxanized rabbits along with decrease in the activity of gluconeogenic enzymes and reversal of pathological changes in the liver initiated during the hyperglycemic phase. Some studies in animals have even reported regeneration of islet cells and an increase in *b*-cell function. Oral administration of aqueous extract of leaves of *G. sylvestre* (20 mg/day) for 20–60 days normalized blood sugar level of STZ diabetic rats through *b*-cell regeneration. Single as well as chronic (32–35 days) oral administration of aqueous extract of *G. sylvestre* leaves (1 g/kg) to 18-h fasted non-diabetic and STZ (30 mg/kg) induced mild diabetic rats showed significant reduction in blood glucose on OGTT (1 g/kg) without any significant effect on immuno-reactive insulin (IRI) levels. In another study, water-soluble fraction of alcoholic extract of the plant significantly lowered the hepatic glycogen content of the glucose fed rats.

Glycyrrhiza glabra L. (Family: Fabaceae)

Glycyrrhiza glabra commonly known as licorice, is a flavorful perennial herb that grows 3–7 ft high and has been used in food and medicinal remedies for thousands of years. The effect of hydrophobic flavonoids from this plant was studied on abdominal fat accumulation and blood glucose level in obese diabetic KK-A (y) mice. The findings indicated that the flavonoids have abdominal fat-lowering and hypoglycemic effects, possibly mediated through activation of peroxisome proliferator-activated receptor-gamma (PPAR-gamma) (Nakagawa *et al.*, 2004).

Hibiscus rosa sinensis L. (Family: Malvaceae)

These are large shrubs or small trees grow to 15 ft high in frost-free climates and are native to southern Asia. The plant was studied extensively by many workers for its hypoglycemic activity in various models of experimental diabetes like glucose-loaded rats, streptozotocin diabetic rats, etc. and it was found that the plant has potent blood glucose lowering activity.

Blood glucose and total lipid levels were determined in streptozotocin induced diabetic rats after oral administration of an ethanol flower extract of *Hibiscus rosa sinensis*. A comparable hypoglycemic effect was evidenced from the data obtained after 7 and 21 days of oral administration of the extract and glibenclamide. Maximal diminution in blood glucose (41-46 per cent) and insulin level (14 per cent) was noticed after 21 days. The extract lowered the total cholesterol and serum triglycerides by 22 and 30 per cent, respectively. The increase in HDL-cholesterol was much higher (12 per cent) under the influence of the extract as compared to that of glibenclamide (1 per cent). The hypoglycemic activity of this extract is comparable to that of glibenclamide but is not mediated through insulin release. Other possible mechanisms are discussed by Sachdewa *et al.* (2003).

Helicteres isora L. (Family: Sterculiaceae)

It is a well-known plant of Indian subcontinent. The root juice of this plant has been used in the treatment of diabetes by several ethnic groups in different parts of India. The root extracts has been reported to possess significant hypoglycemic activity because of the insulin-sensitizing property of the plant.

The antihyperglycemic and hypolipidemic activities of *Helicteres isora* root extracts were investigated in alloxan-induced diabetic rats and a possible mechanism of the blood glucose lowering action was studied. Alloxan-induced diabetic rats experienced 69.13 and 51.14 per cent, 22.60 and 21.89 per cent, 30.12 and 19.96 per cent, and 50.05 and 34.29 per cent reduction in blood glucose, total cholesterol, triglycerides, and urea levels following oral administration of butanol and aqueous ethanol extracts of *H. isora* root, respectively, at 250 mg/kg for 10 days. The beneficial effects of these extracts were supported by evidence from histological examinations of the liver, pancreas, and kidney. Following the treatment with both extracts, the degenerative changes caused by alloxan in pancreatic cells were restored, particularly with the butanol extract. Histological examination convincingly showed the restoration of pancreatic islets, kidney glomeruli, and liver to its normal size. These results suggest that *H. isora* roots possess antidiabetic principles and can be useful for treatment of diabetes (Venkatesh *et al.*, 2010).

Ipomoea batatas (L.) Lam. (Family: Convolvulaceae)

It is a tuberous-rooted perennial plant commonly known as Sweet potato, cultivated in many tropical and subtropical countries and has become an important food crop, especially in India, China, Philippine Islands, and the South Seas Islands.

After treatment with Caiapo, Hb16 decreased significantly ($P < 0.001$) from 7.21 ± 0.15 to 6.68 ± 0.14 per cent, whereas it remained unchanged ($P = 0.23$) in subjects given placebo (7.04 ± 0.17 vs. 7.10 ± 0.19 per cent). Fasting blood glucose levels decreased ($P < 0.001$) in the Caiapo group (143.7 ± 1.9 vs. 128.5 ± 1.7 mg/dl) and did not change in the placebo group (144.3 ± 1.9 vs. 138.2 ± 2.1 mg/dl; $P = 0.052$). A decrease in body weight was observed in both the placebo group ($P = 0.0027$) and in the Caiapo group ($P < 0.0001$), probably due to a better- controlled lifestyle. In the Caiapo group, body weight was related to the improvement in glucose control ($r = 0.618$; $P < 0.0002$). Two-hour glucose levels were significantly ($P < 0.001$) decreased in the Caiapo group (193.3 ± 10.4 *vs.* 162.8 ± 8.2 mg/dl) compared with the placebo group (191.7 ± 9.2 *vs.* 181.0 ± 7.1 mg/dl). Mean cholesterol at the end of the treatment was significantly lower in the Caiapo group (214.6 ± 11.2 mg/dl) than in the placebo group (248.7 ± 11.2 mg/dl; $P < 0.05$). No significant changes in triglyceride levels or blood pressure were observed, and Caiapo was well tolerated without significant adverse effects (Ludvik *et al.*, 2004).

Lantana camara L. (Family: Verbenaceae)

It is a rugged evergreen shrub found throughout India. The leaf juice of this plant at a dose of 1500 mg/kg p.o. daily for 14 days produced significant hypoglycemic activity in rats (Garg *et al.*, 1997). Oral administration of the methanol extract of *Lantana camara* (200 and 400 mg/kg body weight) leaves in alloxan-induced diabetic rats, showed significant ($P<0.01$) reduction in the blood glucose concentration in dose dependent manner (Unpublished results). Treatment with extract (400 mg/kg) decreased blood glucose level to 121.94 mg/dl. Body weight significantly ($P<0.05$) increased to normal after treatment with extract and it was found effective in oral glucose tolerance test as it decreased the elevated level of glucose after one hour. The biochemical parameters like triglycerides (TG), total cholesterol (TC), low density lipoprotein (LDL), very low density lipoprotein (VLDL) and high density lipoprotein were investigated and extract was found effective against diabetes induced hyperlipidemia. Methanol extract of *Lantana camata* leaves exhibit promising anti-hyperglycemic activity against alloxan-induced diabetic rats (Ganesh *et al.*, 2010).

Mangifera indica L. (Family: Anacardiaceae)

It is a well known perennial tree commonly known as Mango, distributed and widely cultivated throughout India. The aqueous leaf-extract (1 g/kg) failed to exert any hypoglycemic activity in normoglycemic as well as streptozotocin-induced diabetic rats upon oral administration (Aderibigbe *et al.*, 1999). Antihyperglycemic activity of the leaf extract at the same dose level was investigated by the same author in different experimental condition along with its antioxidant activity (Martinez *et al.*, 2000). The glucose lowering effect of mangiferin (Figure 17.4, [VI]), a xanthone glucoside, isolated from the leaves of *Mangifera indica* was also studied.

Memecylon umbellatum Burm. f. (Family: Melastomataceae)

Oral administration of an alcoholic extract of the leaves of *Memecylon umbellatum* led to a significant lowering of serum glucose levels in normal and alloxan-induced diabetic mice. Although the mechanism of action is unknown, the magnitude of glucose reduction in both the animal models is encouraging. The results indicate that *M. umbellatum* has interesting possibilities as a source of oral hypoglycaemic agents (Amalraj and Ignacimuthu, 1998b).

Momordica cymbalaria Fenzl ex Naudin (Family: Cucurbitaceae)

It is a well known medicinal plant found in different parts of India. Fruit powder and aqueous fruit extract of *Momordica cymbalaria* was investigated for its effect on blood glucose and other biochemical parameters in alloxan-induced diabetic rats.

Aqueous, ethanolic and hexane fractions of *Momordica cymbalaria* fruits were prepared and given individually at different doses to different batches of rats (both normal and alloxan diabetic rats) after an overnight fast. The blood glucose levels were measured at 0, 1, 3, 5 and 7 h after the treatment. The aqueous extract of *Momordica cymbalaria* at a dosage of 0.5 g/kg b.w. is showing maximal blood glucose lowering effect in diabetic rats. The same dosage did not produce any hypoglycemic activity in normal rats. The antihyperglycemic activity of *Momordica cymbalaria* fruit was compared with the treatment of glibenclamide, an oral hypoglycemic agent (Kameswara Rao *et al.* 2001).

Mucuna pruriens (L.) DC. (Family: Leguminosae)

Mucuna pruriens is one of the popular medicinal plants of India and is constituent of many indigenous drug formulations. The seed and plant extracts were investigated for possible blood sugar lowering activity in different animal models of diabetes and the results indicated a strong hypoglycemic potential of the plant.

Alloxan (120 mg/kg, i.p.) elevated the blood glucose levels which was partially restored or improved upon the administration of chloroform fraction of leaf extract of *Mucuna pruriens.* Glucose levels were found to be significantly increased till 9th day after alloxan administration and thereafter decreased on 12th day. Decrease in Serum glucose may be due to the regeneration of β-cell of the pancreas which was destroyed by alloxan. Administration of the extract produced a significant ($p<0.001$) decrease in the serum glucose as compared to diabetic control group (Anusha Bhaskar *et al.* 2008)

Musa sapientum L. (Family: Musaceae)

It is a perennial herbaceous plant commonly known as 'banana'. It is mainly used in Indian folk medicine for the treatment of diabetes mellitus. Several studies revealed its hypoglycemic activity (Jain, 1968, 1969). Blood glucose lowering activity of flower extract (0.15, 0.20 and 0.25 g/kg p.o. for 30 days) in experimental animals in an oral glucose tolerance test along with a reduction in glycosylated haemoglobin and an increase in total haemoglobin as well as significant antioxidant activity at the same dose levels were investigated and reported (Pari and Maheswari, 1999; Pari and Umamaheswari, 2000).

Momordica charantia L. (Family: Cucurbitaceae)

Momordica charantia goes under a variety of names and is native to some areas of Asia, India, Africa and South America. Marketed as *charantia,* it is also known as *karela* or *karolla* and bitter melon. It is a very common folklore remedy for diabetes. Extract of fruit pulp, seed, leaves and whole plant of *Momordica charantia* has shown hypoglycemic effect in various animal models. The herb may be prepared in a variety of different ways, and may be able to help diabetics with insulin secretion, glucose oxidation and other processes. Acute effects on blood glucose levels have also been reported (Gupta and Seth, 1962; Jayasooriya, 2000).

Several earlier and recent studies have indicated the hypoglycemic activity of various parts of this plant (Sharma *et al.*, 1960; Gupta and Seth, 1962; Vimla Devi *et al.*, 1977; Khanna *et al.*, 1981; Kedar and Chakrabarti, 1982; Welihinda *et al.*, 1982; Ng *et al.*, 1986 a,b, 1987, Karunanayake *et al.*, 1990; Ali *et al.*, 1993; Shibib *et al.*, 1993;Cakici *et al.*, 1994; Sarkar *et al.*, 1996; Sitasawad *et al.*, 2000; Miura *et al.*, 2001, 2004; Kar *et al.*, 2003; Sekar *et al.*, 2005; Yadav *et al.*, 2005).

Figure 17.4. Phyto-constituents (I- XXVIII) with hypoglycemic potential.

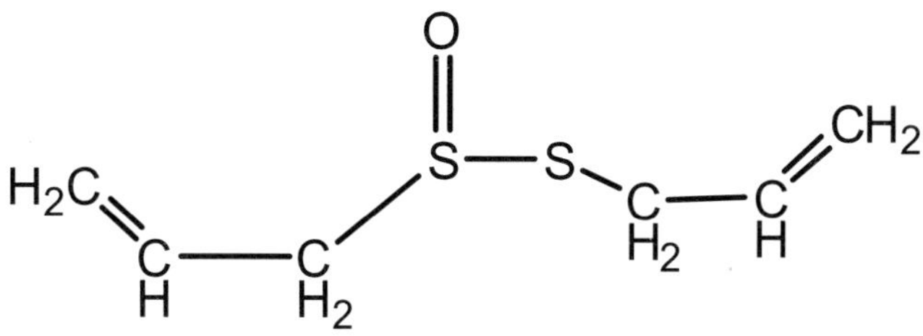

Allicin [I]

Arecolin[II]

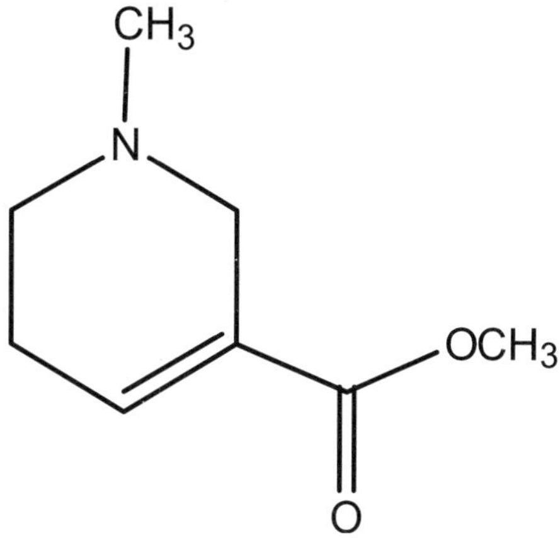

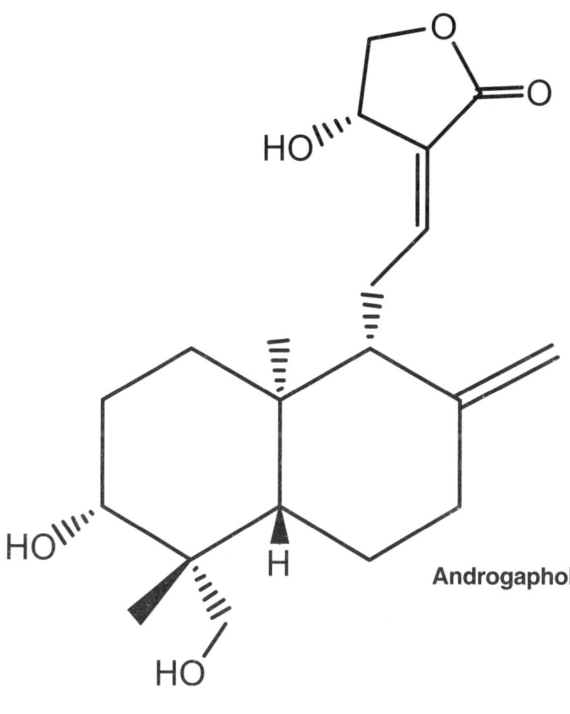

Androgapholide [III]

Contd...

Figure 17.4–*Contd...*

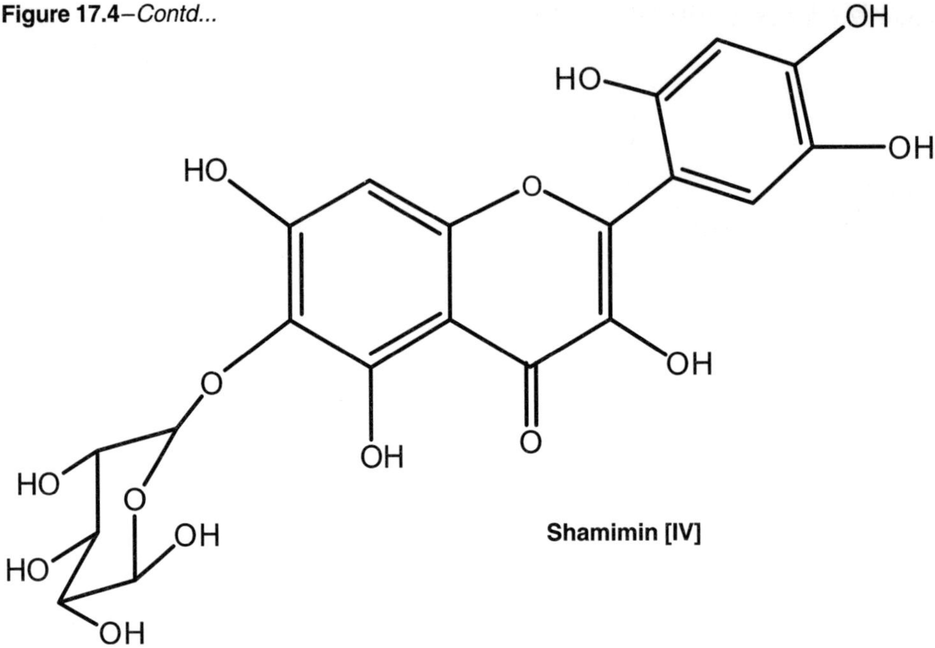

Shamimin [IV]

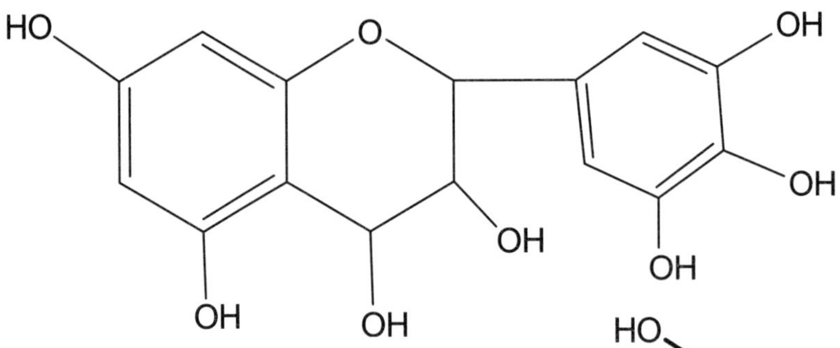

Leucodelphinidine [V]

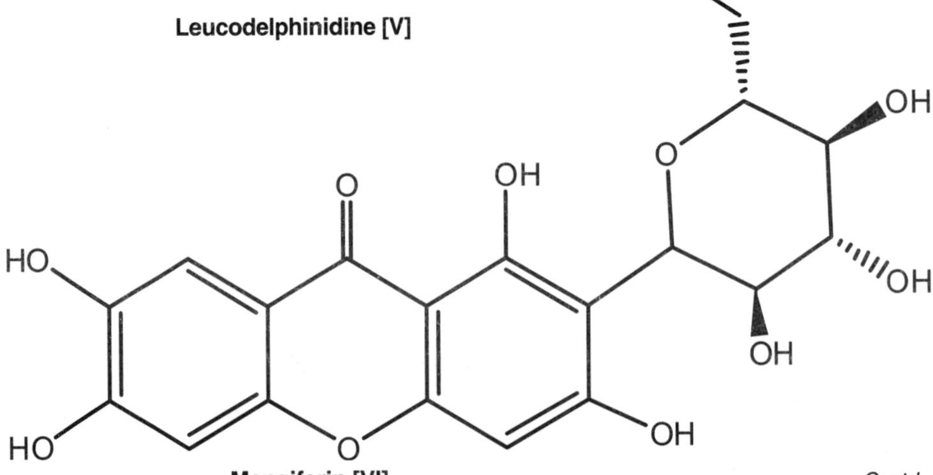

Mangiferin [VI]

Contd...

Figure 17.4–*Contd...*

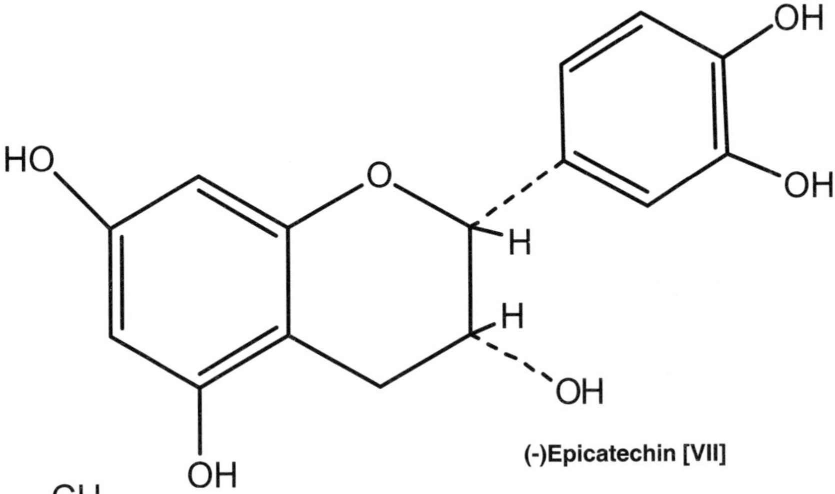

(-)Epicatechin [VII]

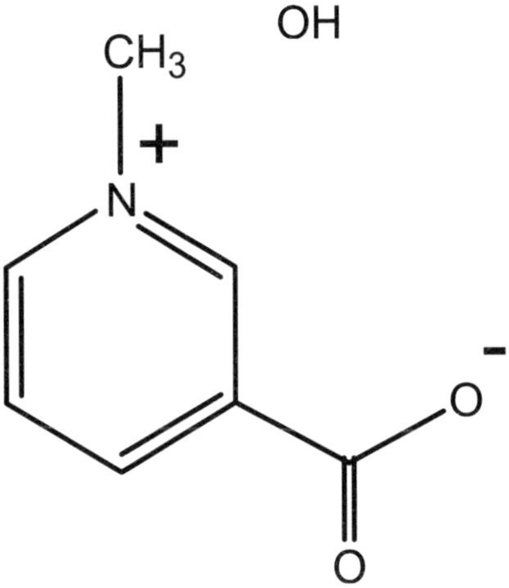

Trigonelline [VIII]

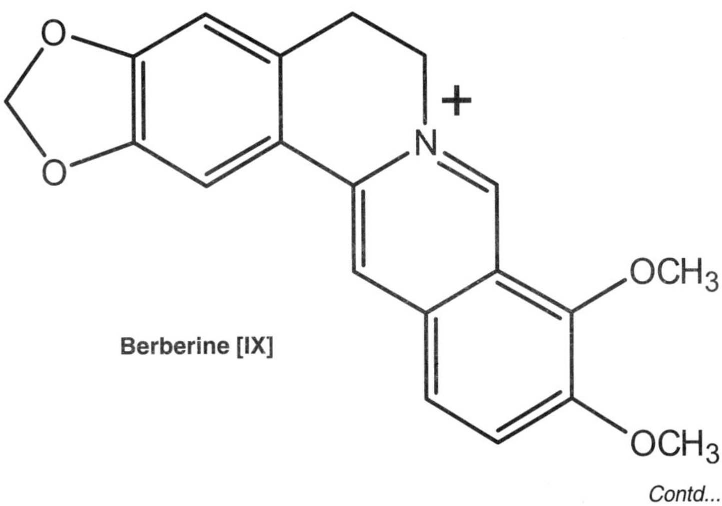

Berberine [IX]

Contd...

Figure 17.4–*Contd...*

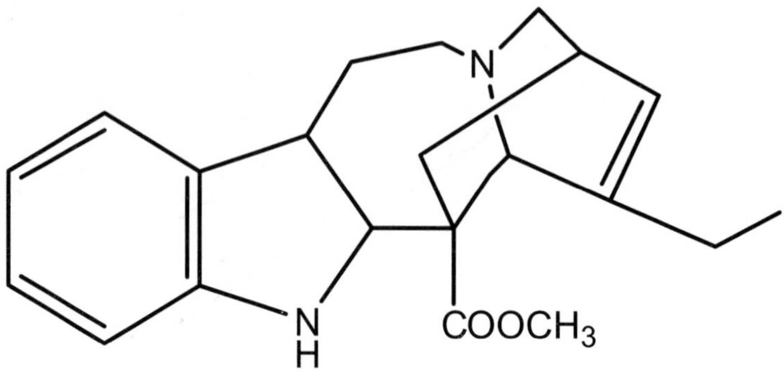

Cathaaranthine [X]

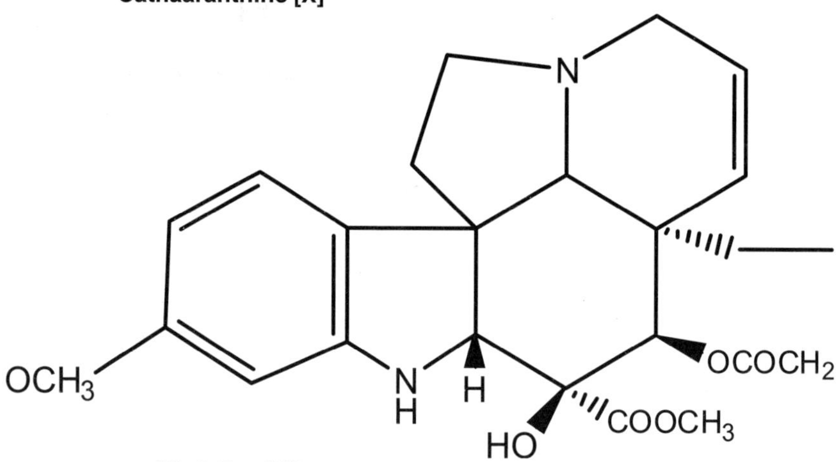

Vindoline [XI]

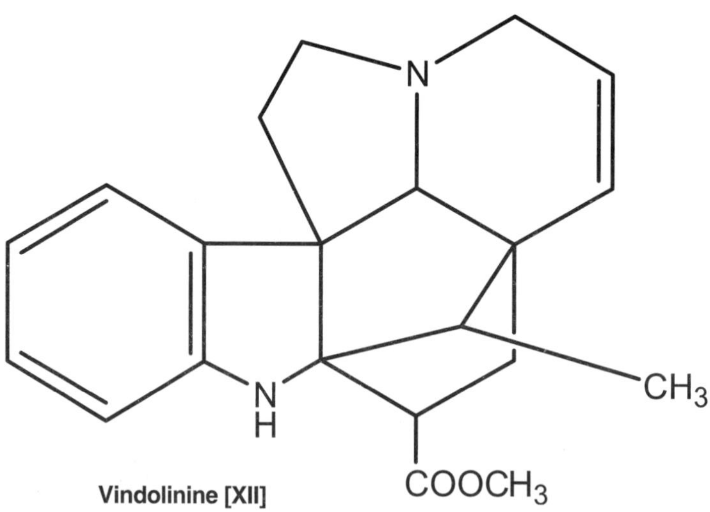

Vindolinine [XII]

Contd...

Figure 17.4–*Contd...*

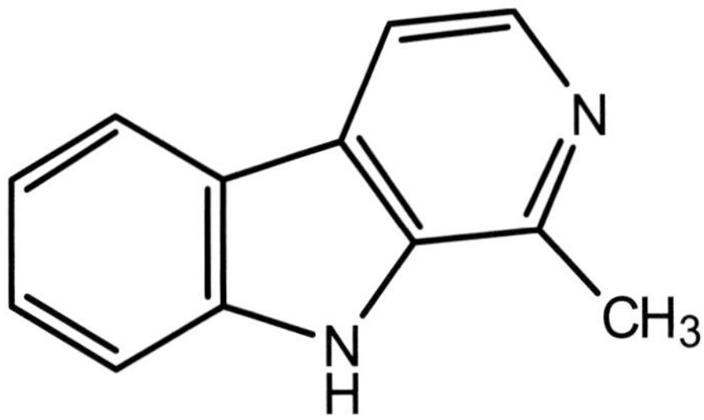

Harmane [XIII]

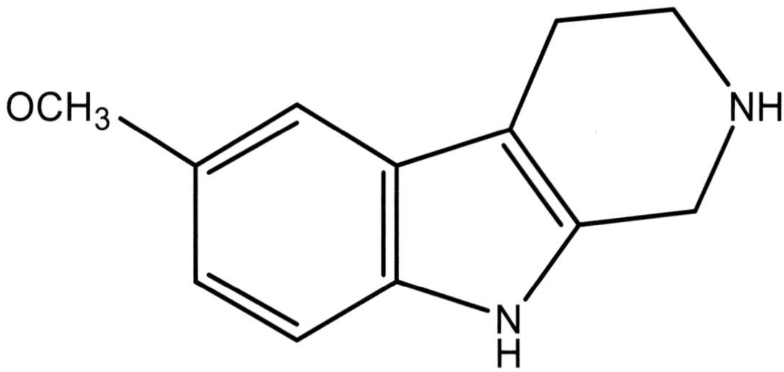

Pinoline [XIV]

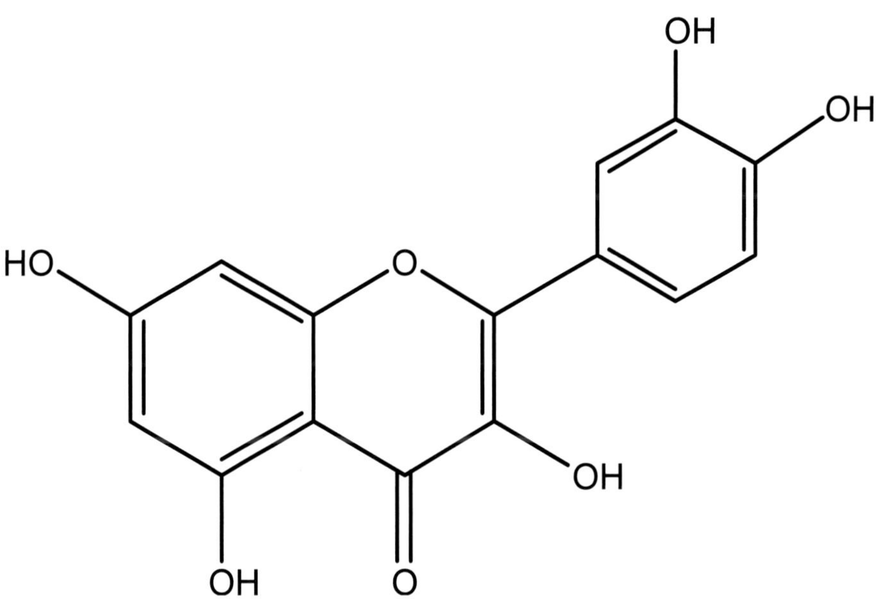

Quercetin [XV]

Contd...

Figure 17.4–*Contd...*

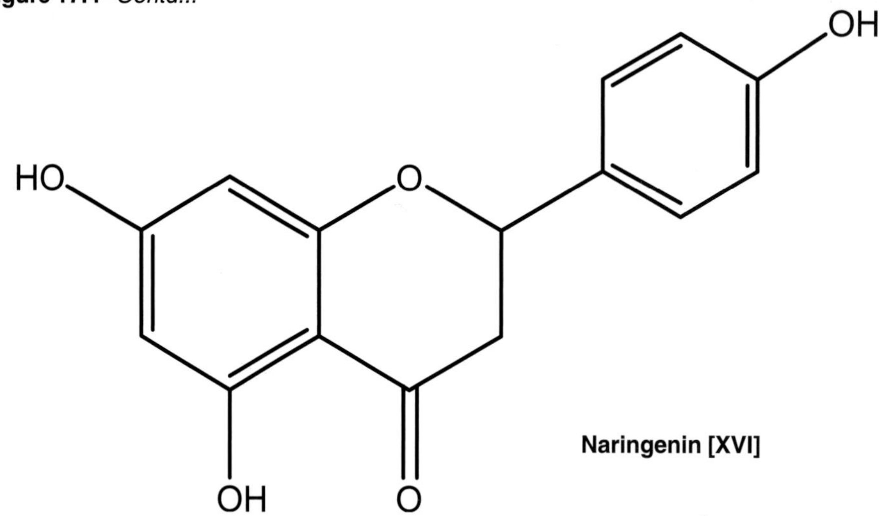

Naringenin [XVI]

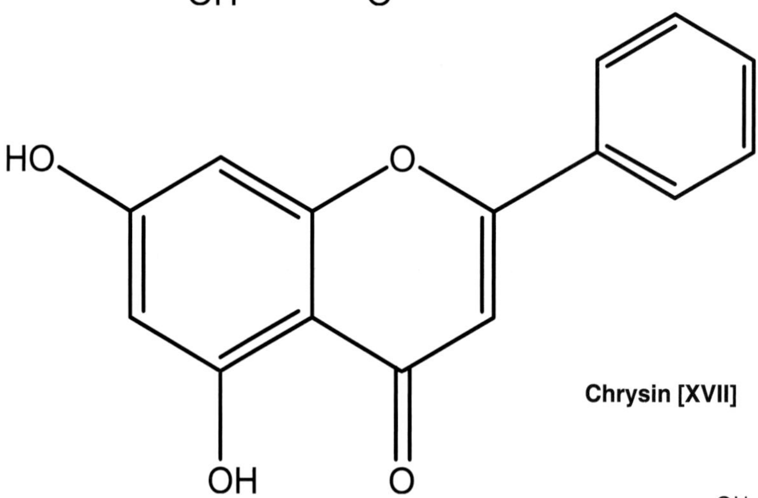

Chrysin [XVII]

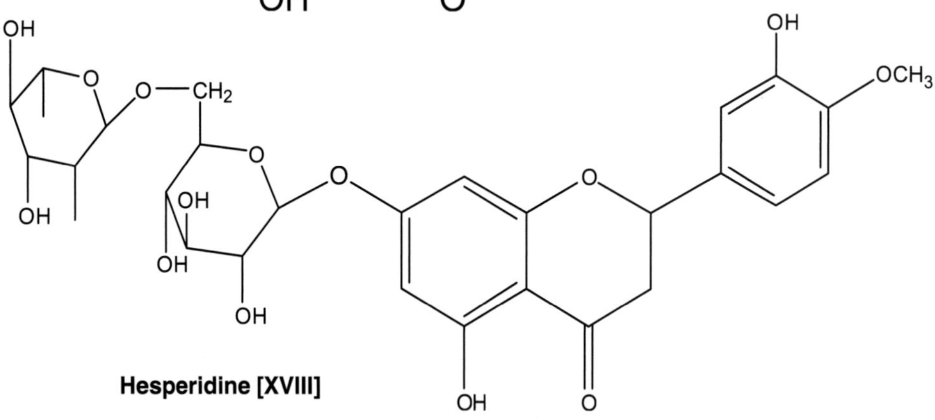

Hesperidine [XVIII]

Contd...

Figure 17.4–*Contd...*

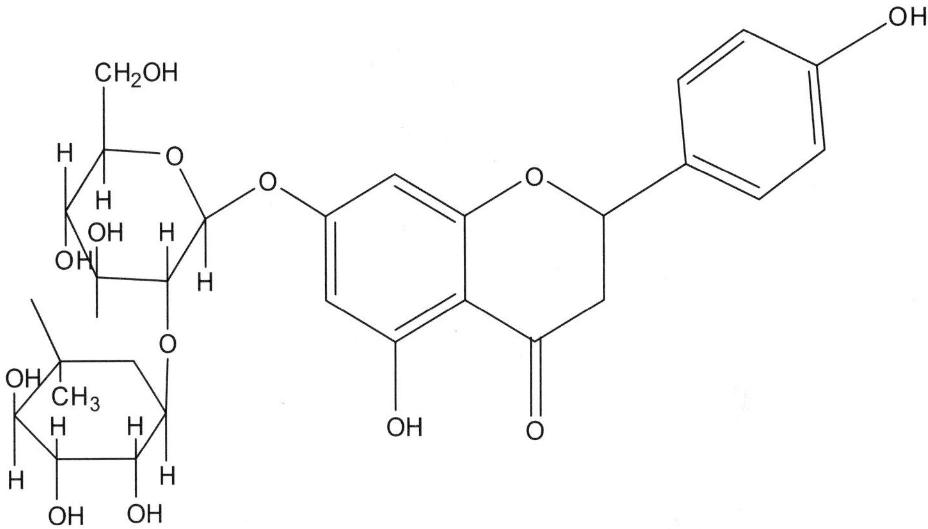

Naringin [XIX]

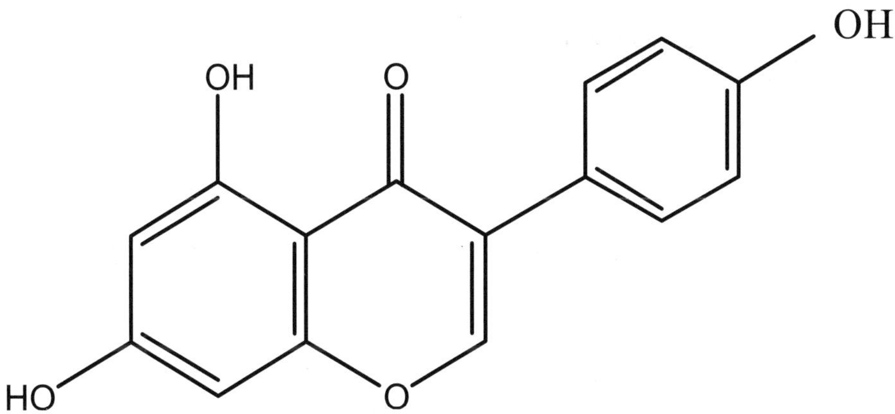

Genistein [XX]

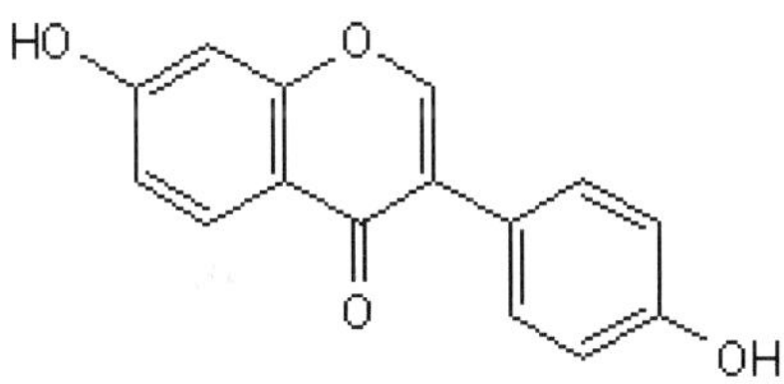

Daidzein [XXI]

Contd...

Figure 17.4–*Contd...*

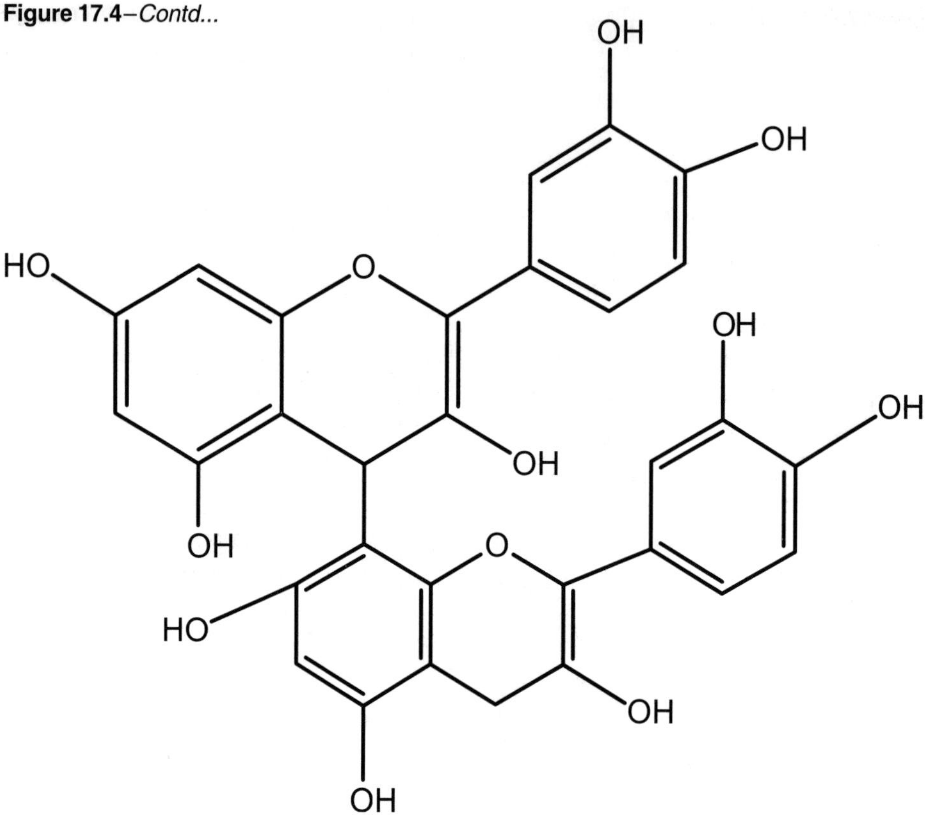

Proanthocyanodine [XXII]

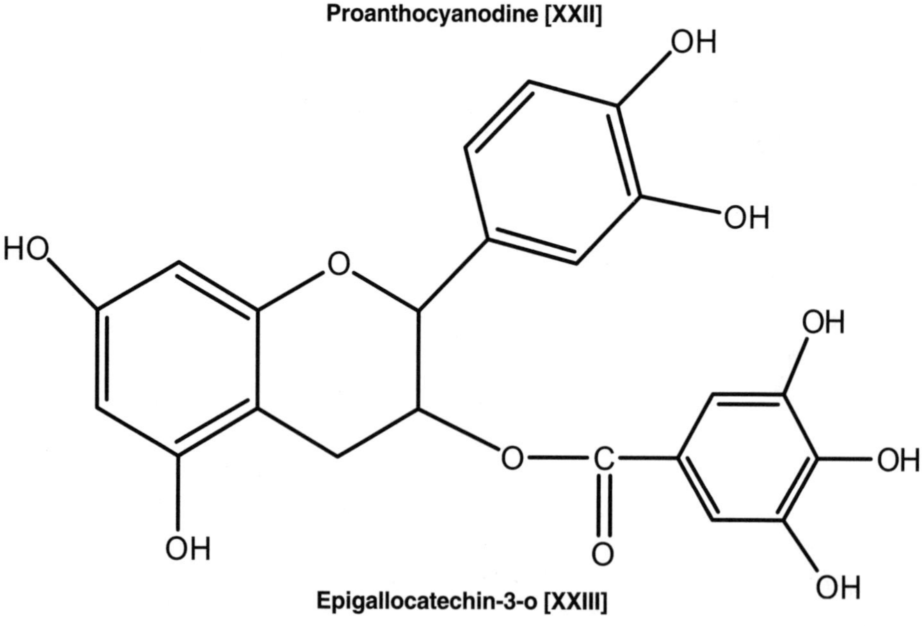

Epigallocatechin-3-o [XXIII]

Contd...

Figure 17.4–*Contd...*

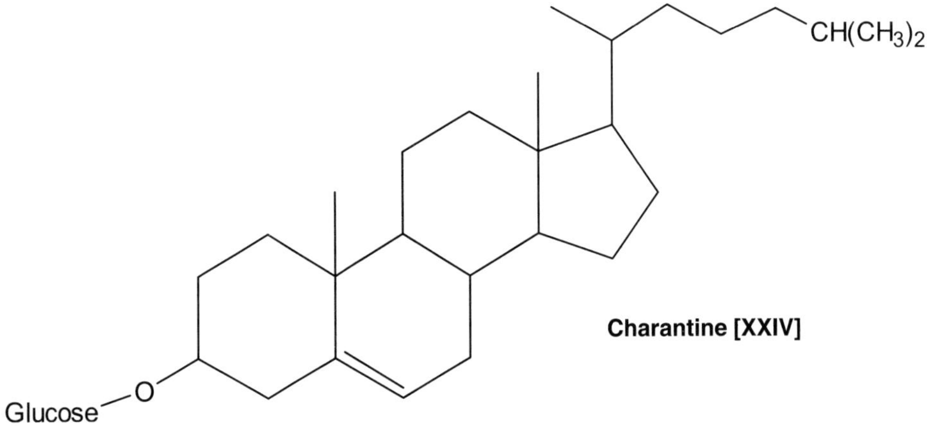

Charantine [XXIV]

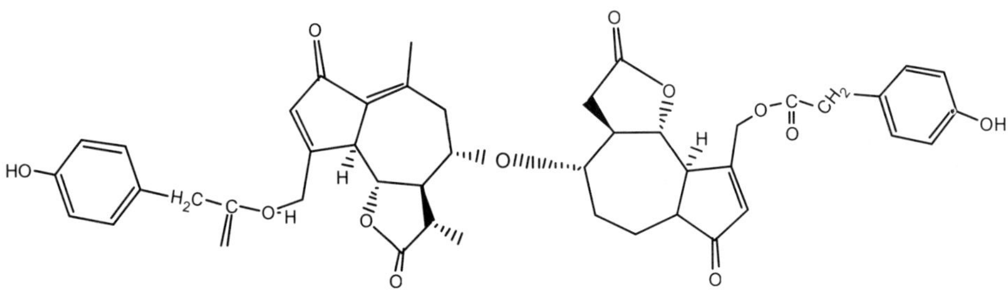

Lactucaine C [XXV]

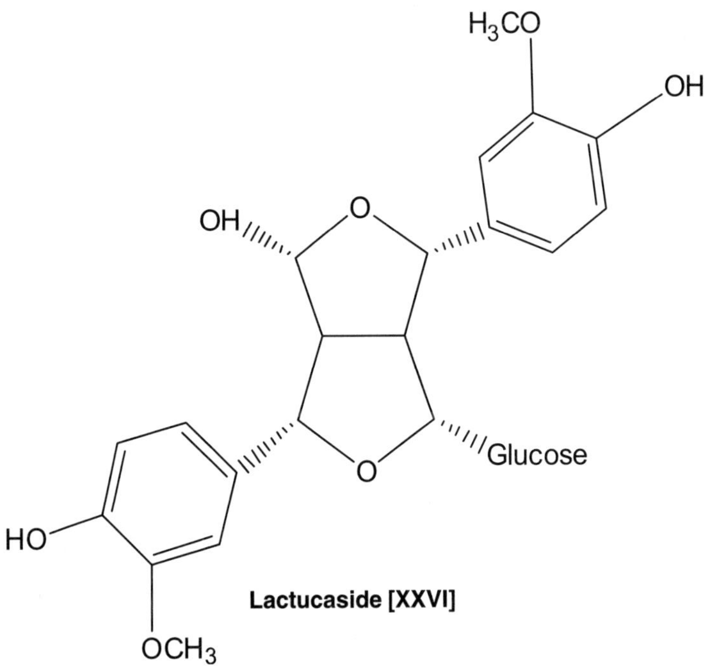

Lactucaside [XXVI]

Contd...

Of the few non-controlled trials that have been carried out on type 2 diabetics, most report improved glycaemic control. The hypoglycemic effect of fenugreek seeds has been demonstrated in experimentally induced diabetic rats, dogs, mice and healthy volunteers (both IDDM and NIDDM). Oral administration of aqueous leaf extract (0.06, 0.2, 0.5, 1 g/kg, i.p. and 1, 2, 8 g/kg p.o.) to normal and alloxanized diabetic rats showed significant anti-hyperglycemic effect while 50 per cent ethanolic extract significantly reduced blood glucose concentration ($P<0.02$) at 2 and 24 h when given i.p. (0.8 g/kg) (Abdel-Barry, 1997).

Terminalia catappa L. (Family: Combretaceae)

It is a large deciduous stately tree from India, growing up to 90 ft tall with horizontal whorls of branches. The effect of petroleum ether, methanol, and aqueous extracts of the fruit was examined on fasting blood sugar levels and serum biochemical parameters in alloxan-induced diabetic rats and produced significant hypoglycemic activity and alleviated the pancreatic necrosis produced by alloxan administration (Nagappa *et al.*, 2003).

Terminalia pallida Brandis (Family: Combretaceae)

It is a well-known plant found in various parts of India. Ethanolic fraction of fruits of *Terminalia pallida* has been reported to exhibit a significant antihyperglycemic activity in alloxan diabetic rats at a dose of 0.5 g/kg orally but failed to reduce the blood sugar level in normal rats (Kameswara Rao *et al.*, 2003b).

Tinospora cordifolia (Willd.) Hook.f. & Thonnson (Family: Menispermaceae)

It is a large climbing shrub found throughout India and used in various ailments. Various extracts of the leaves of this plant were investigated for their blood sugar lowering activity in normal and alloxanized rabbits in graded doses and the findings have proved that the plant has potent hypoglycemic activity (Wadood *et al.*, 1992; Prince and Menon, 1999; Stanely *et al.*, 1999; Grover *et al.*, 2000; Stanely and Menon, 2000, 2001, 2003; Prince *et al.*, 2004b, c).

Zingiber officinale Roscoe (Family: Zingiberaceae)

It is a dietary component widely cultivated in India and commonly known as ginger. The juice of *Zingiber officinale* administered at a dose of 4 ml/kg p.o. daily for 6 weeks significantly prevented hyperglycaemia and hypoinsulinaemia in streptozotocin (STZ)-induced type I diabetic rats. It also produced a significant increase in insulin levels and a decrease in fasting glucose levels in diabetic rats. In an oral glucose tolerance test, the extract was found to decrease the glucose level and to increase the insulin level significantly in STZ-diabetic rats and suggested that hypoglycemic activity of the juice of *Zingiber officinale* in type I diabetic rats possibly involved 5-HT receptors (Akhani *et al.*, 2004).

Zizyphus sativa Gaertn. (Family: Rhamnaceae)

It is a small spreading tree with drooping branches. An alcoholic extract of *Zizyphus sativa* leaves was tested for hypoglycemic activity in normal and alloxan-diabetic rats. Single (100-400 mg/kg) oral doses of extract to normal animals showed a dose-dependent statistically significant lowering of blood glucose 2, 4 and 6 h later. The effect was most pronounced at 6 h with blood glucose returning to control values at 24 h. In alloxan-diabetic rats, no significant effect was observed with extract and tolbutamide. The minimum lethal dose was greater than 3000 mg/kg, orally in mice (Anand *et al.*, 1989).

Phytoconstituents with Hypoglycemic Potentials

Compounds with different structure but with the same therapeutic activity isolated from different plant species act as active moieties for the treatment of various diseases. Some of these active principles originate from edible plants and their inclusion in the diet would undoubtedly be of some value because of their hypoglycemic potential. Several phytomolecules including flavonoids, alkaloids, glycosides, saponins, glycolipids, dietary fibres, polysaccharides, peptidoglycans, carbohydrates, amino acids and others obtained from various plant sources have been reported as potent hypoglycemic agent as has been further explained in the following section. The chemical structures of a few potential phytomolecules with hypoglycemic activity are shown in Figure 17.4.

Alkaloids

Various alkaloids have been isolated from numerous Indian medicinal plants and investigated for their possible hypoglycemic activity in different animal models. Berberine (Figure 17.3, [IX]) is known to have potent hypoglycemic activity. It is obtained from *Tinospora cordifolia* (Singh *et al.*, 2003). The mode of its antihyperglycemic activity was investigated in the CaCo-2 cell line. Berberine effectively inhibited the activity of disaccharidases in CaCo-2 cells, decreased sucrase activity after preincubation with CaCo-2 cells for 72 h but failed to produce any significant effect on gluconeogenesis and glucose consumption of CaCo-2 cells, suggesting that the antihyperglycaemic activity of berberine is at least partly due to its ability to inhibit alpha-glucosidase and decrease glucose transport through the intestinal epithelium (Pan *et al.*, 2003). Alkaloids like catharanthine [X], vindoline [XI] and vindolinine [XII] (Figure 17.4), obtained from *Catharanthus roseus* also lower blood sugar level (Chattopadhyay, 1999).

Imidazoline Compounds

Certain imidazoline compounds are known to have a stimulatory action on insulin secretion by activation of imidazoline I (3) binding sites in the pancreatic beta cell. Beta-carbolines, having activity at imidazoline sites been studied for their effects on insulin secretion. Harmane (Figure 17.4, [XIII]), norharmane and pinoline (Figure 17.4, [XIV]), the beta-carbolines were found to increase insulin secretion two- to three-fold from isolated human islets of Langerhans. Harmane and norharmane obtained from *Tribulus terrestris* L. and may account for the hypoglycemic property of the plant (Nadkarni, 1976; Kirtikar and Basu, 1993). Harmane stimulates insulin secretion in a glucose-dependent manner. The results strongly substantiated the claim of beta-carbolines as potent insulin secretagogues (Cooper *et al.*, 2003).

Polysaccharides

Various Indian hypoglycemic plants like *Aloe vera, Ocimum sanctum, Alpinia galanga* are found to contain polysaccharides. A protein-bound polysaccharide, isolated from water-soluble substances of pumpkin was investigated for hypoglycemic activity in various doses (500 and 1000 mg/kg body weight) in alloxan diabetic rats. The results indicated that the polysaccharides increased the levels of serum insulin, reduce the blood glucose levels and improve tolerance of glucose (Quanhong *et al.*, 2005).

Flavonoids

Flavonoids represent another beneficial group of naturally occuring compounds with hypoglycemic potentials. These are widely distributed in plant kingdom and exhibit distinctive pharmacological properties. The flavonoids can be widely classified into different categories like flavanols, flavones, catechins, flavanones, etc. Some flavonoids have hypoglycemic properties because they improve altered glucose and oxidative metabolisms of diabetic states. Quercetin (Figure 17.4, [XV]) is an important flavonoid known to possess a vast array of pharmacological activities. Intraperitoneal administration of quercetin to normal as well as streptozocin-induced diabetic rats resulted in marked reduction in plasma glucose level of diabetic animals while the glucose level of the normoglycemic rats remained unalterd. Quecrcetin also suppressed the glucose level in diabetic rats in a glucose tolerance test, reduced plasma cholesterol and triglycerides significantly and increased their hepatic glucokinase activity probably by enhancing the insulin release from pancreatic islets of the diabetic rats (Vessal *et al.,* 2003). Some flavonoid molecules like quercetin, naringenin [XVI], chrysin [XVII] (Figure 17.4) significantly enhanced the insulin release from isolated rat islets of Langerhans in presence of 20 mmol glucose/l. Quercetin exerted its stimulatory effect on insulin release partly by changing Ca^{2+} metabolism (Hii and Howell, 1985). Effect of citrus bioflavonoids, hesperidin [XVIII] and naringin [XIX] (Figure 17.4), on blood glucose level, hepatic glucose-regulating enzymes activities, hepatic glycogen concentration, and plasma insulin levels was investigated in male C57BL/KsJ-db/db mice, an animal model for Type II diabetes.

Supplementation of the citrus flavonoids (0.2 g/kg diet) in the diet significantly reduced the blood glucose level as well as increased hepatic glucokinase activity and glycogen concentration in diabetic rats. Naringin also markedly lowered the activity of hepatic glucose-6-phosphatase and phosphoenolpyruvate carboxykinase and the plasma insulin, C-peptide, and leptin levels in the diabetic mice were significantly increased as a result of supplementation. The findings suggested that hesperidin and naringin both play important roles in preventing the progression of hyperglycemia, partly by increasing hepatic glycolysis and glycogen concentration and/or by lowering hepatic gluconeogenesis (Jung *et al.,* 2004). The soy isoflavones genistein [XX] or daidzein [XXI] (Figure 17.4) were investigated for their possible hypoglycemic activity in male and female obese Zucker rats, a model of Type II diabetes.

Peroxisome-proliferator activated receptors (PPAR) are promiscuous nuclear receptors that regulate the transcription of genes involved in lipid and glucose homeostasis and lipid metabolism within the cell. The results of the study indicated that the isoflavones significantly improved lipid and glucose metabolism by acting as an hypoglycemic PPAR agonist (Mezei *et al.,* 2003). Proanthocyanidins (Figure 17.4, [XXII]) the flavonoids with an oligomeric structure, are found to improve the pathological oxidative state of a diabetic situation. An extract of grape seed procyanidins administered orally to streptozotocin-induced diabetic rats produced significant antihyperglycemic activity possibly by its insulinomimetic activity. It also stimulated glucose uptake in insulin sensitive cells*in vitro* (Pinent*et al.,*2004). Another flavonoid glycoside Kaempferitrin (Kaempferol-3,7-*O*-(alpha)-l-dirhamnoside) was found to have an acute lowering effect on blood glucose in diabetic rats and stimulated the glucose uptake, as efficiently as insulin in muscle from normal rats *in vitro,* suggesting that blood glucose lowering activity of the compound attributed to altered intrinsic activity of the glucose transporter (Jorge *et al.,* 2004). The hypoglycemic activity of the compound was also studied along with its antioxidant potential in normal and in alloxan-induced diabetic rats. Oral administration of the compound (200 mg/kg) significantly reduced the blood glucose level in normal rats 1 h after treatment and the antihyperglycemic activity in diabetic rats was observed at all doses tested (50, 100, and 200 mg/kg) throughout the period of the study. Green tea flavonoid, epigallocatechin gallate (Figure 17.4, [XXIII]) is reported to have glucose-lowering effects in animals. It was found to decrease hepatic glucose production and increased tyrosine phosphorylation of the insulin receptor and insulin receptor substrate-1 (IRS-1) like insulin. It also reduces phosphoenolpyruvate carboxykinase gene expression in a phosphoinositide 3-kinase-dependent manner and mimics insulin by increasing phosphoinositide 3-kinase, mitogen-activated protein kinase, and p70 (s6k) activity. These findings suggest that epigallocatechin gallate is an important hypoglycemic agent (Waltner-Law *et al.,*2002). Another flavonoid molecule, (–)-epicatechin (VII), has been reported to possess insulin-like activity. Chakravarthy *et al.* (1981) suggested that the molecule protected the experimental albino rats against the diabetogenic actions of alloxan. This flavonoid molecule mimics insulin in its effect on erythrocyte membrane acetylcholinesterase (AChE) and has a pronounced insulin-like effect on erythrocyte membrane-bound AChE in Type II diabetic patients (Rizvi *et al.,* 1995; Rizvi and Zaid, 2001).

Dietary Fibers

The role of dietary fibers in diabetes has been studied by several workers. Long term dietary treatment with increased amounts of fiber rich low glycaemic index natural foods improves blood glucose levels and reduces the number of hypoglycemic events in type I diabetic patients (Nandini *et al.,* 2003). The hypgolycaemic and antihyperglycaemic actions of fenugreek have been attributed both to gastrointestinal effects of local dietary fibre (Madar *et al.,* 1988). A study investigated the effect of dietary carbohydrate and fiber on mucosal insulin receptors in order to correlate changes in cellular proliferation with hormonal responsiveness. It revealed that insulin binding was significantly affected by the consumption of dietary fiber (MacDonald*et al.,* 1991). A high insoluble fiber diet containing 15 per cent cellulose in dry matter, high soluble fiber diet containing 15 per cent pectin in dry matter and low fiber diet was tested for effect on glycemic control in six dogs with alloxan-induced insulin-dependent diabetes mellitus. High insoluble fiber and soluble fiber diet fed animals showed significant lowering in the mean postprandial plasma glucose concentration in comparison to the low fiber diet fed dogs (Nelson *et al.*, 1991). Effect of soluble (5 per cent guar gum) and insoluble (10 per cent wheat bran) dietary fibre supplementation on glycaemic control and nephropathy was investigated in streptozotocin-treated diabetic rats and the results indicated that both soluble and insoluble dietary fibers ameliorated a significant increase in the activity of GFAT and decrease in the renal content of heparan sulfate in diabetic animals (Nandini *et al.*, 2003). Another study involving insoluble fiber rich fractions including insoluble dietary fiber, alcohol insoluble solid, and water insoluble solid, obtained from the peel of *Citrus sinensis* showed that the fiber rich fraction effectively absorbed glucose, retard glucose diffusion and inhibit the activity of alpha-amylase to different extents and may be responsible for decreasing the rate of glucose absorption and concentration of postprandial serum glucose (Chau *et al.*, 2003).

Saponins: Triterpenoid and Steroidal Glycosides

Triterpenoid and steroidal glycosides, referred to collectively as saponins, are bioactive compounds present naturally in many plants and known to possess potent hypoglycemic activity (Rao and Gurfinkel, 2000). Charantin (Figure 17.4, [XXIV]), a steroidal saponin, obtained from *Momordica charantia* is known to have an insulin-like activity, responsible for its hypoglycemic effect (Ng *et al.*, 1986a). Charantin stimulates the release of insulin and blocks the formation of glucose in the bloodstream, which may be helpful in the treatment of diabetes, particularly in non-insulin-dependent diabetes. Lactucain C (Figure 17.4, [XXV]) and furofuran lignan, lactucaside (Figure 17.4, [XXVI]), obtained from *Lactuca indica* found to produce significant hypoglycemic activity (Hou *et al.*, 2003). β-Sitosterol (Figure 17.4, [XXVII]), a steroid obtained from *Azadirachta indica*, may be responsible for its hypoglycemic property. Andrographolide, another diterpenoid lactone, obtained from *Andrographis paniculata* Nees was found to possess significant hypoglycemic activity (Yu *et al.*, 2003). Gymnemic acid IV, obtained from leaves of *Gymnema sylvestre* exhibits potent hypoglycemic activity in experimental animals models of diabetes (Sugihara *et al.*, 2000).

Ferulic Acid

It is 4-hydroxy-3-methoxycinnamic acid (Figure 17.4, [XXVIII]) found in the leaves and seeds of many plants like *Curcuma longa* L. Oral administration of ferulic acid at low dose produced significant hypoglycemic activity in both types of diabetes as evident from a study on streptozotocin-induced diabetic mice and KK-Ay mice. The study suggested potent antioxidant activity of the compound in addition to its blood glucose lowering activity in experimental hyperglycemia in animals (Ohnishi *et al.*, 2004). An *in vitro* study utilising rat pancreatic RIN-5F cell suggested that amide compounds, derived from ferulic acid have stimulatory effects on insulin secretion (Nomura *et al.*, 2003).

Table 17.1. Chemical constituents from some herbs reported for anti-diabetic activity.

Sl.No.	*Vernacular Name*	*Chemical Constituents*
1.	*Blighia sapida*	Amino acids (Hypoglycin A, Hypoglycin B) (Handa *et al.*, 1989).
2.	*Azadirachta indica*	Quercetin, Quercetrin, Nimboflavone, Nimbin, Rutin (Pillai and Santhakumari, 1981).
3.	*Poterium ancisroides*	Triterpenoids (Tormantic acid) (Chauhan *et al.*, 2010).
4.	*Trigonella foenum graceum*	Trigonellin, Salicylic acid (Shani *et al.* 1974).
5.	*Allium cepa*	Sulphide (Allicin) Allylpropyldisulphide (Augusti, 1976).
6.	*Cantharus roseus*	Alkaloids (Catharanthine), (Leurosine) (Lochnerine), Vindoline etc. (Khosla, 2000)
7.	*Pterocarpus marsupium*	Flavonoid [(–) – epicatechin] (Kuruvilla, 1981)
8.	*Gymnema sylvestre*	Gymnemic acid, Quercetin, Gymnemogenin (Sugihara *et al.*, 2000).
9.	Dioscorea japonica	(Dioscoran A,B,C,D,E,F) (Hikino et al., 1986).
10.	*Momoradica charantia*	Charantin, Polypeptide-p, Ascorbigen, Momordicin (Harinantenaina *et al.*, 1986).

Polyherbal Formulations

Ayurveda is the oldest healing system of medicine. Major formulations used in Ayurveda are based on herbs. The medicinal herbs are used in the form of decoctions, infusions, tinctures, and powders. These are considered as safe since they are natural products. Herbal formulations which have gained widespread acceptability as therapeutic agents in India include anti-diabetics, hepatoprotective and lipid lowering agents. Some polyherbals formulations for diabetes are being marketed in India (Table 17.2). However, there are many limitations regarding safety and efficacy of these preparations.

- ☆ Knowledge about active principles of herbal preparations are not well defined.
- ☆ Information on toxicity and adverse effects of these formulations are lacking.
- ☆ Information regarding pharmacokinetics and bioavailability is not available.

Selection of plant material based on quality, standardization of methods of preparation, enforcement of regulation regarding appropriate labels, are measures which will improve the quality and acceptability of herbal preparations as therapeutic agents.

Today, chromatographic methods HPLC, GC, HPTLC are used for identifying active constituent of medicinal herbs. The modern technology have brought revolution in the field of herbal medicine, particularly in case of single plant based formulation. The concept of standardization is fast catching with herbal products based on active constituent.

Anand, K.K., Singh, B., Chand, D., Chandan, B.K. and Gupta, V.N. (1989). Effect of *Zizyphus sativa* leaves on blood glucose levels in normal and alloxan-diabetic rats. *Journal of Ethnopharmacology*, **27**: 121–127.

Ananthan, R., Latha, M., Pari, L., Ramkumar, K.M., Baskar, C.G. and Bai, V.N. (2003). Effect of *Gymnema montanum* leaves on serum and tissue lipids in alloxan diabetic rats. *Experimental Diabesity Research*, **4**: 183–189.

Ananthan, R., Latha, M., Pari, L., Ramkumar, K.M, Baskar, C.G. and Bai, V.N. (2004). Modulatory effects of *Gymnema montanum* leaf extract on alloxan-induced oxidative stress in Wistar rats. *Nutrition*, **20**: 280–285.

Ananthan, R., Latha, M., Pari, L., Ramkumar, K.M., Baskar, C.G. and Bai, V.N. (2003). Effect of *Gymnema montanum* on blood glucose, plasma insulin, and carbohydrate metabolic enzymes in alloxan-induced diabetic rats. *Journal of Medicinal Food*, **6**: 43–49.

Anonymous (1992). Bangladesh National Formulatory of Ayurvedic medicines. **116**: 20.

Anuradha, C.V. and Ravikumar, P. (2001). Restoration on tissue antioxidants by fenugreek seeds (*Trigonella foenum graecum*) in alloxan-diabetic rats. *Indian Journal of Physiology and Pharmacology*, **45**: 408–420.

Anusha Bhaskar, Vidhya, V.G. and Ramya, M. (2008). Hypoglycemic effect of *Mucuna pruriens* seed extract on normal and streptozotocin-diabetic rats. *Fitoterapia*, **79**: 7-8.

Arai, I., Amagaya, S., Komatsu, Y., Okada, M., Hayashi, T., Kasai, M., Arisawa, M. and Momose, Y. (1999). Improving effects of the extracts from *Eugenia uniflora* on hyperglycemia and hypertriglyceridemia in mice. *Journal of Ethnopharmacology*, **68**: 307–314.

Atkinson, M.A. and Maclaren, N.K. (1994). The pathogenesis of insulin-dependent diabetes mellitus. *N Engl J Med.*, **331**: 1428-1436.

Augusti, K.S. (1976). Chromatographic analysis of onion principles and a study on their hypoglycaemic action. *Indian J Exp Biol.*, **14 (2)**: 110.

Augusti, K.T. (1973). Studies on the effects of a hypoglycemic principle from *Allium Cepa* Linn. *Indian Journal of Medical Research*, **61**: 1066–1071.

Augusti, K.T., Joseph, P. and Babu, T.D. (1995). Biologically active principles isolated from *Salacia oblonga* wall. *Indian Journal of Physiology and Pharmacology*, **39**: 415–417.

Bae, M.A., Rhee, H. and Song, B.J. (2003). Troglitazone but not rosiglitazone induces G1 cell arrest and apoptosis in human and rat hepatoma cell lines. *Toxicol Lett.*, **139**: 67-75.

Bearse, M.A., Jr Han, T. and Schneck, M.E. (2004). Local multifocal oscillatory potential abnormalities in diabetes and early diabetic retinopathy. *Invest Ophthal Vis Sci.*, **45**: 3259-3265.

Bernhard Ludvik., Beatrice Neuffer. and Giovanni Pacini. (2004). Efficacy of *Ipomoea batatas* (Caiapo) on Diabetes Control in Type 2 Diabetic Subjects Treated With Diet. *Diabetes Care,* **27**: 2.

Betterle, C., Zannette, F. and Pedini, B. (1983). Clinical and subclinical organ-specific autoimmune manifestations in type 1 (insulin-dependent) diabetic patients and their first-degree relatives. *Diabetologia,* **26**: 431-436.

Beverley, B. and Eschwège, E. (2003). The diagnosis and classification of diabetes and impaired glucose tolerance. *Textbook of Diabetes,* **3**: 2.1-2.11.

Bischoff, H. (1995). The mechanism of α-glucosidase inhibition in the management of diabetes. *Clin Invest Med.,* **18**: 303-311.

Bisset, N.G. (1994). Herbal Drugs and Phytopharmaceuticals. Boca Raton, FL: CRC Press.

Bolli, G.B. (1997). Hypoglycaemia unawareness. *Diabetes Metab.,* **23(3)**: 29-35.

Borhanuddin, M., Shamsuzzoha, M., and Hussain, A. H. (1994). *Bangladesh Med Res Counc Bul.,* **20(1)**: 24-6.

Bose, S.N. and Sepaha, G.C. (1956). Clinical observations on the hypoglycemic properties of *Pterocarpus marsupium* and *Eugenia jambolana*. *Journal of the Indiana State Medical Association,* **27**: 388–391.

Brahmachari, H.D. and Augusti, K.T. (1964). Isolation of orally effective hypoglycemic compounds from *Ficus bengalensis* Linn. *Indian Jornal of Physiology and Pharmacology,* **13**: 60–64.

Cakici, I., Hurmoglu, C., Tunctan, B., Abacioglu, N., Kanzik, I. and Sener, B. (1994). Hypoglycemic effect of *Momordica charantia* extracts in normoglycemic or cyproheptadine-induced hyperglycemic mice. *Journal of Ethnopharmacology,* **44**: 117–121.

Campos, K.E., Diniz, Y.S., Cataneo, A.C., Faine,L.A., Alves, M.J. and Novelli, E.L. (2003). Hypoglycaemic and antioxidant effects of onion, *Allium cepa*: dietary onion addition, antioxidant activity and hypoglycaemic effects on diabetic rats. *International Journal of Food Sciences and Nutrition,* **54**: 241–246.

Chakrabarti, S., Biswas, T.K., Seal, T., Rokeya, B., Ali, L., Azad Khan, A.K., Nahar, N., Mosihuzzaman, M. and Mukherjee, B. (2005). Antidiabetic activity of *Caesalpinia bonducella* F. in chronic type 2 diabetic model in Long-Evans rats and evaluation of insulin secretagogue property of its fractions on isolated islets. *J. Ethnopharmacol.,* **97(1)**: 117-22.

Chakrabarti, S., Kanti, B. T., Rokeya, B., Ali, L., Mosihuzzaman, M., Nahar, N., Azad Khan, A. K., and Mukherjee, B. (2003). Advanced studies on the hypoglycemic effect of *Caesalpinia bonducella* F. in type 1 and 2 diabetes in Long Evans rats. *Journal of Ethnopharmacology,* **84(1)**: 41-46.

Chattopadhyay, R.R. (1996). Possible mechanism of antihyperglycemic effect of *Azadirachta indica* leaf extract, part IV. *General Pharmacology,* **27**: 431–434.

Chattopadhyay, R.R. (1998). Possible mechanism of antihyperglycemic effect of *Gymnema sylvestre* leaf extract, part I. *General Pharmacology*. **31 (3)**: 495–496.

Chattopadhyay, R.R. (1999). A comparative evaluation of some blood sugar lowering agents of plant origin. *Journal of Ethnopharmacology*, **67**: 367–372.

Chau, C.F., Huang, Y.L. and Lee, M.H. (2003). *In vitro* hypoglycemic effects of different insoluble fiber-rich fractions prepared from the peel of *Citrus sinensis* L. cv. Liucheng. *Journal of Agricultural and Food Chemistry*, **51**: 6623–6626.

Chempakam, B. (1993). Hypoglycemic activity of arecoline in betel nut *Areca catechu* L. *Indian Journal of Experimental Biology*, **31**: 474–475.

Chen, F., Nakashima, N., Kimura, I. and Kimura, M. (1995). Hypoglycemic activity and mechanisms of extracts from mulberry leaves (*folium mori*) and cortex mori radicis in streptozotocin-induced diabetic mice. *Yakugaku Zasshi*, **115**: 476-482.

Cheng, D. (2005). Prevalence, predisposition and prevention of type II diabetes. *Nut Metab.*, **18**: 2-29.

Choudhury, K.D. and Basu, N.K. (1967). Phytochemical and hypoglycemic investigation of *Casearia esculenta*. *Journal of Pharmaceutical Sciences*, **56**: 1405–1409.

Coimbra, T.C., Danni, F.F., Blotta, R.M., Da Periara, C.A., Guedes, M.D. and Graf, R.G. (1992). Plants employed in the treatment of diabetes mellitus, results of an ethnopharmacological survey in Porto Alegre, Brazil. *Fitoterapia*, **63**: 320–322.

Cooper, E.J., Hudson, A.L., Parker, C.A. and Morgan, N.G. (2003). Effects of the beta-carbolines, harmane and pinoline, on insulin secretion from isolated human islets of Langerhans. *European Journal of Pharmacology*, **482**: 189-196.

DeFronzo, R.A. (1999). Pharmacologic therapy for type 2 diabetes mellitus. *Ann Intern Med.*, **131**: 281-303.

Deshmukh, V.K., Shrotri, D.S. and Aiman, R. (1960). Isolation of a hypoglycemic principle from the bark of *Ficus bengalensis* Linn. A preliminary note. *Indian Journal of Physiology and Pharmacology*, **4**: 182–185.

Devi, G., Falco, A. and Patrono, C. (2005). Lipid peroxidation in diabetic mellitus. *Antioxid Redox Signal*, **7**: 256-268.

Dhar, M.L., Dhar, M.M., Dhawan, B.N., Mehrotra, B.N. and Ray, C. (1968). Screening of Indian plants for biological activity. *Indian Journal of Experimental Biology*, **6(4)**: 232–247.

Dolly, Jaiswal., Prashant, Kumar.Rai., Amit, Kumar and Geeta, Watal. (2008). Study of glycemic profile of *Cajanus cajan* leaves in experimental rats. *Indian Journal of Clinical Biochemistry*, **23(2)**: 167-170

El-Demerdash, F.M., Yousef, M.I. and El-Naga, N.I. (2005). Biochemical study on the hypoglycemic effects of onion and garlic in alloxan-induced diabetic rats. *Food and Chemical Toxicology*, **43**: 57–63.

Eriksson, J., Saloranta, C. and Widen, E. (1991). Non-esterified fatty acids do not contribute to insulin resistance in persons at increased risk of developing type 2 (noninsulin- dependent) diabetes mellitus. *Diabetologia*, **34**: 192-197.

Esmaillzadeh, A., Tahbaz, F., Gaieni, I., Alavi-Majd, H. and Azadbakht, L. (2004). Concentrated pomegranate juice improves lipid profiles in diabetic patients with hyperlipidemia. *Journal of Medicinal Food*, **7:** 305–308.

Fushiki, T., Kojima, A., Imoto, T., Inoue, K. and Sugimoto, E. (1992). An extract of *Gymnema sylvestre* leaves and purified gymnemic acid inhibits glucose-stimulated gastric inhibitory peptide secretion in rats. *Journal of Nutrition*, **122**: 2367–2373.

Ganesh, T., Saikat, Sen., Thilagam, E., Thamotharan, G., Loganathan, T. and Raja, Chakraborty. (2010). Pharmacognostic and anti-hyperglycemic evaluation of *Lantana camara* (L.) var. aculeate leaves in alloxan-induced hyperglycemia. I*nt. J. Res. Pharm. Sci.*, **1(3)**: 247-252.

Garg, S.K., Shah, M.A., Garg, K.M., Farooqui, M.M. and Sabir, M. (1997). Antilymphocytic and immunosuppressive effects of *Lantana camara* leaves in rats. *Indian Journal of Experimental Biology*, **35**: 1315–1318.

Genet, S., Kale, R.K and Baquer, N.Z. (2002). Alterations in antioxidant enzymes and oxidative damage in experimental diabetic rat tissues: effect of vanadate and fenugreek (*Trigonella foenum graecum*). *Molecular and Cellular Biochemistry*, **236**: 7–12.

Ghafghazi, T., Sheria,t H.S., Dastmalchi, T., and Barnett, R.C. (1977). Antagonism of cadmium and alloxan-induced hyperglycemia in rats by *Trigonella foenum graecum. Pahlavi Medical Journal*, **8**: 14–25.

Gholap, S. and Kar. (2003). Effects of *Inula racemosa* root and *Gymnema sylvestre* leaf extracts in the regulation of corticosteroid induced diabetes mellitus: involvement of thyroid hormones. *Pharmazie*, **58**: 413–415.

Gomes, A., Vedasiromoni, J.R., Das, M., Sharma, R.M. and Ganguly, D.K. (1995). Anti-hyperglycemic effect of black tea (*Camellia sinensis*) in rat. *Journal of Ethnopharmacology*, **45(3)**: 223-226.

Gray, A.M. and Flat, P.R. (1998). Antihyperglycemic actions of *Eucalyptus globulus* (Eucalyptus) are associated with pancreatic and extra-pancreatic effects in mice. *Journal of Nutrition*, **128(12)**: 2319–2323.

Grossman, E. and Messerli, F.H. (1996). Diabetic and hypertensive heart disease. *Ann Int Med.*, **125**: 304-310.

Grover, J.K., Vats, V. and Rathi, S.S. (2000). Anti-hyperglycemic effect of *Eugenia jambolana* and *Tinospora cordifolia* in experimental diabetes and their effects on key metabolic enzymes involved in carbohydrate metabolism. *Journal of Ethnopharmacology*, **73**: 461–470.

Gulubova, R. and Boiadzhiev, T.S. (1975). Morphological changes in the endocrine pancreas of the rabbit after the administration of a *Morus alba* extract. *Eksperimentalna meditsina i morfologiia*, **14**: 166-171.

Pari, L. and Venkateswaran, S. (2003). Protective effect of *Coccinia indica* on changes in the fatty acid composition in streptozotocin induced diabetic rats. *Pharmazie.*, **58(6)**: 409-412.

Pari, L., Pinent, M., Blay, M., Blade, M.C., Salvado, M.J., Arola, L. and Ardevol, A. (2004). Grape seed-derived procyanidins have an antihyperglycemic effect in streptozotocin-induced diabetic rats and insulinomimetic activity in insulin-sensitive cell lines. *Endocrinology*, **145**: 4985–4990.

Persaud, S.J., Al-Majed, H., Raman, A. and Jones, P.M. (1999). *Gymnema sylvestre* stimulates insulin release *in vitro* by increased membrane permeability. *Journal of Endocrinology*, **163**: 207–212.

Ponnachan, P.T.C., Paulose, C.S. and Panikar, K.P. (1993). Effect of leaf extract of *Aegle marmelos* in diabetic rats. *Indian J Exp Biol.*, **31**: 345-347.

Prakasam, A., Sethupathy, S., and Pugalendi, K.V. (2004). Influence of *Casearia esculenta* root extract on protein metabolism and marker enzymes in streptozotocin-induced diabetic rats. *Polish Journal of Pharmacology*, **56**: 587–593.

Prince, P.S. and Menon, V.P. (1999). Antioxidant activity of *Tinospora cordifolia* roots in experimental diabetes. *Journal of Ethnopharmacology*, **65**: 277–281.

Prince, P.S., Kamalakkannan, N. and Menon, V.P. (2004). Restoration of antioxidants by ethanolic *Tinospora cordifolia* in alloxan-induced diabetic Wistar rats. *Acta Poloniae Pharmaceutica*, **61**: 283–287.

Prince, P.S., Padmanabhan, M. and Menon, V.P. (2004). Restoration of antioxidant defence by ethanolic *Tinospora cordifolia* root extract in alloxan-induced diabetic liver and kidney. *Phytotherapy Research*, **18**: 785–787.

Pushparaj, P.N., Tan, C.H. and Tan, B.K.H. (2001). The mechanism of hypoglycemic action of the semi-purified fractions of *Averrhoa bilimbi* in streptozotocin diabetic rats. *Life Sciences*, **70(5)**: 535–547.

Quanhong, L., Caili, F., Yukui, R., Guanghui, H. and Tongyi, C. (2005). Effects of protein-bound polysaccharide isolated from pumpkin on insulin in diabetic rats. *Plant Foods for Human Nutrition*, **60**: 13–16.

Raffel, L.J., Scheuner, M.T. and Rotter, J.I. (1997). Genetic diabetes. *Porte D Jr, Sherwin RS, eds. Ellenberg and Rifkin's Diabetes Mellitus*, **5**: 401-454.

Rahier, J., Goebbles, R.M. and Henquin, J.C. (1983). Cellular composition of the human diabetic pancreas. *Diabetologia Metab.*, **22**: 153-156.

Ramarao, P. and Kaul, C.L. (1999). Insulin resistance: Current therapeutic approaches. *Drugs Today*, **35**: 895-911.

Ramkumar, K.M., Latha, M., Venkateswaran, S., Pari, L., Ananthan, R. and Bai, V.N. (2004). Modulatory effect of *Gymnema montanum* leaf extract on brain antioxidant status and lipid peroxidation in diabetic rats. *Journal of Medicinal Food*, **7**: 366–371.

Rao, A.V. and Gurfinkel, D.M. (2000). The bioactivity of saponins: triterpenoid and steroidal glycosides. *Drug Metabolism and Drug Interactions*, **17**: 211–235.

Rao, B.K. and Rao, C.H. (2001). Hypoglycemic and antihyperglycemic activity of *Syzygium alternifolium* (Wt.) Walp.seed extracts in normal and diabetic rats. *Phytomedicine*, **8:** 88–93.

Rao, V.V. (1992). Studies on hypoglycaemic activity of some indigenous drugs in normal and alloxan induced diabetic rabbits. M.V.Sc. Thesis, submitted to IVRI Deemed University, Izatnagar, India.

Raphael, K.R., Sabu, M.C. and Kuttan, R. (2002). Hypoglycemic effect of methanol extract of *Phyllanthus amarus* Schum and Thonn on alloxan induced diabetes mellitus in rats and its relation with antioxidant potential. *Indian Journal of Experimental Biology*, **40:** 905–909.

Rawls, R. (1996). Europe's strong herbal brew. *Chem Eng News*, **74(39)**: 53-60.

Ribes, G., Sauvaire, Y., DaCosta, C., Baccou, J.C. and Loubatieres- Mariani, M.M. (1986). Hypoglycemic effects of subfractions from fenugreek seeds in diabetic dogs. *Proceedings of the Society for Experimental Biology and Medicine*, **182:** 159–166.

Rizvi, S.I., AbuZaid, M. and Suhail, M. (1995). Insulin-mimetic effect of (–)-epicatechin on osmotic fragility of human erythrocytes. *Indian Journal of Experimental Biology*, **33:** 791–792.

Rizvi, S.I. and Zaid, M.A. (2001). Insulin-like effect of (–)-epicatechin on erythrocyte membrane acetylcholinesterase activity in type 2 *diabetes mellitus. Clinical and Experimental Pharmacology and Physiology*, **28**: 776–778.

Roman-Ramos, R., Flores-Saenz, J.L. and Alarcon-Aguilar, F.J. (1995). Anti-hyperglycemic effect of some edible plants. *Journal of Ethnopharmacology*, **48**: 25–32.

Sachdewa, A. and Khemani, L.D. (2003). Effect of *Hibiscus rosasinensis* Linn. ethanol flower extract on blood glucose and lipid profile in streptozotocin induced diabetes in rats. *J Ethnopharmacol.*, **89(1)**: 61-6.

Saely, C.H., Aczel,S. and Marte, T. (2004). Cardiovascular complications in type 2 diabetes mellitus depend on the coronary angiographic state rather than on the diabetes state. *Diabetologia*, **47**: 145-146.

Saleem, R., Ahmad, M., Hussain, S.A., Qazi, A.M., Ahmad, S.I., Qazi, M.H., Ali, M., Faizi, S., Akhtar, S. and Husnain. (1999). Hypotensive, hypoglycaemic and toxicological studies on the flavonol C-glycoside shamimin from *Bombax ceiba*. *Planta Medica*, **65:** 331–334.

SamaVenkatesh, B., Madhava Reddy., G. Dayanand Reddy., Ramesh Mullangi. and Lakshman, M. (2010). Antihyperglycemic and hypolipidemic effects of *Helicteres isora* roots in alloxan-induced diabetic rats: a possible mechanism of action. *Journal of Natural Medicines*, **64(3)**: 295-304.

Sarkar, S., Pranava, M. and Marita, R. (1996). Demonstration of the hypoglycemic action of *Momordica charantia* in a validated animal model of diabetes. *Pharmacological Research*, **33:** 1–4.

Sastri, B.N. (1952). The wealth of India, A dictionary of Indian Raw Material and Industrial Products. CSIR, New Delhi, Vol III, **218**: 210.

Saxena, A.M., Bajpai, M.B., Murthy, P.S. and Mukherjee, S.K. (1993). Mechanism of blood sugar lowering by a Swerchirin-containing hexane fraction (SWI) of *Swertia chirayita*. *Indian Journal of Experimental Biology,* **31**: 178–181.

Schafer, G. (1983). Biguanides.A review of history, pharmacodynamics, and therapy. *Diabetes Metab.,* **9**: 148-163.

Sekar, D.S., Sivagnanam, K. and Subramanian, S. (2005). Hypoglycemic activity of *Momordica charantia* seeds on streptozotocin induced diabetic rats. *Pharmazie,* **60:** 383–387.

Seki, M., Tanaka, T. and Nawa, H. (2004). Involvement of brain-derived neurotrophic factor in early retinal neuropathy of streptozotocin-induced diabetes in rats: therapeutic potential of brain-derived neurotrophic factors for dopaminergic amacrine cells. *Diabetes,* **53**: 2412-2419.

Serraclara, A., Hawkins, F., Perez, C., Dominguez, E., Campillo, J.E. and Torres, M.D. (1998). Hypoglycemic action of an oral fig-leaf decoction in type-I diabetic patients. *Diabetes Res clin Prac.,* **39(1)**: 19-22.

Shah, D.S. (1967). A preliminary study of the hypoglycemic action of heartwood of *Pterocarpus marsupium* Roxb. *Indian Journal of Medical Research*, **55:** 166–168.

Shanmugasundaram, E.R., Gopinath, K.L., RadhaShanmugasundaram, K. and Rajendran,V.M. (1990b).Possible regeneration of the islets of Langerhans in streptozotocin-diabetic rats given *Gymnema sylvestre* leaf extracts. *Journal of Ethnopharmacology,* **30**(3): 265–279.

Shanmugasundaram, K.R., Panneerselvam, C., Samudram, P. and Shanmugasundaram, E.R. (1983). Enzyme changes and glucose utilization in diabetic rabbits: the effect of *Gymnema sylvestre*, R.Br. *Journal of Ethnopharmacology,* **7:** 205–234.

Sharma, K.K., Gupta, R.K., Gupta, S. and Samuel, K.C.(1977). Antihyperglycemic effect of onion: effect on fasting blood sugar and induced hyperglycemia in man. *Indian Journal of Medical Research,* **65:** 422–429.

Sharma, V.N., Sogani, R.K. and Arora, R.B. (1960). Some observations on hypoglycemic activity of *Momordica charantia*. *Indian Journal of Medical Research,* **48**: 471–477.

Sheehan, E.W., Zemaitis, M.A., Slatkin, D.J. and SchiffJr, P.L. (183). A constituent of *Pterocarpus marsupium,* (–)-epicatechin, as a potential hypoglycemic agent. *Journal of Natural Products,* **46**: 232–234.

Sheela, C.G. and Augusti, K.T. (1992). Hypoglycemic effects of S-allyl cysteine sulphoxide isolated from garlic *Allium sativum* Linn. *Indian Journal of Experimental Biology,* **30:** 523–526.

Shibib, B.A., Khan, L.A. and Rahman, R. (1993). Hypoglycemic activity of *Coccinia indica* and *Momordica charantia* in diabetic rats: depression of the hepatic gluconeogenic enzymes glucose-6-phosphatase and fructose-1,6-bisphosphatase and elevation of both liver and red-cell shunt enzyme glucose-6-phosphate dehydrogenase. *Biochemistry Journal,* **292:** 267–270.

Shimizu, K., Iino, A., Nakajima, J., Tanaka, K., Nakajyo, S., Urakawa, N., M. Atsuchi, M., Wada, T. and Yamashita, C. (1997). Suppression of glucose absorption by some fractions extracted from *Gymnema sylvestre* leaves. *Journal of Veterinary Medical Science,* **59:** 245–251.

Shukla, N., Angelini, G.D. and Jeremy, J.Y. (2003). Homocysteine as a risk factor for nephropathy and retinopathy in type 2 diabetes. *Diabetologia,* **46**: 766-772.

Singh, S.S., Pandey, S.C., Srivastava, S., Gupta, V.S., Patro, B. and Ghosh, A.C. (2003). Chemistry and medicinal properties of *Tinospora cordifolia* (Guduchi). *Indian Journal of Pharmacology,* **35**: 83–91.

Sinha, A., Formica, C. and Tsalamandris, C. (1996). Effect of insulin on body composition in patients with insulin-dependent and non-insulin-dependent diabetes. *Diabetes Med.,* **13**: 40-46.

Sitasawad, S.L., Shewade,Y. and Bhonde, R. (2000). Role of bittergourd fruit juice in stz-induced diabetic state *in vivo* and *in vitro. Journal of Ethnopharmacology,* **73**: 71–79.

Stanely, P. and Menon, V.P. (2000). Hypoglycemic and other related actions of *Tinospora cordifolia* roots in alloxan-induced diabetic rats. *Journal of Ethnopharmacology,* **70**: 9–15.

Stanely, P. and Menon,V. P. (2001). Antioxidant action of *Tinospora cordifolia* root extract in alloxan diabetic rats. *Phytotherapy Research,* **15**: 213–218.

Stanely, P. and Menon,V.P. (2003). Hypoglycaemic and hypolipidaemic action of alcohol extract of *Tinospora cordifolia* roots in chemical induced diabetes in rats. *Phytotherapy Research,* **17**: 410–413.

Stanely, P., Menon, V.P. and Gunasekaran, G. (1999). Hypolipidaemic action of *Tinosporacordifolia* roots in alloxan diabetic rats. *Journal of Ethnopharmacology,* **64**: 53–57.

Suba, V., Murugesan, T., Arunachalam, G., Mandal, S.C. and Saha, B.P. (2004). Anti-diabetic potential of *Barleria lupulina* extract in rats. *Phytomedicine,* **11**: 202–205.

Suba, V., Murugesan, T., Rao, R.B., Ghosh, L., Pal, M., Mandal, S.C. and Saha, B.P. (2004). Hypoglycemic potential of *Barlerialupulina* extract in rats. *Fitoterapia,* **75**: 1–4.

Sugihara, Y., Nojima, H., Matsuda, H., Murakami, T., Yoshikawa, M. and Kimura, I. (2000). Antihyperglycemic effects of gymnemic acid IV, a compound derived from *Gymnema sylvestre* leaves in streptozotocin-diabetic mice. *Journal of Asian Natural Product Research,* **2**: 321–327.

Svensson, M., Eriksson, J. W. and Dahlquist, G. (2004). Early glycemic control, age at onset, and development of microvascular complications in childhood-onset type 1 diabetes: a population-based study in northern Sweden. *Diabetes Care,* **27**: 955-962.

Thakran, S., Siddiqui, M.R. and Baquer, N.Z. (2004). *Trigonella foenum graecum* seed powder protects against histopathological abnormalities in tissues of diabetic rats. *Molecular and Cellular Biochemistry,* **266**: 151–159.

Tjokroprawiro, A., Pikir, B.S., Budhiarta, A.A., PranawaSoewondo, H.M., Donosepoetro, M., Budhianto, F.X., Wibowo, J.A., Tanuwidjaja, S.J. and Pangemanan, M. (1983). Metabolic effects of onion and green beans on diabetic patients. *Tohoku Journal of Experimental Medicine,* **141**: 671–676.

Tominaga, M., Kimura, M., Sugiyama, K., Abe, T., Igarashi, K., Igarashi, M., Eguchi, H., Sekikawa, A., Ogawa, A. and Manaka, H. (1995). Effects of seishin-renshi-in and *Gymnema sylvestre* on insulin resistance in streptozotocin-induced diabetic rats. *Diabetes Research and Clinical Practice,* **29**: 11–17.

Tunali, T., Yarat, A., Yanardag, R., Ozcelik, F., Ozsoy, O., Ergenekon, G. and Emekli, N. (1998). The effect of chard (*Beta vulgaris* L. var. cicla) on the skin of streptozotocin induced diabetic rats. *Die Pharmazie,* **53**: 638–640.

University Group Diabetes Program. (1975). A study of the effects of hypoglycaemic agents on vascular complications in patients with adult-onset diabetes, V: Evaluation of phenformin therapy. *Diabetes,* **24**(1): 65-184.

Upadhyay, U.M. and Goyal, R.K. (2004). Efficacy of *Enicostemma littorale* in Type 2 diabetic patients. *Phytotherapy Research,* **18**: 233–235.

Vats, V., Grover, J.K. and Rathi, S.S. (2002). Evaluation of antihyperglycemic and hypoglycemic effect of *Trigonella foenum graecum, Ocimum sanctum* and *Pterocarpus marsupium* in normal and alloxanized diabetic rats. *Journal of Ethnopharmacology,* **79**: 95–100.

Vats, V., Yadav, S.P. and Grover, J.K. (2004). Ethanolic extract of *Ocimum sanctum* leaves partially attenuates streptozotocin-induced alterations in glycogen content and carbohydrate metabolism in rats. *Journal of Ethnopharmacology,* **90**: 155–160.

Vats, V., Yadav, S.P., Biswas, N.R. and Grover, J.K. (2004). Anti-cataract activity of *Pterocarpus marsupium* bark and *Trigonella foenum-graecum* seeds extract in alloxan diabetic rats. *Journal of Ethnopharmacology,* **93**: 289–294.

VenkataRao, E. (1997). Scope of plant drugs in modern medicine, *Visakha Sci. J.,* **1**: 47.

VenkataRao, E. (2000). Modern approaches to herbal medicine. *The Eastern Pharmacist,* 35-38.

Venkateswaran, S. and Pari, L. (2003). Effect of *Coccinia indica* leaves on antioxidant status in streptozotocin-induced diabetic rats. *Journal of Ethnopharmacology,* **84**: 163–168.

Venkateswaran, S. and Pari, L. (2003). Effect of *Coccinia indica* leaf extract on plasma antioxidants in streptozotocin-induced experimental diabetes in rats. *Phytotherapy Research,* **17**: 605–608.

Venkateswaran, S., Pari, L., Suguna, L. and Chandrakasan, G. (2003). Modulatory effect of *Coccinia indica* on aortic collagen in streptozotocin-induced diabetic rats. *Clinical and Experimental Pharmacology and Physiology,* **30**: 157–163.

Vessal, M., Hemmati, M. and Vasei, M. (2003). Hypoglycemic effects of quercetin in streptozocin-induced diabetic rats, *Comparative Biochemistry and Physiology C. Toxicology and Pharmacology,* **135C**: 357–364.

Vetrichelvan, T. and Jegadeesan., M. (2002). Anti-diabetic activity of alcoholic extract of *Aerva lanata* (L.) Juss.exSchultes in rats. *Journal of Ethnopharmacology,* **80**: 103–107.

Vimla Devi, M., Venkateswarlu, M. and KrishanaRao, R.V. (1977). Hypoglycemic activity of the leaves of *Momordica charantia. Indian Journal of Pharmacology,* **39**: 167–169.

Wadood, A., Wadood, N. and Shah, S.A. (1989). Effects of *Acaciaarabica* and *Caralluma edulis* on blood glucose levels on normal and alloxan diabetic rabbits. *J. Pakistan Med. Assoc.,* **39**: 208–212.

Wadood, N., Wadood, A. and Shah, S.A. (1992). Effect of *Tinospora cordifolia* on blood glucose and total lipid levels of normal and alloxan-diabetic rabbits. *Planta Medica,* **58**: 131–166.

Wallace, C., Reiber, G. E. and LeMaster, J. (2002). Incidence of falls, risk factors for falls, and fall-related factures in individuals with diabetes and a prior foot ulcer. *Diabetes Care,* **25**: 1983-1986.

Waltner-Law, M.E., Wang, X.L., Law, B.K., Hall, R.K., Nawano, M. and Granner, D.K. (2002). Epigallocatechin gallate, a constituent of green tea, represses hepatic glucose production. *Journal of Biological Chemistry,* **277**: 34933–34940.

Welihinda, J., Arvidson, G., Gylfe, E., Hellman, B. and Karlsson, E. (1982). The insulin-releasing activity of the tropical plant *Momordica charantia. Acta Biologica et Medica Germanica,* **41**: 1229–1240.

World Health Organization Expert Committee on Diabetes Mellitus.(1965). *Second WHO Technical Report, Series 310.* Geneva: World Health Organization,

World Health Organization Technical Report. (1994). Prevention of Diabetes Mellitus, Series No. 844.

Yadav, P., Sarkar, S. and Bhatnagar, D. (1997). Action of *Capparis decidua* against alloxan-induced oxidative stress and diabetes in rat tissues. *Pharmacological Research,* **36**: 221–228.

Yadav, P., Sarkar, S. and Bhatnagar, D. (1997). Lipid peroxidation and antioxidant enzymes in erythrocytes and tissues in aged diabetic rats. *Indian Journal of Experimental Biology,* **35**: 389–392.

Yadav, U.C., Moorthy, K. and Baquer, N.Z. (2005). Combined treatment of sodium orthovanadate and Momordica charantia fruit extract prevents alterations in lipid profile and lipogenic enzymes in alloxan diabetic rats. *Molecular and Cellular Biochemistry,* **268**: 111–120.

Yoshikawa, M., Murakami, T., Kadoya, M., Li, Y., Murakami, N., Yamahara, J. and Matsuda, H. (1997). Medicinal foodstuffs. IX. The inhibitors of glucose absorption from the leaves of *Gymnema sylvestre* R. BR. (Asclepiadaceae). Structures of gymnemosides a and b. *Chemical and Pharmaceutical Bulletin (Tokyo),* **45**: 1671–1676.

Yoshikawa, M., Murakami, T., Yashiro, K. and Matsuda, H. (1998). Kotalanol, a potent alpha-glucosidase inhibitor with thiosugar sulfonium sulfate structure, from hypoglycemic Ayurvedic medicine *Salacia reticulate. Chemical and Pharmaceutical Bulletin (Tokyo),* **46**: 1339–1340.

Yu, B.C., Hung, C.R., Chen, W.C. and Cheng, J.T. (2003). Antihyperglycemic effect of andrographolide in streptozotocin-induced diabetic rats. *Planta Medica,* **69**: 1075–1079.

Zacharias, N.T., Sebastian, K.L., Philip, B. and Augusti, K.T. (1980). Hypoglycemic and hypolipidemic effects of garlic in sucrose fed rabbits. *Indian Journal of Physiology and Pharmacology,* **24**: 151–154.

Zimmet, P., Cowie, C., Ekoe, J.M. and Shaw, J.E. (2004). Classification of diabetes mellitus and other categories of glucose intolerance. *International Textbook of Diabetes Mellitus,* chapter 1(3): 3-14.

Zimmet, P. (2000). Globalization, coca-colonization and the chronic disease epidemic: can the Doomsday scenario be averted. *J Med.,* **247**: 301-310.

Medicinal Plants: Phytochemistry, Pharmacology and Therapeutics Vol. 2 (2012) *Pages* **307–315**
Editor-in-Chief: **V.K. Gupta**
Published by: **DAYA PUBLISHING HOUSE, NEW DELHI**

18

Effects of Soy Protein Supplementation on the Reproductive System of Male Wistar Rats

O. Akinloye[1], O.O. Oguntibeju[1*], A.O. Adaramoye[2], M.O. Oyeyemi[3], O. Jegede[3] and E.J. Truter[1]

ABSTRACT

The adverse effects of soy protein on female reproduction in rodents have been widely investigated, but data of male rats are scarce. This chapter reports on the effects of soy protein supplementation on the biophysical parameters, reproductive hormones and genital tracts in male rats. The semen samples were analyzed by conventional methods and serum testosterone and estrogen levels were determined by the enzyme immunoassay (EIA) technique as proposed by the World Health Organization. The results of our study showed a significant reduction in sperm count, motility, viability and morphology of the sperm of experimental animals (phytoestrogen and estrogen groups) following soy protein supplementation. Consequently, the quality of semen from the experimental animals (phytoestrogen and estrogen groups) was adversely affected when compared with a control group ($p < 0.05$). Also, the serum testosterone levels in the experimental animals were significantly reduced when compared with controls

1 Oxidative Stress Research Centre, Department of Biomedical Sciences, Faculty of Health and Wellness Sciences, Cape Peninsula University of Technology, Bellville Campus, Cape Town, South Africa

2 Department of Biochemistry, College of Medicine, University of Ibadan, Nigeria

3 Faculty of Veterinary Medicine, University of Ibadan, Nigeria

* *Corresponding author*: E-mail: oguntibejuo@cput.ac.za, bejufemi@yahoo.co.uk, Tel: +27219538495, Fax: +27219538490.

($p<0.05$). While there was no significant difference in the serum estrogen levels of the control group and phytoestrogen-treated animals, the serum estrogen levels increased significantly in animals treated with estrogen ($p<0.05$). Our findings demonstrate that soy protein supplementation of the diet of male Wistar rats over a six week period reduces spermatogenesis and testosterone levels significantly.

Keywords: Soy protein, Phytoestrogen, Male reproduction, Wistar rats.

Introduction

Soybeans form important dietary source of protein in Nigeria, China and other countries and has been found to contain naturally occurring phytoestrogens (Anthony *et al.*, 1988; Obatolu and Ashaye, 1999; Brown and Setchell, 2001; Akinloye *et al.*, 2002; Wu, 2002). Loewe *et al.* in 1927 reported that some plant extracts exhibit estrogenic activity and since then it has been shown that many plants demonstrate estrogenic activity or contain estrogenic compounds. Phytoestrogens, in the body affect hormonal activity directly or indirectly and they also vary in chemical structure and plant origin. Phytoestrogens occurring naturally in plants are not actual steroids or hormones but may however interact with estrogen receptor sites in the body. Phytoestrogens also exhibit structural and functional properties similar to the main female sex hormone-17 β-estradiol (Duncan *et al.*, 1999). The phytoestrogens in soybeans have been found to be mainly isoflavones, including genisten (4, 5, 7-trihydroxyisoflavone), daidzein (4, 7-dihydroxyisoflavone) and glycitein (4, 7-dihydroxy-6-methoxyisoflavone). The isoflavones are primarily glucosides, malonyl- and methylglucosides as well as the aglycones (Anthony *et al.*, 1988; Akinloye *et al.*, 2002; Cline *et al.*, 2004)).

The use of herbal prescriptions in the treatment of hormonal imbalances and other diseases has been known for over 2000 years. However, the role of estrogenic substances derived from plants has only been studied over half a century (Setchell *et al.*, 1987). Epidemiologically, the consumption of soybeans or soy-rich diets has been associated with a reduction in the risk of many diseases (*e.g.* cardiovascular disease, cancer and diabetes) and there is evidence indicating a role for the phytoestrogens present in soybeans in mediating other positive effects (Wu, 2002). However experimental studies on the effects of soybeans in the diet of male rats are not common. The present study was designed to investigate the possible estrogenic effect of phytoestrogens present in soybeans (following supplementation) on the male reproductive system of Wistar rats.

Methodology

Chemicals

All chemicals and reagents used in this study were of analytical grade and obtained from Sigma, USA.

Animal Care

All animals used in this study were treated in accordance with the principles of laboratory animal care as indicated in the Guide for the care and Use of Laboratory

Animals of the National Institute of Health (1978). All animals had free access to water and rat chow; they were housed in an animal house at a constant temperature of 27°C and were exposed to a twelve-hour artificial day-night cycle. Male Wistar rats weighing between 125g and 133g were used in the experiment. The animals were divided into three groups of seven per group. The animals in group A (control) were fed normal rat chow (devoid of soyprotein). The chow was purchased from Ladokun Feed Limited, Ibadan, Nigeria. The animals in group B were fed rat pellets and raw soybeans, mixed in a ratio of 1:1 by weight. Animals in group C were also fed rat chow but were injected with estrogen (17 beta estrodiol) (2 mg/kg). The dietary status of all animals was maintained for six weeks. The weights of the animals in each group were recorded before and after the experiment.

Sample Preparation

Blood was obtained from the animals by ear puncture, allowed to clot and then centrifuged at 3000 x g for 10 minutes using an MSE bench macrocentrifuge and the serum collected. The animals were sacrificed by cervical dislocation after six weeks.

The weights of the testes and epididymis as well as their lengths were determined by using either an electronic weighing machine (Mettlar AE 240) or a flexible tape respectively. Semen samples were drawn off with a Pasteur pipette from the epididymis, which was carefully trimmed off the body of the testes. Two to four (2-4) drops of 2.9 per cent sodium citrate was used as the flushing fluid. The semen samples were analyzed by using the method of World Health Organization (WHO) (2000). Serum steroids: testosterone and estrogen levels were determined by the enzyme immunoassay (EIA) technique of WHO (1999).

Results

Animals injected with estrogen showed a significant weight loss when compared with the control and phytoestrogen groups ($p < 0.001$) (Table 18.1). On the other hand, animals supplemented with soy protein showed a significant weight gain (Table 18.1). The testicular weight, the circumference of the testis and length of epididymis of the experimental animals differ significantly from the control group ($p < 0.05$) (Table 18.2). There was a significant reduction in sperm count, motility, viability and morphology of the sperm of experimental animals (phytoestrogen and estrogen groups). Consequently, the quality of semen from the experimental animals (phytoestrogen and estrogen groups) was adversely affected when compared with the control group ($p < 0.05$). These differences were more pronounced in animals to whom estrogen was administered than in the phytoestrogen and control groups (Table 18.3). The serum testosterone levels in the experimental animals were found to be significantly reduced when compared with the controls ($p<0.05$). While there was no significant difference in the serum estrogen levels of control group and animals given phytoestrogen, the serum estrogen level was shown to increase significantly in animals treated with estrogen ($p<0.05$) (Table 18.3). Table 18.4 shows the correlation of spermogram with food intake, weight and measured parameters of reproductive organs in both experimental and control animals.

Table 18.1. Comparison of the effect of estrogen and phytoestrogens in a soyprotein diet on the weight and food intake of wistar rats.

Grouping	*Initial Weight (g)*	*Final Weight (g)*	*Weight Difference (g)*	*F*	*P*	*Food Intake (g)*
Control	125±3.14	188.3±3.22	70.8±2.71			239.18±0.55
Phytoestrogen	133±3.74	188.3±3.52	73.3±3.33*	39.1	0.001	238.3±0.89*
Estrogen	126.7±2.11	101.3± 1.89	–15.42±1.06+			*229.06±0.21+*

Results are expressed as means ± SEM.

Statistical significance between and within groups are expressed as F (ANOVA).

+: Significant difference between controls and test animals (Student 't' test; p <0.05).

*: Significant difference between test animals (Student 't' test; p <0.05).

Table 18.2. Effect of estrogen and phytoestrogens on reproductive organs.

Parameters	*Control*	*Phytoestrogen*	*Estrogen*	*F*	*P*
Weight of testis	1.21±0.06	1.02 ± 0.05+	0.97± 0.08+	7.22	0.006
Circumference of testis	3.20±0.05	3.03 ± 0.02+*	1.30± 0.08+*	112.14	0.001
Length of epididymis	4.70±0.04	4.33 ± 0.08+*	3.47 ± 0.10+*	74.18	0.001
Breadth of epididymis	0.33±0.02	0.31 ± 0.05	0.32 ± 0.04	1.58	0.285

Results are expressed as means ± SEM.

Statistical significance between and within groups are expressed as F (ANOVA).

+: Significant difference between controls and test animals (Student 't' test; p <0.05).

*: Significant difference between test animals (Student 't' test; p <0.05).

Table 18.3. Effect of estrogen and phytoestrogens on spermogram and gonadal hormones.

Parameters	*Control*	*Phytoestrogen*	*Estrogen*	*F*	*P*
Sperm count X 10^6	105.67±1.48	85.67±2.45+*	44.97 ± 0.08+*	251.97	0.001
Motility %	90±0.01	40 ± 0.02+*	20 ± 0.01+*	122.10	0.001
Viability %	83.33±6.67	50.04 ± 0.02+*	30.23 ± 0.09+*	118.75	0.001
Abnormality %	10.17±1.05	20.73 ± 0.72+*	30.65 ± 2.62+*	36.82	0.001
Estrogen (ng/ml)	0.25 ±0.01	0.27±0.02*	1.42±0.04+*	0.87	0.87
Testosterone (ng/ml)	3.68±0.05	3.03 ± 0.02+*	2.43 ± 0.03+*	12.55	0.002

Results are expressed as means ± SEM.

Statistical significance between and within groups are expressed as F (ANOVA).

+: Significant difference between controls and text animals (Student 't' test; p <0.05).

*: Significant difference between text animals (Student 't' test; p <0.05).

Table 18.4. Correlation of spermogram with food intake, weight and measured parameters of reproductive organs.

Spermogam and Groups	*Food Intake*	*Weight Gain/Loss*	*Weight of Testes*	*Circum. of Testes*	*Length of Epididymis*	*Breadth of Epididymis*
			Control			
Sperm counts X10^6	+0.170	+0.459*	+0.342*	+0.789*	+0.990*	+0.011
Motility %	+0.074	+0.107	+0.518*	–0.700*	+0.548*	+0.001
Viability %	+0.159	+0.405*	+0.192	–0.741*	+0.366*	+0.001
Morphology %	+0.032	+0.237	+0.114	–0.773*	+0.866*	+0.031
			Phytoestrogen			
Sperm count X 10^6	–0.470*	–0.858*	+0.840*	+0.497*	+0.423*	+0.180
Motility %	–0.311*	+0.311*	+0.534*	–0.906*	+0.809*	+0.116
Viability %	–0.342*	+0.212*	+0.250*	–0.740*	+0.680*	+0.134
Morphology %	–0.263*	–0.479*	+0.800*	–0.590*	+0.350*	+0.092
			Estrogen			
Sperm count X 10^6	+0.470	–0.660	+0.370	+0.650	+0.638	0.012
Motility %	+0.240	–0.129	+0.406	–0.804	+0.725	0.001
Viability %	+0.237	–0.689	+0.376	–0.652	+0.433	0.001
Morphology %	+0.375	–0.262	+0.299	0.460	+0.256	0.121

Significant correlation; $p < 0.05$.

+: Positive correlation.

–: Negative correlation.

Discussion

To date the mechanisms and potencies of phytoestrogens have not been fully explained and they may be considered to be potential endocrine disrupters, therefore caution should be exercised when consuming phtytoestrogen-rich products. Some concerns have previously been expressed about the risks associated with phytoestrogen consumption. Such concerns or risks include increased plasma concentrations of isoflavones in babies who ingest soymilk, the ability of non-hormonal secondary plant metabolites which are able to modify sex steroid metabolism, and the effects of phytoestrogens on the thyroid (Ibarreta *et al.*, 2001). In addition, a concern is also the genetic toxicity potential of phytoestrogens which has been reported (Kulling *et al.*, 2002).

The phytoestrogens which possess estrogen-like biological activities have been found to influence human and animal reproduction by altering the sexual behavior and function of the reproductive organs (Opalka *et al.*, 2004). It has been reported that sheep consuming large amounts of phytoestrogen-rich diets showed infertility and reproductive disorders (Adams, 1995). Cheetahs in captivity also exhibited reduced fertility rates when consuming a feline diet containing a soybean product, which was reversed by its removal from the diet (Setchell *et al.*, 1987). Toxicities associated with the intake of herbal medicines that include phytoestrogens have also been reported on in the literature (Sheehan, 1998). Our study, therefore substantiates these findings and provide an evidence that phytoestrogens from soy protein influences steroidogenesis and causes spermatogenic defects.

In a previous report, we demonstrated that soy protein caused an increase in uterine weight of female rabbits making it unsuitable for implantation and foetal development (Akinloye *et al.*, 2002). In our current study, we observed a significant reduction in the weight and circumference of the testes and also in the length of the epididymis and consequently a reduction in the quality of semen of rats supplemented with soybeans.

Some animal studies have linked a high consumption of plant-derived estrogens known as isoflavones with infertility (Setchell, 1987; Makela *et al.*, 1990; Adams, 1995; Sheehan, 1998; Robert *et al.*, 2000). It has been shown that a high intake of soy-based foods could lower sperm count (Chavarro, 2008). Chavarro (2008) of the Harvard School of Public Health in Boston, found that men who consumed the highest amounts of soy foods had a lower sperm count compared to those who did not consume soy foods at all. Chavarro (2008) evaluated the intake of 15 soy-based foods in 99 men who attended a fertility clinic. They were questioned on the frequency and amount of soy-rich foods they had taken including: tofu, tempeh, tofu or soy sausages, bacon, burgers and mince, soy milk, cheese, yogurt and ice cream, and other soy products such as drinks, powders and energy bars. Men in the highest soy product intake category had 40 million sperm per milliliter less than men who had eaten no soy foods. A normal sperm count ranges from 80 million to 120 million per milliliter, and a sperm count of 20 million per milliliter or below is considered low. Overweight men tended to have lower sperm counts which could be due to estrogen production by fat cells. It is therefore possible, based on Chavarro's study that a cause of infertility could be linked to a high intake of soy foods.

Phytoestrogens contained in a vegetarian diet are supposed to have beneficial effects on the development and progression of endocrine related diseases and disorders, of which cancer has been widely reported (Krazeisen *et al.*, 2002). Our results however showed a negative influence of soy protein on testicular steroidogenesis. Previous studies have shown that phytoestrogen inhibits the reductive and oxidative activities of the enzyme; 17 β-hydroxysteroid dehydrogenase type 5, a key enzyme in the metabolism of estrogens and androgens. It is also possible that inhibitory effects of isoflavone on spermatogenesis and testosterone synthesis are mediated at the level of the hypothalamo-pituitary system (that is by altering the secretion of luteinizing hormone and follicle stimulating hormone. One other potential mechanism of anti-androgenic effects on males is the inhibition of 5-α reductase activity. It has also been shown that exposure of male rats to phytoestrogens induced persistent reductions in 5-α reductase activity in the prostate (Makela *et al.*, 1990).

These mechanisms may possibly explain the reduced testosterone levels which were observed in our study. Van Veldhuizen *et al.* (2006) performed a pilot study to determine the dose effect of soy supplement on serum hormonal levels, estrogen receptor alpha (ERalpha) and androgen receptor (AR) expression in patients scheduled to undergo prostatectomy. Cohorts of 3-4 eligible patients received doses of a commercial soy supplement, Flavein, from the time of study enrollment until prostatectomy. Serum prostate specific antigen (PSA), testosterone, and estrogen levels were measured at study enrollment and prior to prostatectomy. AR and ERalpha expression was evaluated in the pretreatment biopsy specimen and post-treatment prostatectomy specimen using immunohistochemical analysis. A total of 13 patients were enrolled for this pilot study and 11 patients were assessed for response. With soy supplementation, serum testosterone levels decreased in 9 of 11 patients and estrogen levels decreased in 8 of 10 patients in a dose-dependent manner. There was a variable effect on ERalpha expression with down-regulation of receptor expression seen at the highest dose level. There was no effect on AR expression. The investigators concluded that supplementation with soy products produced a consistent decrease in serum sex hormone levels. The study of Van Veldhuizen and coworkers (2006) further confirms our result which showed a decrease in testosterone levels in soy protein supplemented rats.

Our study and that of Van Veldhuizen*et al.* (2006) disagree with previous reports that exonerated phytoestrogen in reproductive disruption (Robert *et al.,* 2000). Furthermore, our study provides evidence in support of other studies which demonstrated that phytoestrogen affects testicular steriodogenesis (Opalka *et al.,*2004).

The observed estrogenic effects of soy protein have been attributed to the relatively large quantity of isoflavones, especially genistines which are present in soy foods and isoflavones have been implicated in infertility (Adams, 1995, Chavarro, 2008) and genistins have been identified to be an enzyme inhibitor of 17 β-OHsteroid deOHgenase, binding to the hydrophilic cofactor binding pocket of the enzyme (Krazeisen *et al.,* 2002).

In conclusion, our data demonstrate that dietary soy protein supplementation over a six week period in male Wistar rats negatively affects sperm count and quality and reduces testosterone levels. We therefore, implicate phytoestrogen present in a soy protein diet in infertility. Further studies are required to identify and clarify a possible link between soy protein and its effects on the male reproductive system.

References

Adams, N.R. (1995). Detection of the effects of phytoestrogens on sheep and cattle. *J Anim Sci.,* **73**: 1509–1515.

Akinloye, O., Akintunde, C. O., Banjoko, S. O., Adaramoye, A. O., and Adeleye A.O (2002). An assessment of the estrogenic effect of soy protein in female rabbits. *Food Chemistry*, **77**: 67-69.

Anthony, D., Ologhobo, X., and Adejuwon, D.O. (1988). Effect of dietary soybean on total protein content and relative acetylcholisterase activity in rat brain. *Nut Report Intern.,* **37**: 1042.

Brown, N.M., and Setchell, K.D. (2001). Animal models impacted by phytoestrogens in commercial chow: implications for pathways influenced by hormones. *Lab Invest.,* **81**: 735-747.

Chavarro, J.E., Toth, T.L., Sadio, S.M. and Hauser, R. (2008). Soyfood and isoflavone intake in relation to semen quality parameters among men from an infertility clinic. *Human Reprod.*, **23**: 2384-2390.

Cline, J.M., Franke, A.A., Register, T.C., Golden, D.L., and Adams, M.R. (2004). Effects of dietary isoflavones on the reproductive tract of female mice. *Toxicol Pathol.*,**32**: 91-99.

Duncan, A.M., Merz, B.E., Xu, X., Nagel, T.C., Phipps, W.R., and Kurzer (1999). Soy isoflavones exert modest hormonal effects in premopausal women. *J Clin Endocrinol metab.*, **84:** 192-197.

Ibarreta, D., Daxenberger, A., and Meyer, H.H.D. (2001). Possible health impact of phytoestrogens and xenoestrogens in food. *APMIS.*, **109**: 161–184.

Krazeisen, A., Breitling, R., Moller, G., and Adamski, J. (2002). Human 17 beta-hydroxysteroid dehydrogenase type 5 is inhibited by dietary flavonoid. *Adv Exp Med Biol.*, **505**: 151-161.

Kulling, S.E., Lehmann, L., and Metzler, M. (2002). Oxidative metabolism and genotoxic potential of major isoflavone phytoestrogens. *J Chromatogr and Analyt Technol.*, **777**: 211–218.

Loewe, S., Lange,F., and Spohr, E. (1927). Female sex hormones (Thelytropine). *Biochem.*, **180**: 1-26.

Makela, S., Santti, R., Martikainen, P., Nienstetd, W., and Paranko, J. (1990). The influence of steroidal and nonsteroidal estrogens on the 5-alpha reduction of testosterone by the ventral prostate of the rat. *J Steroid Biochem.*, **35:** 249-256.

Obatolu, V.A., and Ashaye, O.A. (1999). Assessing the contribution of soybean utilisation on the nutritional status of children from low-income families: Lagos State, Nigeria as a case study. *Int J Food Sci Nutr.*, **50(6):** 375-81.

Opalka, M., Kaminska, B., Ciereszko, R., and Dusza, L, (2004). Genistein affects testosterone secretion by Leydig cells in roosters (*Gallus gallus domesticus*). *Reproductive Biol.*, **4 (2)** : 185 – 195.

Robert, D., Veeramachaneni, D.N., Schalaff, W.D., and Awoniyi, C.A. (2000). Effect of chronic dietary exposure to genistein, a phytoestrogen, during various stages of development on reproductive hormones and spermatogenesis in rats. *Endorcine.*, **13**: 281-286.

Setchell, K.D.R., Gosselin, S.J., and Welsh, M.B. (1987). Dietary estrogens – a probable cause of infertility and liver disease in captive cheetahs. *Gastroenterology*, **93**: 225–233.

Sheehan, D.M. (1998). Herbal medicines, phytoestrogens and toxicity: risk: benefit considerations. *Proc Soc Exp Biol Med.*, **217**: 379–385.

Van Veldhuizen, P.J., Thrasher, J.B., Ray, G., Cherian, R., Ward, J., Holzbeierlein, J., Gutow, S., and Banerjee, S.K. (2006). Effect of soy supplement on serum hormonal levels, estrogen receptor alpha and androgen receptor. *Oncol Reprod.*, **16**: 1221-1224.

WHO (2000). Collection and examination of human semen In: WHO laboratory manual for the examination of human semen and sperm–cervical mucus interaction, 4th ed., WHO Cambridge University Press, Cambridge, pp. 4–33.

WHO (1999). Enzyme immunoassay technique In: WHO special program research in human reproduction. Program for provision of matched assay reagents for immunoassay of hormones, immunometrics (UK), London.

Wu, A.H. (2002). Phytoestrogens and cancer: epidemiologic evidence. Phytoestrogen and Health, G Gilani and J Anderson. AOCS Press Champaign, IL.

Medicinal Plants: Phytochemistry, Pharmacology and Therapeutics Vol. 2 (2012) *Pages* **317–330**
Editor-in-Chief: **V.K. Gupta**
Published by: **DAYA PUBLISHING HOUSE, NEW DELHI**

19

Herbals and Androgenic Activity: Antioxidant Effect of Ginger, Carrot Seed, *Allium cepa*, Quercetin and *Danae racemosa* in Spermatogenesis

Arash Khaki[1]*

ABSTRACT

Many of the herbs and spices used by humans to season food, yield useful medicinal compounds. Medicinal use of these herbs can be traced back to ancient China, India and Iran. The herbs and there constituents are stated to have antiemetic, antithrombotic, antihepatotoxic, anti-inflammatory, stimulant, cholagogic and antioxidant properties. The antioxidant properties of herbs have a beneficial effect on spermatogenesis and sperm quality. In the present study, Wistar male rats were kept in standard conditions and allocated into control and test groups. Test groups received either ginger rhizome powder (100mg/kg/day), carrot seed extract (200mg/kg/day), fresh juice of Allium cepa (1cc/rat/day), Quercetin (15mg/kg/day) or Danae racemosa powder (400mg/kg/day) for 20 consecutive days. Serum total testosterone was significantly increased in the groups that had received herbs ($p<0.05$) in comparison to the control group. In addition, sperm concentration, viability and motility was significantly increased ($p<0.05$) in both test groups in comparison to the control group, whereas LH and FSH hormone profiles, sperm concentration, morphology and testes weight were similar in the experimental and control groups. Results revealed that administration of

1 Tabriz Branch, Islamic Azad University, Tabriz, Iran.

* *Corresponding Address*: No.1 Ettekali La, South Shariati Street, 5138815941, Tabriz, Iran.

E-mail: arashkhaki@yahoo.com,
Tel: (Mobile) +98-914-3138-399, +44-7924-517599

these herbs significantly increased sperm percentage, viability, motility and serum total testosterone. This suggests that they may have value in enhancing traits associated with sperm health.

Keywords: Antioxidant, *Allium cepa,* Carrot seed, *Danae racemosa,* Ginger, Quercetin, Spermatogenesis.

Introduction

Herbalism is a traditional or folk medicinal practice based on the use of plants and plant extracts. Herbalism is also known as botanical medicine, medical herbalism, herbal medicine, herbology, and phytotherapy. The scope of herbal medicine is sometimes extended to include fungal and bee products, as well as minerals, shells and certain animal parts (Aitken *et al.,* 1989). Pharmacognosy is the study of medicines derived from natural sources. The traditional use of medicines is recognized as a way in which to identify and develop potential future medicinal products. In 2001, researchers identified 122 compounds used in mainstream medicine which were derived from "ethno medical" plant sources, 80 per cent of which were used in the same or related manner as their traditional use (Sharma and Agarwal, 1996). Many plants synthesize substances that are useful to the maintenance of health in humans and other animals. These include aromatic substances, most of which are phenols or their oxygen-substituted derivatives such as tannins. Many are secondary metabolites, of which at least 12,000 have been isolated; a number estimated to be less than 10 per cent of the total. In many cases, substances such as alkaloids serve as plant defense mechanisms against predation by microorganisms, insects, and herbivores. Many of the herbs and spices used by humans to season food yield useful medicinal compounds (de Lamirande *et al.,* 1997; Tremellen, 2008). However, in the same manner as prescription drugs, a number of herbs are thought to have adverse side-effects (Aziz and Agarwal, 2008). Furthermore, excessive use, inappropriate formulation, or lack of understanding of plant and drug interactions have led to adverse reactions that are sometimes life threatening or lethal (Griveau and Lannou, 1997). People on all continents have used hundreds or thousands of indigenous plants for treatment of ailments since prehistoric times. Medicinal herbs were found in the personal effects of Ötzi the Iceman, whose body was frozen in the Swiss Alps for more than 5,300 years. These herbs appear to have been used to treat the parasites found in his intestines. Anthropologists theorize that animals evolved a tendency to seek out bitter plant parts in response to illness. Indigenous healers often claim to have learned their skills by observing the way in which sick animals change their food preferences to consume bitter herbs that they would normally reject (Jones *et al.,* 1979). Field biologists have provided corroborating evidence based on observations of a diverse range of species, such as chimpanzees, chickens, sheep and butterflies. Lowland gorillas obtain 90 per cent of their food intake from the fruits of *Aframomum melegueta*, a relative of the ginger plant, that is a potent antimicrobial and apparently keeps shigellosis and similar infections under control (Aitken *et al.,* 1992; Zalata *et al.,* 1995; Lenzi *et al.,* 2000; Cocuzza *et al.,* 2007). The study of herbs dates back over 5,000 years to the Sumerians, who described well-established medicinal uses for such plants as laurel, caraway, and thyme. Ancient Egyptian medicines of 1000 B.C. are known to have used garlic, opium, castor oil, coriander, mint, indigo, and other herbs and the Old Testament also mentions herb use and cultivation, including mandrake, vetch, caraway, wheat, barley, and rye. Indian Ayurveda medicine used herbs such as turmeric possibly as early as 1900 B.C. (Alvarez *et al.*, 1987; Storey, 1997; Garrido *et al.*, 2004; Acharya and Shrivastava, 2008). Many other herbs and minerals used in Ayurveda were later described by ancient Indian herbalists such as Charaka and Sushruta during the 1st millennium B.C. The Sushruta Samhita, attributed to Sushruta in the 6th century B.C., describes 700 medicinal plants, 64 preparations from mineral sources, and 57 preparations based on animal sources (Fabricant and Farnsworth, 2001). The first Chinese herbal book, the Shennong Bencao Jing, compiled during the Han Dynasty but dating back to a much earlier date, possibly 2700 B.C., lists 365 medicinal plants and their uses. These include ma-Huang; the shrub that introduced the drug ephedrine to modern medicine. Succeeding generations built on the Shennong Bencao Jing, as in the production of the Yaoxing Lun (Treatise on the Nature of Medicinal Herbs); a 7th century Tang Dynasty treatise on herbal medicine. The ancient Greeks and Romans also made medicinal use of plants. Greek and Roman medicinal practices, as preserved in the writings of Hippocrates and especially Galen, provided the pattern for later western medicine. Hippocrates advocated the use of a few simple herbal drugs along with fresh air, rest, and a proper diet. Conversely Galen recommended large doses of drug mixtures including plant, animal, and mineral ingredients. The Greek physician compiled the first European treatise on the properties and uses of medicinal plants, known as De Materia Medica. In the first century A.D., Dioscorides prepared a compendium of more than 500 plants that remained an authoritative reference into the 17th century. Similarly important for herbalists and botanists of later centuries was the Greek book that founded the science of botany, Theophrastus' Historia Plantarum, written in the fourth century B.C. Thyme from Project Gutenberg EBook of Culinary Herbs: Their Cultivation Harvesting Curing and Uses, by M. G (Lai and Roy, 2004). All plants produce chemical compounds as part of their normal metabolic activities. These are arbitrarily divided into primary metabolites, such as sugars and fats which are found in all plants, and secondary metabolites. The latter are compounds not essential for basic functions and are found in a smaller range of plants. It is these secondary metabolites and pigments that can have therapeutic actions in humans and which can be refined to produce drugs. Some of the most useful secondary metabolites are produced by a single genus or species. Pigments harvest light, protect the organism from radiation and display colors to attract pollinators. Many common weeds, such as nettle, dandelion and chickweed, have medicinal properties (Talalay and Talalay, 2001; Huffman, 2003; Tapsell *et al.*, 2006). The functions of secondary metabolites vary from toxins used to deter predators, to pheromones used to attract insects for pollination. As specific examples, phytoalexins protect against bacterial and fungal attack whilst allelochimicals inhibit rival plants that are competing for soil and light. Plants up and down regulate their biochemical pathways in response to the local mix of herbivores, pollinators and microorganisms (Castleman, 2001; Diane, 2002; Aggarwal *et al.*, 2007). The chemical profile of a single plant may vary over time as it reacts to changing conditions. Plants synthesize a be wildering variety of phytochemicals but most are derivatives of a few biochemical motifs. Fruit and vegetables are the main dietary sources of vitamins for humans, but they can also be taken as supplements. Infertility is one of the principal health conditions affecting human populations and approximately 30 per cent of cases result from problems in the man rather than the woman (Huff, 2003; Khaki *et al.*, 2009a). Spermatogenesis can be compromised by a variety of routes, resulting in reduced sperm quality and production. These routes include drug treatment, chemotherapy, toxins, air pollutants and insufficient vitamin intake (Khaki *et al.*, 2009c,d). Several studies have reported that antioxidants and the dietary intake of vitamins A, B, C, and E can protect sperm DNA from free radicals and increase the stability of the blood testis barrier (Khaki *et al.*, 2009e; Nouri *et al.*, 2009). In modern times, ginger rhizome (*Zingiber officinale* R., family: Zingiberaceae) is used worldwide as a spice and is reported to have both antioxidant (Nassir *et al.*, 2009) and androgenic activity in model animal. The antioxidant properties of *Z. officinale* can be assigned to all of its major active ingredients, such as zingerone, gingerdiol, zingibrene, gingerols and shogaols (Khaki *et al.*, 2009b). Furthermore, other research has demonstrated that ginger oil has a major protective effect from DNA damage induced by H_2O_2 and might therefore act as a scavenger of oxygen radicals and have value as an antioxidant (Khaki *et al.*, 2010). *Daucus carota*, commonly known as the carrot, belongs to the family Apiaceae and is cultivated throughout the world as a useful vegetable. The plant has also been used in folk medicine for the treatment of a broad spectrum of ailments including kidney dysfunction, asthma, worm infections, inflammation and leprosy (Fabricant and Farnsworth, 2001; Talalay and Talalay, 2001; Khaki *et al.*, 2010). According to some studies, carrot extract also offers some protection against myocardial infarction (de Lamirande *et al.*, 1997) and lindane-induced hepatotoxicity. The chemical composition of the plant has been extensively studied and a large number of active ingredients such as volatile oils, steroids, tannins, flavonoids, and caroten have been isolated (Cocuzza *et al.*, 2007). Recently, however, pharmacological studies have shown that *Daucus carota* seeds exhibit fertility-suppressing properties in females (Aitken *et al.*, 1992; Lenzi *et al.*, 2000). Majumder *et al.* have shown that the petroleum ether extract and fatty acids of carrot seeds are able to arrest the normal estrus cycle of adult mice and significantly reduce weight (Zalata *et al.*, 1995). These authors also found that treatment with carrot seed extract (CSE) can lead to a significant inhibition of delta 5,3-β-hydroxy steroid dehydrogenase and glucose-6-phosphate dehydrogenase in mouse ovaries; the two key enzymes involved in ovarian steroidogenesis. In another *in vitro* study performed using an isolated rabbit ovarian perfusion system, progesterone and human chorionic gonadotropin-induced progesterone secretions were found to be acutely and significantly diminished after the feeding of carrots (Nouri *et al.*, 2009). The effects of carrots on human fertility have also been highlighted in traditional Iranian medicine. In the Zakhireh Kharazmshahi (Kharazmshahi's Treasure), a book written by Seyyed-Esmail Jorjani born in the 11th Century, one chapter has been allocated to the properties of carrots.

The onion (*Allium cepa*) has long been used in traditional medicine and one of the important *Allium* species commonly used as human food has recently been a source of much interest because of its antithrombotic, hypolipidaemic, hypotensive, diaphoretic, antibiotic, antidiabetic, antiatherogenic and anticancer medicinal properties (Aitken *et al.*, 1989; Tapsell *et al.*, 2006). For example, the administration of onion products to diabetic rats has been found to significantly reduce hyperglycemia (Lai and Roy, 2004). The biological action of *Allium* products is ascribed to organosulfur and phenolic compounds. Onion has been shown to contain exogenous and endogenous antioxidants such as selenium, glutathione, vitamins A, B, and C, and well-known flavonoids such as quercetin and isorhamnetin (Castleman, 2001). Quercetin (QR) has strong antioxidant properties capable of reducing oxidative stress in the long-term treatment of streptozotocin (STZ)-induced diabetes in animals. *Danae racemosa* is used worldwide as a spice and has been reported to have both antioxidant (Jones *et al.*, 1979) and antinociceptive activity (Cocuzza *et al.*, 2007) in animal models. Like ginger oil, it appears to offer significant protection from cell damage induced by H_2O_2 and its antioxidant properties might result from its ability to scavenge oxygen free-radicals (Cocuzza *et al.*, 2007). Antioxidants protect DNA and other important molecules from oxidative damage, and can improve sperm quality and consequently increase the male fertility rate. Therefore, understanding the role of nutritional and biochemical factors in reproduction and the treatment of sub-fertility is highly important. The present study examined the ability of ginger, carrot seed, *Allium cepa*, quercetin and *Danae racemosa* to promote sperm quality and to modulate follicle stimulating hormone (FSH), luteinizing hormone (LH) and serum testosterone concentration in rats.

Materials and Methods

Preparation of Onion Juice

The underground yellowish-white bulbs of *Allium cepa* (onion) were collected during August 2007 from Ilkhchi in the province of East Azerbaijan-Iran. The skin was removed and fresh juice was prepared using a Tefal fruit juicing machine prior to the experiments.

Analysis of Onion Juice

The flavonoid content of the onion juice was determined using a Shinoda test kit. Qualitative thin-layer chromatography (TLC) was employed for assessing the quercetin content as the main flavonoid in onion. For the TLC, 10ml fresh onion juice was dried under vacuum and the resulting residue was dissolved in 1ml methanol. 20 µl of the methanolic solution was spotted onto a silica gel plate (10×20 cm, silica gel 60 GF254, Merck, Darmstadt, Germany) with a solvent system of EtOAc/MeOH (80:20). Quercetin (Sigma Chemical Co., St. Louis, MO, USA) was used as a control. After developing and drying, the TLC plate was sprayed with a 2 per cent AlCl3 solution in methanol. Quercetin appeared as a yellow spot at RF=0.6. Separation of quercetin was performed with further purification by preparative TLC on silica gel and quantitative determination was performed with a Model 2100 Spectrophotometer (Shimadzu, Japan) at 370 nm by comparison to a pure quercetin standard curve. The amount of quercetin found in fresh onion was 12mg/100g.

Ginger Preparation

Indian Ginger was purchased from Porcina Herbal Shopping Center in Tabriz-Iran. After mixing the ginger rhizome powder, it was dissolved in distilled water and 100mg/kg of it given daily to the experimental animals by gavage.

Quercetin Preparation

Quercetin (QR) was dissolved in 20 per cent glycerol in 0.9 per cent normal saline, mixed vigorously and stored in a dark bottle at 4 °C. The solution was prepared freshly each week.

Carrot Seed Preparation

The seeds of *Daucus carota* were obtained from a local market in Tabriz city (Iran) and used for the extraction. Finely ground carrot seeds (88 g) were macerated in 2 liters of ethanol (95.5 per cent) for 24 h in a procedure repeated three times. After filtration, the filtrate was concentrated in a vacuum in a rotary evaporator (Heidolph, Laborta 4003) at 50°C yielding 24.31 per cent ethanolic extract of carrot seeds. The required concentrations of CSE were prepared by dissolving the ethanolic extract in a mixture of normal saline and DMSO (4:1) and then used for administration to the animals.

Danae racemosa Preparation

Fresh *Danae racemosa* extract was given to animals by gavage at a concentration of 400mg/kg/rat/day.

Experimental Animals

Adult Wistar albino male rats weighing 200 + 10g were 8 weeks old and were obtained from the animal facility of the Pasture Institute of Iran. The animals were housed in temperature controlled rooms (25°C) with constant humidity (40-70 per cent) and a 12h/12h light/dark cycle prior to experimental protocols. All animals were treated in accordance with the Principles of Laboratory Animal Care and the protocols were approved by the Animal Ethical Committee in accordance with the Guide for the Care and Use of Laboratory Animals prepared by Tabriz Medical University.

The rats were provided with water and fed a standard diet. Daily water intake per animal was monitored for at least one week prior to the start of the treatments in order to determine an appropriate amount of water to offer during the experiments. Thereafter, the rats received herbal treatments by gavage for 20 consequence days whilst the control group only received 4cc distilled water.

Surgical Procedure

On the twentieth day at the end of the treatment period, the rats were killed with diethyl ether and the testes in both control and experimental groups were immediately removed and weighed (NIH).

Epididymal Sperm Motility, Viability, Counts and Abnormalities

Sperm from the caudal epididymis were obtained by cutting of the epididymis and release of the sperm into 2 ml of medium (Hams, F10) containing 0.5 per cent bovine serum albumin (Acharya and Shrivastava, 2008). After 5 min of incubation at 37°C with 5 per cent CO_2, the sperm number was determined using the standard hemocytometric method and sperm motility was analyzed using a microscope (Olympus IX70) at 10X magnification. Results were reported as the mean number of motile sperm following the WHO method. Sperm abnormalities were evaluated according to a standard method described by Khaki *et al.*(2009d). Briefly, smears of sperm suspension were made on clean glass slides and stained with periodic acid-Schiff's reaction hematoxylin. The stained smears were observed under a light microscopic at 40X magnification. Sperm were classified normal or abnormal and the rate of abnormal sperm was expressed as a percentage of all sperm observed.

Serum Total Testosterone, LH and FSH

Serum concentrations of FSH and LH were determined in duplicated samples using radioimmunoassay (RIA). Rat FSH/LH kits were obtained from Biocode Company (Belgium) and the protocol provided with each kit was followed. The hormone concentration detected per assay tube was associated with sensitivities of 0.2ng/ml and 0.14ng/ml for FSH and LH, respectively. The concentration of total serum testosterone was measured by using a double antibody RIA kit from Immunotech Beckman Coulter Company (USA). Quantification of testosterone concentration per assay tube was sensitive to 0.025ng/ml (Alvarez *et al.*, 1987).

Total Antioxidant Capacity (TAC) and Malondialdehyde (MDA) Concentration Measurement in Serum

A TAC detecting kit was obtained from Nanjing Jiancheng Bioengineering Institute, China. The adopted method utilized the ability of enzymatic and non-enzymatic antioxidants to reduce Fe^{3+} to Fe^{2+}. TAC was measured by the reaction of phenanthroline and Fe^{2+} using a spectrophotometer at 520 nm. A unit of TAC was defined as the amount of antioxidants required to increase absorbance by 0.01 in 1 ml of serum at 37°C (Lenzi *et al.*,2000). Free radical damage was determined by measuring the concentration of malondialdehyde (MDA). MDA, which is formed as an end product of lipid peroxidation, was treated with thiobarbituric acid to generate a colored product that was measured at 532 nm using an MDA detecting kit from Nanjing Jiancheng Bioengineering Institute, China (Khaki *et al.*, 2009e).

Results

Allium cepa Treatment

The quantity of serum total testosterone was significantly increased in all groups treated with onion juice ($p<0.05$) whilst the level of LH was significantly increased only in the group that received the high dose of juice ($p<0.05$). However, the level of FSH did not differ between experimental and control animals. Sperm viability and motility was higher in both test groups than the controls ($p<0.05$), but only the treatment with the high concentration of onion juice was significantly associated with an increased concentration of sperm ($p<0.05$) (Table 19.1).

Table 19.1. The effect of treating rats with either 0g (controls), 0.5g or 1g onion/animal on sperm parameters, serum FSH, LH, total testosterone, testes weight and the diameter of the seminiferous tubules.

Parameter	*Control (n=10)*	*Onion (0.5g/kg/day) (n=10)*	*Onion (1g/kg/day) (n=10)*
Weight of the testes (g)	1.40±0.821	1.26±0.355	1.42±0.829
Sperm concentration (total count) (No. of sperm/rat $\times 10^6$)	48.68±7.70 (0.319)	57.35±5.36 (0.219)	75.70±2.34* (0.008)
Motility (per cent)	33.75±6.88 (0.112)	73±9.43* (0.003)	87±5.14* (0.002)
Viability (per cent)	66.25±4.73 (0.281)	93.60±1.83* (0.006)	96.20±1.20* (0.009)
Serum testosterone concentration (µg/ml)	1.60±0.091 (0.189)	3.908±0.221* (0.004)	5.017±0.949* (0.003)
Sperm abnormalities (per cent)	6.27±0.711	5.20±0.618	5.12±0.656
LH concentration (µg/ml)	1.51±0.138 (0.371)	2.01±0.197 (0.315)	2.94±0.473* (0.002)
FSH concentration (µg/ml)	20.37±1.788	23.49±1.894	26.61±1.597
Total antioxidant capacity (TAC)	0.53±0.777 (0.151)	0.53±0.138 (0.211)	0.88±0.033* (0.001)
Malondialdehyde (MDA)	4.80±0.212 (0.105)	3.30±0.228* (0.002)	2.43±0.182* (0.006)

Data are presented as mean±SE.

Significance levels with respect to the control group are presented in parentheses, as calculated using the Dunnett homogeneity test. Few significant differences existed. Indeed, testes weight, the diameter of the seminiferous tubules, the percentage of abnormal sperm and the FSH levels did not differ statistically between groups (p value 0.491, 0.381, 0.467 and 0.501, respectively).

Treatment with Ginger

The serum total testosterone concentration was significantly increased in the experimental group that received 100 mg/kg/day of ginger ($p<0.05$) in comparison to the control group. Furthermore, the percentage of viable and motile sperm was higher in both test groups ($p<0.05$) compared to the controls. However, the concentrations of LH, FSH, and sperm together with the morphology and weight of the testes were unaffected by treatment with ginger (Table 19.2).

Treatment with Carrot Seed

Carrot seed administration caused a marked increase with respect to the controls in both testosterone and LH concentrations in spite of receiving 400 mg/kg/day carrot seed (Table 19.3).

Table 19.2. The effect of providing ginger at 0 (control), 50 or 100 mg/kg/rat on sperm parameters, testes weight and serum FSH, LH and total testosterone concentrations.

Parameter	*Control (n=10)*	*G. 1 Ginger Rhizome (50mg/kg/day) (n=10)*	*G.2 Ginger Rhizome (100mg/kg/day) (n=10)*
Weight of the testes (g)	1.40±0.821	1.47±0.373	1.41±0.479
Sperm concentration (total count) (No. of sperm/rat ×10^6)	48.68±7.70	51.90±5.36	61.60±2.34*
Motility (per cent)	33.75±6.88	73±4. 35*	81±5.33*
Viability (per cent)	66.25±4.73	95.80±1.68*	98.80±80*
Serum testosterone concentration (μg/ml)	1.60±0.091	2.91±0.349	3.71±0.387*
LH concentration (μg/ml)	1.51±0.138	1.66±0.316	2.23±0.453
FSH concentration (μg/ml)	20.37±1.788	21.59±2.69	21.68±2.11
Total antioxidant capacity (TAC)	0.53±0.777	0.92±0.016*	0.88±0.341*
Malondialdehyde (MDA)	4.80±0.212	2.64±0.193*	0.81±0.192*

Data are presented as mean ± SE.

* Significantly different from the control group at p< 0.05.

Table 19.3. Caudal epididymal sperm reserves (CESR) and sperm motility of rats exposed to carrot seed extract (CSE)*

Parameter	*Control*	*CSE (200 mg/kg)*	*CSE (400 mg/kg)*
CESR (×10^6)	28.2±1.8 (24.2-32.8)	32.1±2.2 (26.8-37.2)	45.1±2.0* (39.6-51.4)
Motility (per cent)	41.8±2.6 (35.1±47.9)	45.7±2.8 (39.4±52.6)	46.4±3.1 (39.5-53.5)

n: 5 rats per group. Data are presented as means ±SE (95 per cent CI for mean).

*: Different superscripts in a row indicate significant variation at the specified level of probability.

Treatment with Quercetin

The total serum testosterone concentration and sperm concentration, viability and motility were significantly higher in the QR-treated rats ($P < 0.05$) compared to those in the control groups (Table 19.4).

Treatment with Danae racemosa

Sperm viability and motility was increased in both test groups compared to the controls ($p<0.05$), but the sperm concentration was increased only in the group that received the high dose of *Danae racemosa* extract ($p < 0.05$). Treatment with the extract had no affect on sperm morphology or the weight of the testes. With respect to the hormone concentrations, serum total testosterone was significantly increased in the experimental groups (p<0.05), whereas LH and FSH remained similar to the controls (Table 19.5).

Table 19.4: The effect quercetin on sperm parameters, serum total testosterone, total antioxidant capacity, malondialdehyde concentration and testes weight. P values are shown in parentheses.

Parameter	*Control (n=10)*	*Quercetin 15 mg/kg (i. p.) (n = 10)*
Weight of the testes (g)	1.40±0.821 (0.092)	1.36±0.821
Body weight (g)	251±0.365 (0.867)	252.3±0.761
Epididymal sperm count/rat × 10^6	48.68±7.70 (0.301)	47.05±5.70
Motility (per cent)	33.75±6.88 (0.231)	35.42±6.88
Viability (per cent)	66.25±4.73 (0.403)	67.05±5.11
Serum testosterone concentration (μg/ml)	4.01±0.50 (0.301)	4.50±0.45
Total antioxidant capacity (TAC) (μmol/ml)	0.70±0.03 (0.006)	0.75±0.03*
Malondialdehyde (MDA) (nmol/ml)	0.25±0.04 (0.004)	0.30±0.212*

Table 19.5. The effect of treating rats with 0 (control), 200 or400mg/kg/animal/day of *Danae racemosa* on sperm parameters and serum TAC and MDA.

Parameter	***Control*** *(n=10)*	*Danae racemosa (D1) (200mg/kg/rat/day) (n=10)*	*Danae racemosa (D2) (400mg/kg/rat/day) (n=10)*
(TAC) (μmol/ml)	0.70±0.03	0.80±0.03* (0.006)	0.83±0.04* (0.003)
(MDA) (μmol/ml)	0.25±0.04	0.24±0.212* (0.004)	22±0.06* (0.008)
Sperm concentration (total count) (No. of sperm/rat ×10^6)	45.68±7.70	54.90±5.36	66.60±2.34*
Motility (per cent)	31.75±6.88	72±4. 35*	77±5.33*
Viability (per cent)	66.25±4.73	95.80±1.68*	97.80±80*

Data are presented as mean ± SE.

*: p-values of less than 0.05 were considered to represent significant differences compared to the control groups and are presented in parentheses.

Discussion

Reactive oxygen and nitrogen species (ROS and RNS), a group of highly reactive oxidants most of which contain unpaired electrons, are usually known as ROS or free radicals. At physiological levels, they have important roles in the metabolism of all aerobic organisms. However, excessive ROS production which can not be effectively controlled by antioxidants leads to oxidative stress (OS) and has been linked to many pathological processes including male infertility (Aitken *et al.*, 1989, Sharma and Agarwal, 1996; Tremellen, 2008). In the genital tract, low levels of ROS are necessary for normal functioning of human spermatozoa (de Lamirande *et al.*, 1997), including their capacitation, acrosomal reaction and sperm-oocyte fusion. Conversely, excessive OS may cause lipoperoxidation of sperm membranes resulting in DNA damage and spermapoptosis. Standard semen analysis is often inadequate to explain conception failure as the routine microscopic evaluation can not reveal subtle disorders at the molecular level which may be caused by OS (Aziz and Agarwal, 2008). This situation often leads to the diagnosis of idiopathic infertility. Since the appearance of the first reports in the early 1990s (Aitken *et al.*, 1989; Sharma and Agarwal, 1996; Fabricant and Farnsworth, 2001; Lai and Roy, 2004), the role of OS in the pathophysiology of male infertility has been gradually accepted. The importance of seminal ROS production has already been stressed in the WHO Manual (1999) and several methods of ROS detection in semen have been reported (Alvarez *et al.*, 1987; Lenzi *et al.*, 2000; Tapsell *et al.*, 2006; Cocuzza *et al.*, 2007). Aerobic metabolism of human sperm produces various reactive oxygen species, which are potentially harmful to the sperm plasma membrane with its high content of polyunsaturated fatty acids (Aitken *et al.*, 1989; Sharma and Agarwal, 1996; Tremellen, 2008). There is growing evidence that damage to the plasma membrane of spermatozoa by lipid peroxidation plays an important role in the mechanism of male infertility (de Lamirande *et al.*, 1997; Aziz and Agarwal, 2008). The toxic lipid peroxides are known to cause various impairments of the sperm cell, such as membrane damage and decreases in motility (Cocuzza *et al.*, 2007). Control of lipid peroxidation in the male reproductive tract is exerted by antioxidant molecules and protective enzymes within the spermatozoa and seminal plasma (Lenzi *et al.*, 2000). The latter contains enzymatic ROS scavengers such as superoxide dismutase (SOD), glutathione peroxidase (GPX) and catalase (CAT). These enzymes act as antioxidants and inhibitors of lipid peroxidation. Thus, the risk and extent of peroxidative damage in spermatozoa depends not only on ROS production but also on sperm and seminal plasma antioxidant defenses. Whether the protective role of seminal antioxidant enzymes against peroxidation can affect the products of spermatozoa or seminal plasma remains unknown.

Conclusions

Ginger is a strong antioxidant substance and may either mitigate or prevent the generation of free radicals. It is considered a safe herbal medicine with few and insignificant adverse side effects (Khaki *et al.*, 2009c; Nouri *et al.*, 2009). A study by Khaki *et al.* (2009c) has demonstrated that ginger possesses an antioxidant and androgenic activity in doses of 50 and 100mg/kg/rat and has a useful effect on spermatogenesis and sperm quality in these animals. Onion and garlic contain a wide variety of phytochemicals and micro-nutrients such as trace elements, vitamins,

Table 20.1. Characteristics details and uses of the study plants.

Plant Name	*Local Name*	*Family*	*Feature*	*Therapeutic Use*	*Parts Used*
Acorus calamus L.	Bach	Araceae	Perennial herb with extensive rhizomatic clumps. Grown in marshy areas	Plant rhizome is an age old remedy for fever, bronchitis, rheumatism, dyspepsis and for flatulence	Rhizome
Asparagus racemosus Willd.	Satawar	Liliaceae	Extensively branched, spiny, climbing shrub. Found in forest areas	Plant is tonic, diuretic and galacto-gogue. Fresh root juice with honey given for dyspepsia and enhances milking of moth.	Tuber
Costus speciosus (J. Koenig) Sm.	Keokand	Zingibera-ceae	Succulent herb with tuberous rhizomes. Inhabitant of forest areas, field bunds	Rhizomes astringent, purgative, depurative, stimulant, antispasmodic, diuretic and used in constipation	Rhizome
Crinum latifolium L.	Geloch	Liliaceae	Large herbs, globose bulbs. Found along streams	Bulbs are useful in rheumatic troublesand in earache	Bulb
Curcuma caesia Roxb.	Shyama haldi	Zingibera-ceae	Annual herb, blue rhizome. Growth sites are forest areas	Rhizome applied externally in sprains and bruises, used for asthma and tuberculosis, skin diseases	Rhizome

hot plate (45-50 min) to prepare hot water extract. To prepare organic solvent extracts acetone, chloroform, hexane, methanol, and petroleum ether were used. Plant materials were dipped in required quantity of respective solvents (1:1 w/v) and kept overnight at room temperature for extraction. In each case, after soaking the pulp of the plant tissue along with the extracts were squeezed through three layers of muslin cloths followed by low speed centrifugation (5000 rpm for 5 min) to get the clear supernatant (Priya and Ganjewala, 2007). Plant extracts thus obtained were crude stock solution (100 per cent) and stored at 4°C until use (Tiwari *et al.*, 2005).

In vitro Antibacterial Activity of Crude Plant Extract Against X. oryzae

'Well in agar' method was applied for this experiment (Devillers *et al.*, 1989; Onkar *et al.*, 1995). Bacterial inoculum size was standardized following the procedure as described by Andrews (2001). In brief, 24 hrs old single colony of *X. oryzae* was dissolved in 5 ml of Mueller Hinton broth (Hi-Media manual, 2003). The bacterial suspension was adjusted by supplementing Mueller Hinton broth to match the density of 0.5 McFarland standards (McFarland, 1907). The suspension thus obtained contained approximately 10^8 cfu/ml (colony forming units/ml) which served as inoculum. Using a micropipette, an aliquot of 0.1 ml of inoculum was aseptically added to 100 ml of sterilized semisolid PAB media at a temperature of 40°-45°C. The flasks were swirled manually to homogenize the inoculum to the media and dispensed in Petri plates (approximately 25 ml in each plate). After solidification a hole was punched at the center using a sterile cork borer of 7 mm diameter.

Plant extracts were used at two concentrations (50 per cent and 100 per cent). Using a micropipette, 0.1 ml of plant extract of different concentrations was dispensed aseptically in the bored well. Media with same volume of sterile distilled water and extraction solvents were served as control and solvent control respectively whereas media with Streptocycline (500 ppm) served as antibiotic control. The treated Petri plates were incubated at 37±1°C for 48 hrs (McCuen and McCuen, 1988; Bradshaw, 1992). Diameter of inhibition zone formed around the well was measured twice perpendicularly, using a transparent millimeter ruler.

In vivo Application of Crude Plant Extract to Control Bacterial Leaf Blight Disease

In vivo, plant extracts were evaluated for controlling bacterial leaf blight disease following leaf detached technique described by Akhtar *et al.* (2008) and Xie and Mew (1998). Rice plants of cultivar IR24 were grown on sterile soil in plastic pots at green house conditions (average temperature of 34°C/24°C at day/night with 14 hrs of light period and ≥70 per cent humidity). Plants were uprooted at 45 days and healthy rice leaves were cut into 6.5 cm segments from the apical portion. The leaf segments were carefully washed twice by sterile distilled water. Filter paper (Watman no.1) was placed inside sterilized Petri plate and moistened with sterile distilled water. Inoculation of leaf segments were done by 'clipping method' (Kauffman *et al.*, 1973; Koch *et al.*, 1991). Inoculum suspension of *X. oryzae* was made as described earlier (*in vitro* study). Stainless steel scissor was surface sterilized with 70 per cent alcohol and dipped in the bacterial suspension. Leaves were cut 1 cm form the top using the inoculum coated scissors. Three inoculated leaf segments were put inside each Petri plates keeping the abaxial side up. Petri plates were kept in BOD incubator for incubation at 37±1°C.

Plant extracts were applied 24 hrs after inoculation. Leaf segments were directly sprayed with plant extract using a plastic hand sprayer. The plastic sprayer was washed thoroughly each time after every application of plant extract. Plants sprayed with Streptocycline (500 ppm) served as negative control whereas plants sprayed with sterile distilled water served as control. Petri plates were incubated in BOD incubator at 37±1°C. After 5 days and 7 days of inoculation lesion length was measured. Per cent disease severity caused by the pathogen and per cent disease suppression brought by the extracts was calculated (Okigbo and Nmeka, 2005).

$$\%\ \text{disease severity} = \frac{\text{Lesion length}}{\text{Leaf length}} \times 100$$

$$\%\ \text{disease suppression} = \frac{\text{Lesion length}_{(\text{control})} - \text{Lesion length}_{(\text{treatment})}}{\text{Lesion length}_{(\text{control})}} \times 100$$

Qualitative and Quantitative Phytochemical Evaluation

Phytochemical tests were performed to detect the major constituents qualitatively present in plant extracts using standard procedures described by Harborne (1973), Trease and Evans (1989) and Sofowara (1993). Quantitative determination of phenol, alkaloid, tannin, saponin and flavonoid were carried out following the protocol of Harborne (1973) and Edeoga *et al.* (2005) and was expressed in percentage.

Experimental Design and Statistical Analysis

All the experiments were arranged in completely randomized design with three replications. Data were analyzed by mixed model using CropStat version 7.0 software (IRRI, 2007) and means were compared by least significant difference (LSD) at 5 per cent level. Average values were calculated from the data gathered for *in vitro* and *in vivo* experiments to find out the most effective medicinal plant species active against the pathogens and also the solvent which showed the superior activity.

Results

In vitro Antibacterial Activity of Crude Plant Extract Against X. oryzae

The study revealed that almost all extracts were found to inhibit the bacterial growth and produced significant zone of inhibition. Data presented in Table 20.2 indicated that 100 per cent concentration of solvent based plant extracts caused greater zone of inhibition than the 50 per cent concentration. Moreover, significantly ($P \leq 0.05$) greater zone of inhibition was brought by extracts of *A. calamus* used at 100 per cent concentration than the Streptocycline 500 ppm. Similarly, methanol and hexane extracts of *A. racemosus* and *C. speciosus* were also found significantly more effective in producing higher zone of inhibition. Amongst different solvents used for extraction, acetone extract of *A. calamus* produced highest zone of inhibition (31.7 mm). However, hexane was found to be the most effective solvent as it has given comparatively higher zone of inhibition for most of the plant species (29.9 mm - 22.2 mm). Average of trial means of solvent extracts revealed that *A. calamus* showed noticeably higher zone of inhibition (26.9 mm) followed by *C. caesia* (18.2 mm), *A. racemosus* (15.6 mm), *C. speciosus* (14.8 mm), *C. latifolium* (11.5 mm) (Figure 20.1A). Average of solvent extracts in descending order were found as methanol (22.2 mm) > hexane (19.0 mm) > acetone (18.4 mm) > petroleum ether (17.8 mm) > hot water (14.4 mm) > chloroform (12.6 mm) (Figure 20.1B).

Table 20.2. *In vitro* antibacterial efficacy of extracts of five medicinal plant species prepared in different solvents against *Xanthomonas oryzae*.

Plant Species	*Plant Extracts*	*Zone of Inhibition (mm)**		*Mean*
		50 per cent	*100 per cent*	*(per cent)*
Acorus calamus	Acetone	20.7 ± 0.16	42.7 ± 0.52	31.7
	Chloroform	14.8 ± 0.50	34.0 ± 0.33	24.4
	Hexane	19.5 ± 0.61	40.3 ± 0.33	29.9
	Hot water	14.7 ± 0.44	30.7 ± 0.57	22.7
	Methanol	16.8 ± 0.70	35.0 ± 0.54	25.9
	Petroleum Ether	18.0 ± 0.62	36.0 ± 0.41	27.0
	Trial mean	**17.4 ± 0.73**	**36.4 ± 0.56**	**26.9**
	$LSD_{0.05}$	**1.0**	**0.8**	
Asparagus racemosus	Acetone	9.3 ± 0.62	19.0 ± 0.61	14.2
	Chloroform	nd	14.0 ± 0.44	14.0
	Hexane	14.3 ± 0.42	30.0 ± 0.62	22.2
	Hot water	8.5 ± 0.57	18.3 ± 0.71	13.4
	Methanol	11.8 ± 0.33	25.0 ± 0.33	18.4
	Petroleum Ether	9.8 ± 0.39	21.0 ± 0.16	15.4
	Trial mean	**10.0 ± 0.45**	**21.2 ± 0.81**	**15.6**
	$LSD_{0.05}$	**1.2**	**0.9**	
Costus speciosus	Acetone	10.7 ± 0.43	21.7 ± 0.50	16.2
	Chloroform	nd	12.3 ± 0.62	12.3
	Hexane	15.7 ± 0.33	31.7 ± 0.52	23.7
	Hot water	6.8 ± 0.53	15.0 ± 0.42	10.9
	Methanol	11.8 ± 0.63	25.0 ± 0.33	18.4
	Petroleum Ether	7.0 ± 0.71	15.3 ± 0.62	11.2
	Trial mean	**9.4 ± 0.39**	**20.2 ± 0.75**	**14.8**
	$LSD_{0.05}$	**1.2**	**1.1**	

Contd...

Table 20.2–*Contd...*

Plant Species	*Plant Extracts*	*Zone of Inhibition (mm)**		*Mean*
		50 per cent	*100 per cent*	*(per cent)*
Crinum latifolium	Acetone	8.1 ± 0.62	17.0 ± 0.51	12.6
	Chloroform	nd	10.3 ± 0.39	10.3
	Hexane	8.3 ± 0.53	18.0 ± 0.49	13.2
	Hot water	nd	12.0 ± 0.50	12.0
	Methanol	7.2 ± 0.33	15.7 ± 0.61	11.5
	Petroleum Ether	9.8 ± 0.71	21.0 ± 0.43	15.4
	Trial mean	**7.2 ± 0.57**	**15.7 ± 0.65**	**11.5**
	$LSD_{0.05}$	**1.3**	**1.4**	
Curcuma caesia	Acetone	12.0 ± 0.23	23.3 ± 0.71	17.7
	Chloroform	8.0 ± 0.63	16.3 ± 0.33	12.2
	Hexane	14.9 ± 0.71	29.7 ± 0.51	22.3
	Hot water	11.0 ± 0.45	21.3 ± 0.62	16.2
	Methanol	14.2 ± 0.54	27.7 ± 0.44	21.0
	Petroleum Ether	13.5 ± 0.39	26.3 ± 0.24	19.9
	Trial mean	**12.3 ± 0.62**	**24.1 ± 0.71**	**18.2**
	$LSD_{0.05}$	**1.1**	**0.9**	
Control		nd		
Solvent control		nd		
Streptocycline (500 ppm)		22.0 ± 0.01		

*: Inhibition zone including the well (7 mm diameter).

nd: Not detected.

In vivo Application of Crude Plant Extract to Control Bacterial Leaf Blight Disease

Results from *in vivo* experiments indicated that extracts of *A. calamus* specially prepared in methanol and acetone closely followed by chloroform were significantly more effective in checking the lesion length as well as suppressing disease severity and were at par ($P \leq 0.05$) with Streptocycline 500 ppm (Table 20.3). Extracts of *A. racemosus* prepared in hexane whereas, extracts of *C. caesia* and *C. speciosus* prepared in methanol were found to check the lesion length considerably. Most of the extracts of *C. latifolium* were less effective except petroleum ether which suppressed the disease severity. Maximum of bacterial leaf blight disease severity was observed in *A. calamus* (61.0 per cent) followed by *A. racemosus* (48.9 per cent), *C. caesia* (44.3 per cent), *C. speciosus* (38.0 per cent) and *C. latifolium* (29.5 per cent) (Figure 20.2A). Amongst solvent extracts methanol was found to be highly effective (69.8 per cent) followed by

Table 20.3. *In vivo* efficacy of extracts of five medicinal plant species prepared in different solvents against bacterial leaf blight.

Plant Extracts	*Acorus calamus*			*Asparagus racemosus*			*Costus speciosus*			*Crinum latifolium*			*Curcuma caesia*		
	LL (cm)	*DSv (%)*	*DSp (%)*	*LL (cm)*	*DSv (%)*	*DSp (%)*	*LL (cm)*	*DSv (%)*	*DSp (%)*	*LL (cm)*	*DSv (%)*	*DSp (%)*	*LL (cm)*	*DSv (%)*	*DSp (%)*
Acetone	0.5±0.13	7.2	92.8	2.9±0.78	44.9	55.1	3.3±0.66	50.0	50.3	4.0±0.45	61.5	38.5	2.8±0.57	42.3	57.7
Chloroform	1.6±0.35	24.4	75.6	4.8±0.40	73.1	26.9	5.8±0.42	88.5	11.5	5.9±0.30	91.0	9.3	4.4±0.60	67.9	32.1
Hexane	3.7±0.48	56.4	43.6	0.8±0.33	12.8	87.2	2.3±0.01	35.9	64.1	5.1±0.71	78.2	21.8	5.2±0.88	79.5	20.5
Hot water	4.0±0.84	61.5	38.5	3.6±0.88	55.1	44.9	5.5±0.41	84.6	15.4	5.7±0.85	87.2	12.8	4.0±0.71	61.5	38.5
Methanol	0.6±0.08	9.1	91.5	2.4±0.90	37.2	62.8	1.7±0.54	25.6	74.4	3.7±0.59	56.4	43.6	1.5±0.18	22.8	77.2
Petroleum Ether	4.9±0.47	75.6	24.4	5.4±0.71	83.3	16.7	5.7±0.40	87.2	12.8	3.2±0.49	48.7	51.3	3.9±0.56	60	40.4
Strepto-cycline	0.2±0.09	3.0	96.9												
Control	6.5±0.00	100.0	0.0												
Trial mean	2.5	39.0	61.0	3.3	51.1	48.9	4.0	62.0	38.0	4.6	70.5	29.5	3.6	55.7	44.3
$LSD_{0.05}$	0.3	13.6	17.1	1.7	20.1	24.1	1.4	21.7	13.3	1.2	18.2	10.6	1.2	12.3	14.7

LL: Lesion length; DSv: Disease Severity; DSp: Disease Suppression.

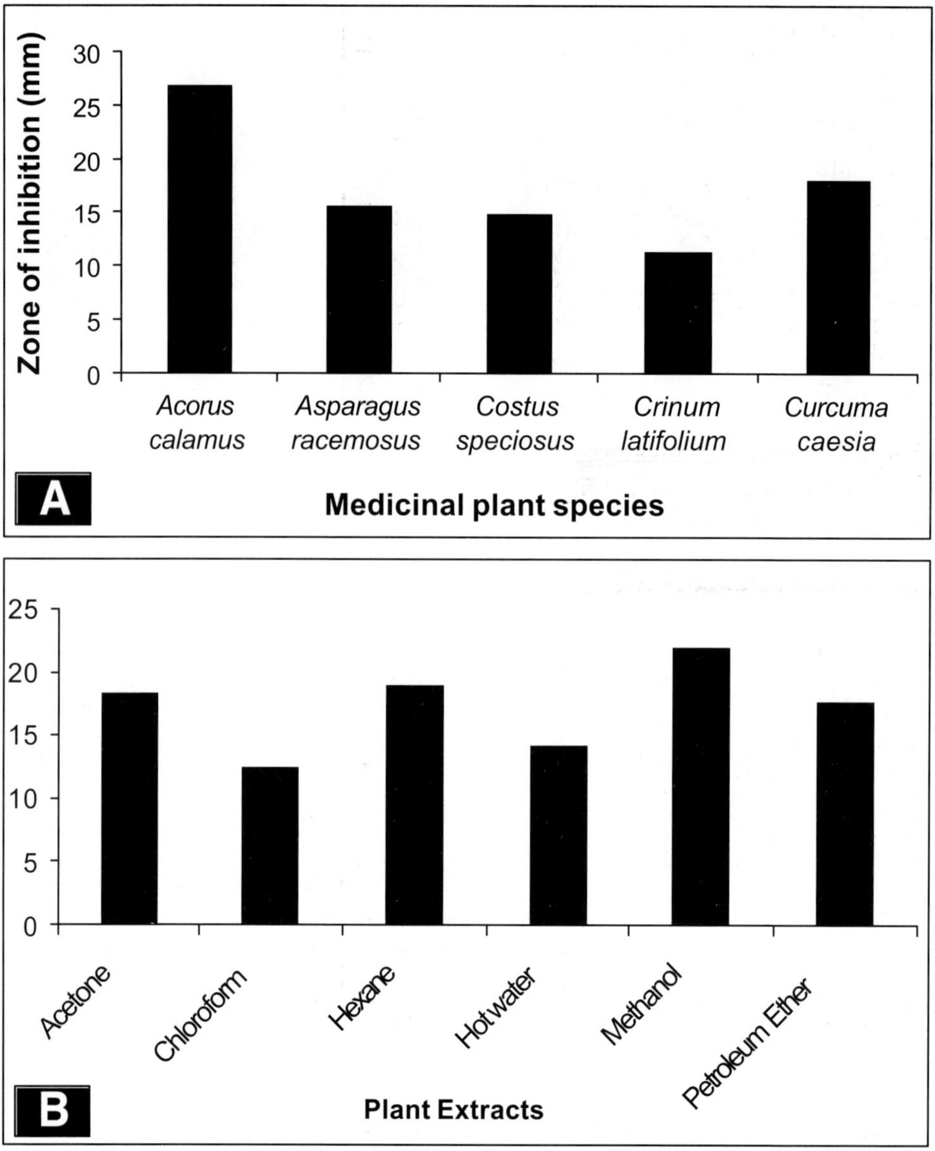

Figure 20.1. Bars represent average zone of inhibition exhibited by different medicinal plant species (A) prepared in different solvents (B) *in vitro* against *Xanthomonas oryzae.*

acetone (58.8 per cent), hexane (47.4 per cent), chloroform (31.0 per cent), hot water (30.0 per cent) and petroleum ether (29.0 per cent) (Figure 20.2B).

Qualitative and Quantitative Phytochemical Evaluation

Phytochemical analysis presented in Table 20.4 indicated that all major phytochemical groups were eluted from the extracts of medicinal plant species

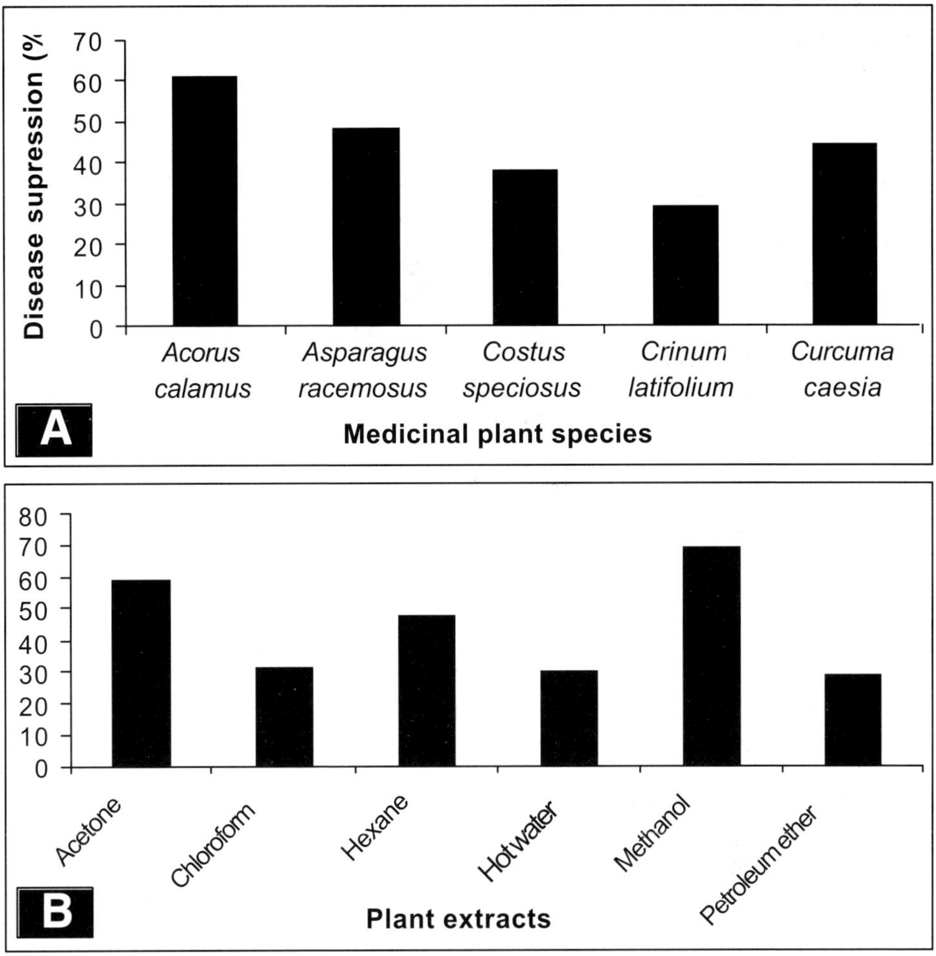

Figure 20.2. Bars represents average percent disease suppression of bacterial leaf blight exhibited by five medicinal plant species (A) prepared in different solvents (B) employing leaf detached technique.

prepared in different organic solvents. However, some of the important phytochemical groups were eluted from particular species by most of the solvents. Tannin was eluted by methanolic extracts as well as hot water extracts from most of the species whereas, phlobatannin was sparingly detected in methanol and hot water among the plant species. Similarly, saponin was also eluted by methanol from most of the species except *C. caesia*. Methanol based extract of *A. calamus* eluted almost all phytochemical groups except cardiac glycoside whereas, acetone extract yielded flavonoid and alkaloid. Moreover, most of the *A. calamus* extracts eluted terpenoid and alkaloid. Methanolic extract was found to elute almost all groups except cardiac glycoside Saponin was the main group being eluted by most of the solvent extracts of *C. speciosus* and *A. racemosus*. Flavonoid and terpenoid were common in extracts of

Table 20.4. Qualitative analysis of the phytochemical groups present in the investigated medicinal plant species.

Plant	*Solvent Extracts*	*Phytochemical Groups*						
		Tannin	*Saponin*	*Flavo-noid*	*Terpe-noid*	*Alkaloid*	*Cardic glycoside*	*Phloba-tanin*
Acorus calamus	Methanol	+	+	+	+	+	–	+
	Acetone	–	–	+	–	+	–	–
	Petrol. Ether	–	–	–	+	+	+	–
	Hexane	–	–	–	+	+	+	–
	Chloroform	–	–	+	+	+	–	–
	Hot Water	+	+	–	+	–	–	–
Asparagus recaemosus	Methanol	+	–	–	–	+	+	–
	Acetone	–	+	–	–	–	–	–
	Petrol. Ether	–	+	–	+	+	–	–
	Hexane	–	+	–	–	–	–	–
	Chloroform	–	+	–	+	–	–	–
	Hot Water	+	+	–	–	–	+	–
Costus speciosus	Methanol	+	+	–	–	–	+	–
	Acetone	–	+	+	–	–	–	–
	Petrol. Ether	–	+	–	+	+	–	–
	Hexane	–	+	–	–	–	–	–
	Chloroform	–	–	–	+	–	–	–
	Hot Water	+	+	+	+	–	+	+
Crinum latifolium	Methanol	+	+	+	–	+	+	+
	Acetone	–	–	–	–	–	+	–
	Petrol. Ether	–	–	–	+	+	–	–
	Hexane	–	–	+	–	–	+	–
	Chloroform	–	+	–	+	+	–	–
	Hot Water	–	+	+	–	–	+	+
Curcuma caesia	Methanol	+	–	+	+	–	+	+
	Acetone	–	–	+	–	–	–	–
	Petrol. Ether	–	+	–	+	+	+	–
	Hexane	–	+	–	+	–	–	–
	Chloroform	–	–	+	+	+	–	–
	Hot Water	+	+	+	–	–	–	+

+: Present; –: Absent.

Table 20.5. Percentage of crude alkaloids, phenols, tannin, flavonoids and saponin present in the studied medicinal plant species.

Plant Species	*Major Phytochemical Groups*				
	Alkaloids (per cent)	*Phenols (per cent)*	*Tannins (per cent)*	*Flavonoids (per cent)*	*Saponin (per cent)*
Acorus calamus	0.65 ± 0.22	0.80 ± 0.22	4.12 ± 0.22	0.56 ± 0.22	1.91 ± 0.22
Asparagus racemosus	0.41 ± 0.22	0.16 ± 0.22	3.25 ± 0.22	0.10 ± 0.22	6.04 ± 0.22
Costus speciosus	0.34 ± 0.22	0.30 ± 0.22	5.50 ± 0.22	0.18 ± 0.22	4.86 ± 0.22
Crinum latifolium	0.52 ± 0.22	0.13 ± 0.22	3.01 ± 0.22	0.15 ± 0.22	3.05 ± 0.22
Curcuma caesia	0.45 ± 0.22	0.81 ± 0.22	3.65 ± 0.22	0.96 ± 0.22	2.82 ± 0.22

C. caesia whereas, extracts of *C. latifolium* mostly yielded cardiac glycoside, alkaloid and flavonoid. The percentage of major phytochemical constituents in different plant species are summarized in Table 20.5. Perusal of table revealed that the crude percentage yield of alkaloids (0.65 per cent) and tannin (4.12 per cent) was in higher amount in *A. calamus* whereas, saponin was precipitated in higher amount from *A. racemous* (6.04 per cent) and *C latifolium* (3.05 per cent) whereas, tannin was detected in higher quantity (5.50 per cent) in*C. speciosus* whereas, higher quantity of flavonoid (0.96 per cent) was yielded from *C. caesia*.

Discussion

Summary of results revealed that *A. calamus* found to have greater antibacterial activity in terms of producing zone of inhibition (*in vitro*) as well as cheking lesion length and suppressing disease severity (*in vivo*). Antibacterial activity and disease controlling ability showed by *A. racemosus*, *C. speciosus* and *C. caesia* were almost similar whereas, *C. latifolium* was least effective in both *in vitro* and *in vivo*. Earlier, Mukherjee and Biswas (1981) tested crude extracts of 25 selected medicinal plants and some were found significantly effective against *Xanthomonas* sp. Similarly, Madhiazhagan *et al.* (2002) found that bacterial leaf blight caused by *Xanthomonas campestris* pv. *oryzae* can be controlled by spraying leaf extract of *Adahatoda vasica*. In our present investigation, there is a strong correlation existed between the activity of different solvent based plant extracts recorded *in vitro* and *in vivo*. Among different solvents used for extraction acetone in particular (for *A. calamus* and *C. caesia*) and hexane in general (for most of the plant species) were found to be more effective in terms of higher antibacterial activity both *in vitro* and *in vivo*. These findings can be explained in the light of Cowan (1999) who reviewed that successful determination of biologically active compound from plant material is largely dependent on the type of solvent used in the extraction procedure. Moreover, intrinsic bioactivity of plant extract depends on their ability to dissolve or diffuse in the media used for the assay (Green, 2004). Moreover, organic solvent based extracts were found more effective than aqueous extract in causing inhibition of *X. oryzae* colonies and greater disease suppression. Among different solvents methanol based plant extracts were found more effective both*in vivo* and *in vitro* irrespective of plant species. Previously, Kagale *et al.* (2004) found that methanol extracts of *Datura metel* exhibited best control of BLB after foliar application under greenhouse condition. Similarly, Satish *et al.* (2007) reported that antimicrobial property of *Polyalthia longifolia* extract prepared in methanol was more effective than chloroform, petroleum ether and hot water.

A wide variability was observed in terms of presence of different phytochemical groups (tannin, saponin, flavonoid, terpenoid, alkaloid, cardiac glysoside and phlobatanin) in the plant extracts prepared in different solvents. This was also reflected in inconsistent antifungal activity of different plant extracts obtained *in vitro* and *in vivo*. Fokunang (2000) suggested that antifungal activity of solvent based plant extracts depends on the nature and amount of active phytochemicals present in it. In the present study majority of phytochemical groups were eluted in methanol irrespective of plant species which may be correlated with its efficacy of the methanolic extract in general for all the medicinal plant species. Similarly, Parekh *et al.* (2005) found that the methanolic extract exhibited more consistent antimicrobial activity compared to aqueous extract. Alkaloids were eluted by methanol and petroleum ether of most of the plant species which was similar to the report of Ramkumar *et al.* (2005) who found that methanol and hexane extracts of *Gymnema montanum* showed the presence of alkaloids. Terpenoid was eluted in petroleum ether and chloroform extract of all plant species. Similarly, Cowan (1999) reviewed that terpenoids can be best extracted in petroleum ether and chloroform. Cardiac glycoside and phlobatanin were mostly present in hot water extract which was align with the report of Vaghasiya and Chanda (2007) who found that cardiac glycosides was mostly found in hot water among fourteen plants.

Presence of high amount of alkaloid in *A. calamus* indicated its possible role of superior antifungal activity. Similarly, Yang *et al.* (1979) also reported that the volatile oil of *A. calamus* rhizome contained six constituents: β-asarone, asarone, duasarone, asaronaldehyde, cis-methylsoeugenol and elemicine possessing strong antimicrobial activity. The trend of various phytochemicals eluted from different organic solvents as well as aqueous extracts of *C. caesia* indicated that the flavonoid alone or in combination with other groups might play an important role in exhibiting the higher antifungal properties. An antimicrobial property of flavonoid was also reported by Alan and Miller (1996). The antifungal activity of *A. racemosus* extracts may be due to the presence of saponin as it was eluted by most of the solvents. The antifungal efficacy of *A. racemosus* due to the presence of saponin was already reported by Shimoyamada *et al.* (1999). Considerable antifungal activity of hexane and methanolic extracts of *C. speciosus* might be due to the presence of saponin and tannin as the earlier reports also indicated the presence of steroidal saponins, sapogenins, oxalates, furans, furan derivatives and starches in genus *Costus* (Oliver, 1986). Activity *C. latifolium* extracts can be aligned with the action of one or more phytochemical groups in combinations as most of them were eluted except terpenoid. Recently Thi Ngoc Trama (2002) in a study found that GC-MS analysis leaves of *Crinum latifolium* the identified 15 alkaloids.

Acknowledgements

We are grateful to Dr. Casiana Vera Cruz of International Rice Research Institute (IRRI) for critical revision of the English and valuable scientific suggestions for the manuscript.

References

Akhtar, M. A., Rafi, A., and Hameed, A. (2008). Comparison of methods of inoculation of *Xanthomonas oryzae* pv. *oryzae* in rice cultivars. *Pakistan Journal of Botany,* **40(5):** 2171-2175.

Alan, L., and Miller, N. D. (1996). Antioxidant flavonoids: Structure, function and clinical usage. *Alternative Medicine Review,* **1(2):** 103-111.

Andrews, J. M. (2001). Determination of minimum inhibitory concentration (MIC). *Journal of Antimicrobial Chemotherapy,* **48(51):** 5-16.

Bradshaw, L. J. (1992). *Laboratory microbiology.* (Fourth edition). Saunders College Publishing. Fort Worth.

Cowan, M. M. (1999). Plant products as antimicrobial agents. *Clinical Microbiology Review,* **12:** 564-582.

Daayf, F., Schmitt, A., and Be´langer, R. R. (1995). The effects of plant extracts of *Reynoutria sachalinensis* on powdery mildew development and leaf physiology of long English cucumber. *Plant Disease,* **79:** 577-580.

Dev, S., and Koul, O. (1997). *Insecticides of natural origin.* Harwood Academic Publishers, Amsterdam, Netherlands, pp. 377.

Devadath, S. (1989). Chemical control of bacterial blight of rice. In: *Bacterial blight of rice.* International Rice Research Institute, Manila, Philippines, pp. 89-98.

Devillers, J., Steiman, R., and Seigle-Murandi, F. (1989). The usefulness of the agar-well diffusion method for assessing chemical toxicity to bacteria and fungi. *Chemosphere,* **19(10-11):** 1693-1700.

Duke, S. O. (1993). Natural pesticides from plants. In: *Advances in new crops* (Janick, J. and Simon, J.E. Eds.). Timber Press, Portland, pp. 511-517.

Edeoga, H. O. Okwu, D. E., and Mbaebie, B. O. (2005). Phytochemical constituents of some Nigerian medicinal plants. *African Journal of Biotechnology,* **4(7):** 685-688.

Enikuomehin, O. A., and Peters, O. T. (2002). Evaluation of crude extracts from some Nigerian plants for the control of field diseases of sesame (*Sesamum indicum* L.). *Tropical Oilseeds Journal,* **7:** 84-93.

Ezuka, A., and Kaku, H. (2000). *A Historical Review of Bacterial Blight of rice.* National Institute of Agrobiological Resources Bulletin, Japan, pp. 207.

Fokunang, C. N., Ikotun, T., Dixon, A. G. O., Akem, C. N., Tembe, E. A., and Nukenine, E. N. (2000). Efficacy of antimicrobial plant crude extracts on the growth of *Colletotrichum gloeosporioides* f. sp. *manihotis. Pakistan Journal of Biolological Science,* **3(6):** 928-932.

Green, R. J. (2004). Antioxidant Activity of Peanut Plant Tissues. *Masters Thesis.* North Carolina State University. USA.

Hall, F. R., and Menn, J. J. (1999). *Biopesticides: use and delivery*. Humana Press Inc., Totowa, N.J., pp. 626.

Harborne, J. B. (1973). *Phytochemical methods.* London. Chapman and Hall, Ltd., pp. 49-188.

Hewitt, H. G. (1998). *Fungicides in crop protection.* CAB International, U.K., pp. 221.

Hickey, K. D. (1986). *Methods for evaluating pesticides for control of plant pathogens.* APS Press, MN, USA, pp. 312.

Huang, H. C., and Acharya, S.N. (2003). *Advances in plant disease management* (Eds.). Research Signpost, Kerala, India, pp. 443.

IRRI. (2007). *CropStat Version 6.1*. International Rice Research Institute, Los Banos, Philippines.

Ishiyama, S. (1922). Studies on bacterial leaf blight of rice. In: *Report of Agricultural Experiment Station. Tokyo*, **45:** 233-261.

Joseph, B., Dar, M. A., and Kumar, V. (2008). Bioefficacy of plant extracts to control *Fusarium solani F.* sp. *melongenaeincitant* of brinjal wilt. *Global Journal of biotechnology and biochemistry*, **3(2),** 56-59.

Kagale, S., Marimuthu, T., Thayumanavan, B., Nandakumar, R., and Samiyappan, R. (2004). Antimicrobial activity and induction of systemic resistance in rice by leaf extracts of *Datura metel* against *Rhizoctonia* and *Xanthomonas oryzae* pv. *oryzae*. *Physiological and Molecular Plant Pathology*, **65(2):** 91-100.

Kauffman, H. E., Reddy, A. P. K., Hsieh, S. P. Y., and Merca, S. D. (1973). An improved technique for evaluating resistance of rice varieties to *Xanthomonas oryzae. Plant Disease Reporter*, **57**: 537-541.

Koch, M., Parllevliet, J. E., and Mew, T. W. (1991). Assesment of quantitative resistance of rice cultivars to *Xanthomonas campestris* pv. *oryzae*: a comparison of inoculation methods. *Euphytica*, **54:** 169-75.

Kurucheve, V., Gerard, E. J., and Jayaraj, J. (1997). Screening of higher plants for fungitoxicity against *Rhizoctonia solani in vitro. Indian Phytopythology*, **50(2):** 235-241.

Madhiazhagan, K., Ramdoss, N., and Anuradha, R. (2002). Effect of botanicals on bacterial blight of rice. *Journal of Mycology and Plant Pathology*, 32: 68-69.

May, R. M. (1985). Evolution of pesticide resistance. *Nature*, **15 :** 12-13.

McCuen, D., and McCuen, P. (1988). *Manual of BBL products and Laboratory procedures.* (Sixth edition). Maryland, pp. 67-72.

McFarland, J. (1907). The nephelometer: an instrument for estimating the number of bacteria used for calculating the opsonic index for vaccines. *Journal of American Medical Association*, **49:** 1176-1907.

Mew, T. W. (1987). Current status and future prospects of research on bacterial blight of rice. *Annual Review of Phytopathology*, **25**: 259-382.

Mew. T. W., Alvarez, A. M., Leach J. E., and Seillgs. J. (1993). Focus on bacterial blight of rice. *Plant Disease*, **77**, 5-12.

Mizukami, T. (1956). Studies on the bacterial leaf blight of rice plant on the entrance and multiplying portion of the pathogen upon the rice plant leaves (preliminary report). *Agricultural Bulletin of Saga University*, **4:** 169-175.

Mukherjee, N., and Biswas, P. (1981). Control of bacterial disease of plants with plant crudes. *Proceedings of Fifth International Conference on Plant Pathogenic bacteria*. CIAT, University of Missouri-Columbia, pp. 549-558.

Nahunnaro, H. (2008). Effects of different plant extracts in the control of Yam rot induced by *Rhizopus stolonifer* on stored Yam (*Dioscorea* sp.) in Yola, Adamawa State Nigeria. *Agricultural Journal*, **3(5):** 382-387.

Okigbo, R. N., and Emoghene, A. O. (2003). Effect of leaf extract of three plant species on *Mycosphaerella fijiensis* Morelet, the causal organism of Black Sigatoka disease of Banana (*Musa acuminata*). *Nigerian Journal of Plant Protection*, **20:** 101-110.

Okigbo, R. N., and Nmeka, I. A. (2005). Control of Yam tuber rot with leaf extracts of *Xylopia aethiopica* and *Zingiber officinale*. *African Journal of Biotechnology*, **4(8):** 804-807.

Oliver, B. B. (1986). *Medicinal plants in Tropical West Africa*. Cambridge University press, Cambridge, pp. 198-199.

Onkar, D. D., and Sinclair, J. B. (1995). *Basic Plant Pathology Methods.* (Edition 2nd). Boca Raton, Florida: CRC Press, Inc.

Ou, S. H. (1985). *Rice Diseases*. 2nd ed. Commonwealth Mycological Institute, Kew, Surrey, England, pp. 61-96.

Parekh, J., Jadeja, D., and Chanda, S. (2005). Efficacy of Aqueous and Methanol Extracts of Some Medicinal Plants for Potential Antibacterial Activity. *Turkish Journal of Biology*, **29**: 203-210.

Pimentel, D., and Levitan, L. (1986). Pesticides: Amounts applied and amounts reaching pests. *BioScience*, **36**: 86-91.

Priya, K., and Ganjewala, D. (2007). Antibacterial activities and phytochemical analysis of different plant parts of *Nyctanthes arbortristis* (Linn.). *Research Journal of Phytochemistry*, **1(2):** 61-67.

Pushpangadan, P. (1995). *Ethnobiology in India: a status report*. GOI, New Delhi.

Ramkumar, K. M., Latha, M., Ashokkumar, N., Pari, L., and Ananthan, R. (2005). Modulation of impaired cholinesterase activity in experimental diabetes: Effect of *Gymnema montanum* leaf extract. *Journal of Basic Clinical Physiology and Pharmacology*, **16:** 17-34.

Satish, S., Mohana, D. C., Ranhavendra, M. P., and Raveesha, K. A. (2007). Antifungal activity of some plant extracts against important seed borne pathogens of *Aspergillus* sp. *Journal of Agricultural Technology*, **3(1):** 109-119.

Shimoyamada, M., Suzuki, M., Maruyama, M., and Watanabe, K. (1999). An antifungal saponin from white Asparagus (*Asparagus officinalis* L.) bottoms. *Journal of the Science of Food and Agriculture*, **72(4):** 430-434.

Sofowara, A. (1993). *Medicinal plants and Traditional medicine in Africa*. Spectrum Books Ltd, Ibadan, Nigeria, pp. 289.

Swain, T. (1977). Secondary compounds as protective agents. *Annual Review of Plant Physiology*, **28:** 479-501.

Tabei, H., and Mukoo, H. (1960). Anatomical studies of rice plant leaves affected with bacterial leaf blight, in particular reference to the structure of water exudation system. *Bulletin National Institute of Agricultural Science*, **11**: 37-43.

Tagami, Y., and Mizukami, T. (1962). Historical review of the researches on bacterial leaf blight of rice caused by *Xanthomonas oryzae* (Uyeda et Ishiyama) Dowson. Special report of the plant diseases and insect pests forecasting service No. 10. Plant protection Division, Ministry of Agriculture and Forestry, Tokyo, Japan, pp. 112.

Thi Ngoc Trama, N., Mitovab, M., Bankovab, V., Handjievab, N., and Popovb, S. S. (2002) GC-MS of *Crinum latifolium* L. Alkaloids. *Zeitschrift für Naturforschung*, **57**: 239-242.

Tiwari, R. K. S., Chandravanshi, S. S., and Ojha, B. M. (2005). Efficacy of extracts of medicinal plant species on growth of *Sclerotium rolfsii* root rot in tomato. *Journal of Mycology and Plant Pathology*, 34(2): 461-464.

Trease, G. E. and Evans, W. C. (1989). *Pharmacognsy*. (Edition 11th). Brailliar Tiridel Can. Macmillian publishers.

Urech, P. A., Staub, T., and Voss, G. (1997). Resistance as a concomitant of modern crop protection. *Pesticides Science*, **51**: 227-234.

Vaghasiya, Y., and Chanda, V. S. (2007). Screening of methanol and acetone extracts of fourteen Indian medicinal plants for antimicrobial activity. *Turkish Journal of Biology*, **31:** 243-248.

Williams, R. J., and Heymann, D. L. (1998). Containment of antibiotic resistance. *Science*, **279**: 1153-1154.

Witte, W. (1998). Medical consequences of antibiotic use in agriculture. *Science*, **279**: 996-997.

Xie, G. L., and Mew, T. W. (1998). A leaf inoculation method for detection of *Xanthomonas oryzae* pv. *oryzicola* from rice seed. *Plant Disease*, **82**: 1007-1011.

Yang, J. S., He, Z. Y., and Chen, Y. W. (1979). Studies on volatile oil constitutions of *Acorus gramines*. *Chinese Traditional and Herbal Drugs*, **4**: 4.

Medicinal Plants: Phytochemistry, Pharmacology and Therapeutics Vol. 2 (2012) *Pages* **349–368**
Editor-in-Chief: **V.K. Gupta**
Published by: **DAYA PUBLISHING HOUSE, NEW DELHI**

21

Pharmacology and Therapeutics of Red Palm Oil Dietary Supplementation in Oxidative Stress Related Diseases: Cardiovascular Disease

O.O. Oguntibeju[1]*, O.B.L. Alinde[1] and A.J. Esterhuyse[1]

ABSTRACT

While it is possible to have nutrition without health it is infinitively impossible to think of health without nutrition. In actual times, the potential of diet in oxidative stress event has motivated many industries to intensify a particular concern toward the impact of dietary components on health. A well established number of studies have documented beneficial effects of natural dietary supplementation against oxidative stress: a condition which represents the impairment of the balance occurring between antioxidants and reactive oxygen and nitrogen species (ROS/RNS) in favour of the reactive species. Health professionals have identified oxidative stress as an underlying metabolic condition which favors the occurrence of a wide variety of diseases, and intensive focus in nutrition research has more than ever brought natural dietary supplementation as a cost-effective therapy. Among the wide diversity of dietary plants and vegetables, red palm oil has captured our interest. In fact, with the recent explosion of red palm oil production obtained from the tropical palm Elaeis guineensis in Southeast Asia, interesting researches in the field are on the rise and the more it is known, the closer palm oil appears as a golden gift of nature. Interesting findings have documented red palm oil potential in health issues and many researches support the hypothesis of crude (fresh,

1 Oxidative Stress Research Centre, Department of Biomedical Sciences, Faculty of Health and Wellness Sciences, Cape Peninsula University of Technology, Bellville, South Africa.

* *Corresponding author*: E-mail: oguntibejuo@cput.ac.za, bejufemi@yahoo.co.uk, Tel: +27 21 953 8495, Fax: +27 21953 8490.

red) palm oil as a good dietary fat and excellent antioxidants source for prevention and/or potential therapy of cardiovascular diseases (an oxidative stress related condition) in human and animals. We aim to overview the knowledge and current understanding on palm oils but more specifically to red palm oil dietary supplementation with special regard to its dietary composition and health implications in the area of oxidative stress related conditions such as cardiovascular diseases.

Keywords: Cardiovascular disease, Red palm oil, Supplementation, Oxidative stress.

Introduction

Taxonomists, throughout the world, have classified up to date an outstanding variety of palm species, about 3000-3700, grouped among 240-387 genera (Bora *et al.*, 2003). Palms are cultivated in mild temperate to warm temperate, subtropical to tropical climates in various part of the world (Australia, Caribbean, China, Japan, Madagascar, Malaysia, Mexico, New Guinea, Nigeria etc). For centuries, people have found many uses of palm trees and their derived products, potentially, as sources of foods (coconuts, dates), as edible products (palm oil, alcoholic beverages) (Ellison and Ellison, 2001). Among this wide variety of palms, a recent explosion of studies and interests concerning the African oil palm known as *Elaeis guineensis* has fuelled the attention of research in many fields. The African oil palm in the scientific classification is a plant of the Palmae (Arecaceae) family, Arecoideae subfamily, Cocoeae tribe, Elaeidinae subtribe, *Elaeis* genus and *guineensis* species (Price *et al.*, 2007). This plant was first illustrated by Nicholas Jacquin in 1763 hence its generic name *Elaeis guineensis* Jacq. *Elaeis* derives etymologically from the Greek *elaia* which means olive and refers to a fruit rich in oil and *guineensis* refers to the site of origin: the guinea's rain forest of West Africa (Henderson and Osborne, 2000). Oil palm has been well distributed in the tropical belt of Africa (Angola, Benin, Burundi, Cameroon, Nigeria etc) and Madagascar (Henderson and Osborne, 2000; Chopra and Peter, 2005). At present, this tropical crop is recorded as one of the most rapidly expanding plant in the world since a phenomenal growth has been reported in the tropical Southeastern Asia particularly in Indonesia and Malaysia. In the later, oil palm plantings have expanded from 60000 hectares in the 1960s to 3.5 millions hectares in 2001 and future prospects even estimate this growth to reach 5.1 millions hectares in 2020 (Jalani *et al.*, 2002). This index made Malaysia to be at current stage as the world's largest producer and exporter of palm oil with an oil yield of 11.80 million tons in 2001, estimates to reach 18.81 million tons in 2020 (Jalani *et al.*, 2002). The outstanding crops expansion seen in Malaysia and Indonesia has drawn the attention of experts of many industries. In fact, interests have been directed not only to the oil production but also to the subsequent solid waste by-products (empty bunch fruit, nut, shell). For instance, in chemical and mechanical engineering, it has been revealed that hybridizing of palm oil empty fruit bunch fibers with phenol-formaldehyde-based composites reinforced with glass does strengthen the mechanical performance of the composites; a finding which could be used for materials in aerospace, automotive parts, boats and office, machinery (Sreekala *et al.*, 2002). Nomanbhay and Palanisamy (2005) have shown that oil palm shell charcoal treated with chitosan acid is highly efficient and eco-friendly to remove heavy metal from industrial wastewater. Another study reveals that the oil palm shell is a useful tool to adsorb hydrogen sulfide (a toxic gaseous compound) emitted from sewage treatment facilities (Guo *et al.,* 2007). A study on the combustion of RPO waste product has also emphasized the use of ash derived from oil palm waste incineration as a cement replacement material (Tay and Show, 1995). Also, palm kernel meal can be useful in animal feedstocks (Onwudike, 1986; Sundu *et al.,* 2006) and palm oil mill effluent can be used as organic fertilizer to enhance considerable growth and yields of crops such as maize (*Zea mays*) (Nwoko and Ogunyemi, 2010). New findings are constantly being discovered. In the transportation sector, Leng and co-workers (2009) demonstrated that 40-70 per cent of palm oil can be converted in a range of hydrocarbons such as gasoline, diesel, and light gases. Therefore, palm oil can be used as an alternative biofuel (Ooi *et al.,* 2004). Increasing data have also identified palm oil as a renewable energy which could be used to generate electricity (Yusoff, 2006). In environmental and civil engineering, due to many of the eco-friendly properties of palm oil and derivatives, the Malaysian palm oil industry is now getting mobilized against the challenge of global warming through projects which could serve in reductions of greenhouse gases emissions (Wahid *et al.,* 2006).

However, notwithstanding the growing interest of those industries, the main application of palm oil production remains in food and oleo-chemical industry. In those industries, two distinct oil by-products are extracted from palm crops: palm kernel oil (PKO) and crude (red) palm oil (RPO) commonly called palm oil. Both oils have gained significant interest in the world market although red palm oil is the most valued in the food industry. Palm kernel oil, the minor oil component (32 per cent), is obtained from the oil-rich seed of the palm fruit (Bora *et al.,* 2003). Palm kernel oil is characterized by a high level of saturated fatty acids (SFA: fatty acids with no double bonds between carbon atoms), about 92 per cent, and a low melting point. PKO is similar to the coconut oil both in color (white to slightly yellow) and in a high content of saturated lauric acid (Bora *et al.,* 2003). Though a vast majority of PKO is used for non-edible products for the manufacturing of detergent and soaps, or biodiesel (Edem, 2002; Jitputti *et al.,* 2006), PKO can be used in confectioneries (margarine, creamy fill of biscuit, chocolate coating), in high-energy sports drinks and infant formulations (Berger, 2007, Murphy, 2007). Red palm oil, the principal oil component (73 per cent) is extracted from the mesocarp of the mature fruit from which it acquires its unusual orange-red color (Bora *et al.,* 2003; Murphy, 2007). Red palm oil is mainly employed for edible applications. Red palm oil has been recorded as the second largest oil consumed and as one of the major vegetable oil sources (Bayorh *et al.,* 2005). Red palm oil is a dietary fat (vegetable oil) with a large fraction of fatty acids and a minor fraction reputed for an excellent phytonutrients content (α- and β-carotene, lycopenes, α-, β-, δ- tocotrienols and tocopherol, and ubiquinone). Red palm oil can be used for home cooking (baking, frying, cooking) and for industrial frying (potatoe chips, instant noodles, snacks) (Ong and Goh, 2002). Al-Saqer *et al.* (2004) demonstrated that functional foods in bakery products can be developed using red palm oil olein (RPOL) and red palm oil stearin (RPOS): fractions of red palm oil obtained after refining. Shyu and co-workers, (1998) emphasized on RPO admirable frying properties. They demonstrated that RPO has a superior thermal stability compared to that of other oil (soybean oil) in vacuum frying: a deep frying method (180°C) that protect frying oil from oxidative degradation (Aladedunye and Przybylski, 2009). However, it is an important notice not to confuse crude (fresh) palm oil/red palm oil with the oxidized palm oil. In fact the crude palm oil mostly refers to the fresh pressed oil that has not been heat processed completely (Tan and Chu, 1991). This concern is raised because oxidised palm oil has been reported to induce rise in blood pressure and cardiac necrosis in heart muscles of experimental rats (Leong *et al.*, 2008).

With the current dietary shift characterized by more fat-intake, more added caloric sweeteners, more animal product consumption, chronic alcohol intake and lack of fitness and weight maintenance, the correlation between diet and oxidative stress related diseases is more than ever established (Popkin, 2003; Popkin, 2006). As health and nutrition are highly correlated, awareness for the relationship between diet and diseases is on the rise. More concerns have lately been raised in the medical and pharmacological fields towards RPO consumption. On-going investigations are archiving reports and several studies have emphasized a link between RPO and oxidative stress related disorders. In the past decades, oxidative stress has been revealed as a major underlying risk factor in the occurrence of chronic diseases such as cardiovascular diseases.

Oxidative Stress and Antioxidant: Relationships

Although oxygen is essential to aerobic life, overwhelming evidence indicate that it is paradoxally involved in toxic reactions which are generative of oxidative stress *in vivo*. Therefore, numerous studies have emphasized the need of a proper balance between oxygen-derivatives and antioxidants as fundamental to maintain health and longevity. However, in the onset of some pathological conditions and mostly with the adoption of a more westernised lifestyle worldwide (reduced physical activity, cigarette smoking, industrialisation, increase of pollution, hypercholesterolemic and improper diet etc.); natural antioxidant defence mechanisms have become unperfected giving a rise to oxidative stress metabolic conditions with subsequent cell and tissue injuries. Oxidative stress represents an overall dysfunction of the balance between the production of reactive oxygen species (ROS) and the antioxidant defence mechanism in favour of ROS production. A wide range of documentations has identified excessive ROS production as a key aspect in severe molecular, cellular and histological damages which arise constantly in the living system. Consequently, oxidative stress in the past decades has appeared as a major underlying risk factor in the occurrence of important diseases such as type 2 diabetes mellitus, metabolic syndrome, cancers, degenerative diseases of the nervous system (Alzheimer disease), degenerative diseases of ageing, cardiovascular diseases (CVD) and inflammatory diseases. Cardiovascular diseases, a generic term which refer to any disorders of the cardiovascular system (stroke, heart failure, ischemic heart diseases etc) represent a major public health problem. It has been reported that a third of the global population is affected (Oguntibeju *et al.*, 2009). A recent review (Oguntibeju *et al.*, 2009) reported that oxidative stress, through lipid peroxidation represents an important risk factor in the development of CVD by induction of vascular dysfunction and inflammation such as atherosclerosis. Indeed, lipid peroxidation has been implicated in a variety of pathological conditions especially in the initiation and promotion of atherosclerosis, an underlying pathology of most CVD. The key aspect identified has been the oxidation of low density lipoprotein (LDL): a major carrier of cholesterol in the blood stream often referred as "bad cholesterol". The formation of oxidized LDL induces the onset of endothelial dysfunction via diverse modifications in the blood arteries as described by Oguntibeju and co-workers (2009). The fact that excessive ROS can generate major health disorders led to the proposal of an increased intake of antioxidants to compensate the depleted stock of antioxidants and to restore the impaired oxidative balance. Thus, growing interest is seen in the field of natural dietary supplementation which indeed serves as supplier of natural antioxidants. Natural dietary supplementation is seen as an improved nutrition strategy to supply natural antioxidants to the depleted stock and therefore can be used for prevention and/or potential therapy of oxidative stress related conditions in human and animals.

Antioxidants play an important role in biological systems. They constitute effective and powerful defence mechanisms against the toxic damages of oxygen by-products *in vivo*. In physiological condition, antioxidants help to equilibrate the oxidative status balance and protect against the onset of carcinogenesis and other oxidative stress related health disorders. Antioxidants can either be natural or synthetic; water soluble (ascorbic acid, gluthathione) or lipid soluble (ubiquinone, vitamin E, carotenoids, retinoids, flavonoids) (Frei, 1994); enzymatic or nonenzymatic; each antioxidant having a specific function. Antioxidants in the human being can be derived from endogenous and exogenous sources. Endogenous antioxidants alone (superoxide dismutase, catalase) however do not totally prevent total reactive species damage *in vivo*, thus, most antioxidants are acquired from our daily diet. Exogenous antioxidants derived from various sources: cereals, oilseeds, legumes, animal products, microbial sources, vegetables, fruits, herbs, spices and teas (Porkorny *et al.*, 2001). Synthetic antioxidants also exists, however natural antioxidants are preferred source as they are readily available, safer and more efficient (Porkorny *et al.*, 2001). Endogenous antioxidants are insufficient to completely prevent oxidative damages *in vivo*. Thus, medical experts and nutritionists have now agreed on the necessity of an adequate fruit and vegetable consumption to supply enough antioxidant defences against incidence of cancers, heart disease, and brain dysfunction. Natural antioxidants are natural defence mechanism against oxidative stress*in vivo*. Natural dietary supplementation is seen as a source of extra natural antioxidants and is achieved from the dietary intake of fruits and vegetables (tomato, spinach, carrots, and red palm oil), or derived food and beverage (rooibos tea, honey bush tea). Natural antioxidant intake has strongly been associated with reduced risk of chronic diseases such as cardiovascular diseases, cancers, diabetes, Alzheimer disease, cataracts and age related degenerative disease (Cao *et al.*, 1996; Wang *et al.*, 1996; Velioglu *et al.*, 1998; Marnewick *et al.* 2000; Knekt *et al.*, 2002; Sweeney *et al.*, 2002; Esterhuyse *et al.*, 2006; Liu *et al.*, 2010). Each antioxidant has a specific line of defence against oxidative stress and acts at a different level to quench oxidative stress related-event. Natural antioxidants may inhibit the formation of reactive oxygen species (sequestration of metal ions, reduction of hydroperoxides and hydrogen peroxide, direct combination with superoxide and singlet oxygen) (Hu and Kitts, 2000), scavenge radicals and inhibit lipid chain breaking reaction initiation and propagation (Nicolle, 2003), or repair damage molecules (DNA, proteins, lipids) and reconstitute enzymes (Porkorny *et al.*, 2001). Natural antioxidants occur in diverse representation: vitamins, enzymes, trace element, proteins and a certain variety of foods product are now well-known as reference source of antioxidants. Some of them are summarized in Table 21.1.

Table 21.1. Natural antioxidants identified in various food products.

Sources	*Antioxidants*	*References*
Animal product (muscles)	Glutathione peroxidase, catalase or superoxide dismutase	Chan and Decker,1994
Nut (peanuts)	Polyphenols, resveratrol and tocopherol	Tosun and Inkaya, 2010
Cereals:		
– Buckwheat	Purified flavonoids fraction	Watanabe *et al.*1997
– Corn	Carotenoids (α-, β-carotene) and tocopherol, sterol	Chen and Yang 1992, Kurilich and juvik,1999,
– Rice bran	Tocols (tocopherols,tocotrienols), oryzanol	Hu *et al.*, 1996; Bergman and Xu, 2003
– Wheat	Tocopherol	
Root (*Echinacea*)	Phenolic acids, echinacoside	(Hu and Kitts, 2000)
Tuberous crop:		
– Carrots	Carotenoids (α-, β-carotene, lutein)	Nicolle *et al.*, 2003
– Potatoes	Carotenoids(lutein, zexanthin, violaxanthin), phenolic compound, flavonoids	Brown, 2005
Cruciferous vegetables (broccoli)	Phenolics, carotenoids, ascorbic acid	Zhang and Hamauzu, 2004
Green leafy vegetables (lettuce, spinach)	Ascorbic acid, vitamin A	Ogunlesi *et al.*, 2010

Seeing that findings have highlighted benefits of natural dietary supplementation in the field of oxidative stress, many studies currently debate the view of RPO as a useful tool in preventive medicine. Thus, the interest of the present work to overview the current knowledge and understanding of red palm oil dietary supplementation in the onset of oxidative stress related conditions such as cardiovascular disease with a special focus on red palm oil dietary composition (fatty acids and antioxidants).

RPO Dietary Fat

Fats are derived from vegetable (vegetable oils) or animal (dairy fats, fish oil, and butter) sources (Zevenbergen *et al.*, 2009). Fats can be classified according to their chain length and the level of saturation. In that order, fats are classified as short, medium and long chain triglycerides (SCT, -MCT, and -LCT) and as saturated, monounsaturated and polyunsaturated fatty acids (SFA, MUFA, and PUFA) (Grundy and Denke,1990; Han *et al.*, 2007; Roynette *et al.*, 2008; Poppit *et al.*, 2010). Fats are important components of a human diet. Fatty acids not only serve for food appeal (texture, flavour, and aroma) and meal satiety, but also intervene in essential body function such as fat-soluble vitamins consumption, gene regulation, and immune function. Moreover, dietary fats are an important source of energy (9 Kcal or $37kJg^{-1}$) for cellular metabolism (Crook, 2000). However, the fat composition of foods determine whether or not their intakes are suitable for a recommended nutrition (Ong and Goh, 2002). It is therefore of great concern since the type of fats consumed has the ability to enhance or reduce blood cholesterol and influence the onset of oxidative stress event such as cardiovascular diseases. In fact, on the subject of fat management, increasing data suggest that the quality of dietary fat-intake worth more than the quantity in the onset of cardiovascular events and other oxidative stress related conditions. Despite the fact that many studies have condemned the role of high intake of SFA, *trans* fatty acids fats in the onset of cardiovascular diseases (Han *et al.*, 2002; Zevenbergen *et al.*, 2009), other studies on fats have also emphasized and recognized the existence of healthy fats such as MCTs, MUFAs, and PUFAs (omega-3, omega-6).

In the 90s, Manorama and Rukmini (1992) evaluated the nutritional value of palm oil and consider it safe for human consumption. However, it is important to remember that red palm oil and palm kernel oil are nutritionally different. Red palm oil constitutes a better choice because of its fatty acids composition (polyunsaturated and monounsaturated fatty acid are higher, saturated fatty acid are lower), and because of its other minor component which gives the later a nice oxidative stability. Bayorh *et al.* (2005) showed that RPO has an unsaturated–to-saturated fatty acid ratio close to one being composed of saturated palmitic acids (40-45 per cent), mono-unsaturated omega-9 oleic acids (35-40 per cent), polyunsaturated omega-6 linoleic acid (10 per cent) and trace of polyunsaturated omega-3 linolenic acid. Palm oil may contain 2-5 per cent of free fatty acids (Matthan *et al.*, 2009; Akusu *et al.*, 2000).

RPO and its Fatty Acids Content

Several reports have acknowledged *trans* fatty acids as an important risk factor for CVD. *Trans* fatty acids also called trans fat are a neo-synthesized type of fatty acid which is derived from SFA and is obtained during the industrial hydrogenation of liquid vegetable oil. Consumption of diet high in hydrogenated fat is reported to increase the production of inflammatory cytokines which have been associated with the pathophysiology of atherosclerosis, an underlying condition of most cardiovascular events (Han *et al.*, 2002). *Trans* fat bears an hypercholesterolemic effect due to the increase of serum levels of lipoprotein a (a strong risk factor for vascular diseases such as coronary heart diseases, stroke) (Mensink *et al.*, 1992; Lichtenstein *et al.*, 1999; Milionis *et al.*, 2000; Vega-López *et al.*, 2006; Zevenbergen *et al.*, 2009). It is therefore important to reduce consumption of diet rich in saturated fatty acids and *trans* fatty acids. With a semi solid texture, an attractive property, red palm oil does not undergo hydrogenation process and therefore is a *trans* fat free oil (Chiu *et al.*, 2009). Hence, red palm oil could be seen as a good substitute for hydrogenated oils. A previous study (Vega-López *et al.*, 2006) investigated if substitution could be useful but study was limited to only older and moderately hypercholesteromic subjects. Intense research towards an RPO substitution of hydrogenated oil is still requested. However, with a low level of saturated acids, the use of RPO came out more attractive than the use of highly saturated oils such as coconut and palm kernel oil. Therefore, in that regard, red palm oil could be seen as potent beneficial oil in the prevention of cardiovascular diseases as a hypocholesterolemic oil (Ladeia *et al.*, 2008).

Mono-unsaturated fatty acids and PUFA can be seen as preventive medicine against CVD since polyunsaturated fatty acids have long been documented for their hypocholesterolemic property characterized by decrease in LDL cholesterol (bad cholesterol) and an increase in HDL cholesterol levels (good cholesterol) (Mattson and Grundy, 1985; Arbonés-Mainar *et al.*, 2007). Ong and Goh (2002) reported that the blood levels of cholesterol and triglycerides depend on the attachment site of the fatty acid to the glycerol backbone (sn 1, 2, 3), with the fatty acids at the 2-position of the glycerol backbone being the most absorbed in humans and animals.

Although dietary palm oil has a similar content of unsaturated and saturated fatty acids, the position sn -2 of the triglycerides of the total fatty acids has been reported essentially occupied (87 per cent) by MUFA, PUFA with a high proportion of mono-unsaturated oleic acid (Ong and Goh, 2002). Fatty acids of the sn-2 position being the most absorbed, such condition enable the dietary palm oil to behave mostly as PUFA instead. This might also explain palm oil potential cholesterol –lowering properties in nutritional studies towards CVD cases and add more credit to its potential preventive performance against CVD events (Ong and Goh, 2002; Bayorh *et al.*, 2005).

Red Palm Oil: A Cocktail of Antioxidants

As previously mentioned, RPO is a dietary vegetable oil with a large fraction of fatty acids and a minor fraction reputed for excellent phytonutrients. A well established number of studies have investigated the beneficial effects of natural alternative against oxidative stress on health. Research in the minor components of RPO has also highlighted promising phytonutrients performance. Red palm oil has been described as a rich cocktail of lipid-soluble antioxidants (carotenoids (α- and β-carotene, lycopenes), vitamin E (α-, β-, δ- tocotrienols and tocopherol) and ubiquinone) (Ebong *et al.*, 1999; van Rooyen *et al.*, 2008). Other minor components are sterols, phospholipids, squalen, tripternic and aliphatic hydrocarbons. The carotenoids, tocopherols and tocotrienols are the most important of these minor components and constitute major antioxidants. The unrefined crude oil is characterized by high level of nutritionally desirable carotenoids and tocols (Murphy, 2007): at least 500-700ppm of carotene of which 90 per cent is mainly alpha (35 per cent) and beta carotene (56 per cent) (Rao, 2000). The vitamin E content is about 800ppm and 70 per cent are tocotrienols (alpha, beta, and gamma) and 30 per cent are tocopherols with α tocopherol and γ tocotrienol for the major portions of the total tocopherols and tocotrienols. Carotenoids are removed in the refining process of crude palm oil (Ong *et al.*, 1999) nd the carotene rich refined palm oil retains up to 80 per cent of the carotene and tamin E originally present in the crude palm oil. Other minor components are quinones and phytosterols, the main sterols present are β- sitosterol (63 per cent), pesterol (21 per cent), and stigmasterol (21 per cent) (Boateng *et al.*, 2006). Recently the minor components sterols and ubiquinols are also gaining positive repute with β- sitosterol found to be cholesterol-lowering agent and ubiquinol (co-enzyme 10) recognised as a more potent antioxidant agent than vitamin E.

Carotenoids

Carotenoids were first isolated from carrots in 1831 by Wakenroder and have been investigated thoroughly since (Krinsky, 1993). Carotenoids derived from animal sources (retinol) and from vegetable sources (mostly as β- carotenoids) are the direct precursors of the essential micronutrient vitamin A. Effectiveness of supplementation with vegetables rich in pro-vitamin A carotenoids has long been adopted as preventive against vitamin A deficiency in children (Tang *et al.*, 2000). In the developing countries, report is made that the main victims of the micro-nutrient deficiency are young children and infants. The vitamin deficiency causes a general impairment of the immune system which renders the children impotent to fight common childhood infections and therefore causes subsequent associated-mortality. The lack of vitamin A daily micronutrient intake also result in the impairment of eye health and vision (Faber and Jaarsveld, 2007). Diverse strategies to improve Vitamin A status of children in developing countries have led many to adopt red palm oil as a readily available and cost effective and natural dietary supplement. Red palm oil content of carotenoids (α- β- γ-) has long been investigated (Hunter and Krakenberger, 1946) and edible crude palm oil is established as one of the richest natural sources of pro-vitaminα- β-carotenes (Lietz *et al.*, 2001). An animal study on Wistar rats conducted by Manomara and Rukmini in the early 1990s signalled that crude palm oil has a high potential to combat vitamin A deficiency in developing countries; an assumption confirmed by many nutritional studies conducted many years later in Honduras, Tanzania, India, South Africa etc (Canfield and Kaminsky, 2000; Lietz *et al.*, 2000; Rao, 2000; Stuijvenberg and Benade, 2000). In South Africa, a national intervention programme of the medical research council in deficient school children showed that fortified biscuits baked with palm oil shortening of approximately 400ppm of total carotenoids were not only effective against the deficiency but also reported as effective as biscuits made of synthetic β- carotene (Stuijvenberg and Benade, 2000). Therefore, palm oil has been adopted to fight vitamin A deficiency in children but also in infants, pregnant and lactating women. A study by Lietz *et al.* (2001) revealed that supplementation with red palm oil increases α- and β-carotenes concentrations both in plasma and breast milk of pregnant women and recommended increasing consumption of the vegetable oil with mild cooking procedures. Other studies in lactating women reported similar findings such as the studies of Canfield and co-workers (2000, 2001) that respectively demonstrated that red palm oil in the maternal diet increased provitamin A carotenoids in breast milk but also improves the vitamin A status of lactating mothers and their infants in many developing countries. The urge for preventive action against vitamin A deficiency, a major public health condition of developing countries has mobilised researchers throughout the world and nutrition potential of red palm oil as an excellent tool for combating vitamin A deficiency (Scrimshaw, 2000). Moreover, RPO carotenoids have also been reported as potent inhibitor of carcinogenesis (Manorama *et al.*, 1993) and powerful antioxidants (Farombi and Britton, 1998).

Vitamin E

In 1922, HM Evans and KS Bishop reported the existence of vitamin E as an unknown factor "factor X" from their reproductive studies on pregnant rats and in 1937, the antioxidant activity of vitamin E was first revealed. Vitamin E is a generic term which refers to a family of eight stereoisomeric compounds. Vitamin E are subdivided in tocopherols and tocotrienols and possess similar chemical structure containing a chromanol ring with a 16-carbon hydrophobic side chain (phytyl in the case of tocopherols, isoprenyl in the case of tocotrienols) (Schwartz *et al.*, 2008; Banks *et al.*, 2010). Diverse representations: α- β- γ- δ- tocopherols and α- β- γ- δ- tocotrienols have been identified and isolated. Both tocopherols and tocotrienols display antioxidant activity due to the hydroxyl group on the chromanol ring (Banks *et al.*, 2010) although in the human body, α-tocopherol has been identified as the more abundant vitamin isomers in the plasma and tissues (Schwartz *et al.*, 2008; Feng *et al.*, 2010).

Biological activities of vitamin E have captured the interest of the world from a health promoting view. In 1981, Burton and Ingold reported α-tocopherol as one of the most active in vitro chain-breaking antioxidants and at present, vitamin E, especially α- tocopherol isomer, is referred to as a superior lipid soluble radical scavenging and chain-breaking antioxidant. Vitamin E is an essential vitamin in diet and its deficiency at a cellular level increase oxidation of cellular membrane hence vitamin E protective effect against lipid peroxidation of cell membrane, oxidative stress damage strongly associated with CVD. Many studies have reported the importance of a diet rich in vitamin E towards oxidative stress related diseases and strong evidences are being collected concerning their important anti-oxidative activity. For instance, Witt *et al.* (1991) showed that supplementation with tocopherols and tocotrienol have protective effect against oxidative protein damage induced during physical exercise. Allard *et al.* (1998) revealed that supplementation with vitamin E and C can significantly decrease oxidative stress in HIV infected individuals and even produce a trend towards reduction of the viral load. Gumustekin and co-workers (2010) indicated both vitamin E and HRe-1 (a hexane extract of *H. rhamnoides*, a plant rich in tocols and vitamin C) as good agent in protecting the heart against nicotine-induced oxidative stress; a finding which support vitamin E as an excellent dietary supplement to prevent nicotine-induced oxidative stress in heart tissue of smokers. Moreover, Vitamin E has been shown to attenuate oxidative stress induced by intravenous iron in patients on hemodialysis (Roob *et al.*, 2000) and therefore appears, as first suggested by Cristol and collaborators (1997), as an appropriated agent to decrease hemodialysis-induced oxidative stress. Another study demonstrated that vitamin E and selenium, an essential micronutrient, promote wound healing activity (Varoglu *et al.*, 2010). A recent study of Seppanen and co-workers (2010), reported the important role of tocopherols and tocotrienols in the shelf life and stability of most vegetables oils, fats and food systems.

The beneficiary effects of supplementation with vitamin E have been widely documented in oxidative stress related diseases and dietary red palm oil has been reported as one of the major sources of vitamin E (Al-Saqer *et al.*, 2004; Muharis *et al.*, 2010). However, contrary to most edible oils, palm oil vitamin E composition is unique. Red palm oil is not only composed of tocopherols but more specifically abounds in tocotrienols, a unique feature. In fact, RPO appears today as one of the unique tocotrienols enriched oils. Intensive researches have lately been oriented on health benefit of tocotrienols. Recent research reveals that tocotrienols have potent anti-carcinogenic properties (Banks *et al.*, 2010; Samant *et al.*, 2010). Recently, Samant *et al.* (2010) explored the molecular mechanisms involved in anti-proliferative effects of γ- tocotrienol in highly malignant mammary cells. They suggested that γ- tocotrienol can be a therapeutic in treatment of breast cancer because of its tumour cells -stopping activity. On a study of inhibition of tumor promotion Goh and colleagues (2006) revealed that γ- and δ- tocotrienols derived from palm oil exhibit a strong activity against tumour promotion. Liu and colleagues (2010) also documented the inhibitory effects of γ- tocotrienol on invasion and metastasis of human gastric adenocarcinomic cells. Tappeiner and colleagues (2010) demonstrated that all tocotrienols may also have antifibrotic effects and could serve in postoperative fibrosis. In a recent study, Muharis *et al.* (2010) provide the evidence of palm oil beneficial tocotrienol cardiovascular properties. They showed that palm oil tocotrienol fractions could restore endothelium dependent relaxation in aortic rings of diabetic –induced and spontaneously hypertensive rats. A research study conducted by Uto-Kondo (2009) has investigated potent action of tocotrienols on adipocytes accumulation, an obesity and CVD risk factor. They concluded that tocotrienols (α- and γ-) can be seen as anti-adipogenic vitamins. Kooyenga *et al.*, 1997 investigated palm oil antioxidant effects in patients with hyperlipidaemia and carotid stenosis. They revealed both palm oil γ- tocotrienol and α- tocopherrol antioxidants potential to prevent and possibly reverse the course of carotid atherosclerosis.

Red Palm Oil in Cardiovascular Diseases

Many investigations in nutrition research have highlighted palm oil health benefits in CVD. Feeding experiment using various animal models have highlighted that RPO is beneficial to health in reducing oxidative stress (Ebong *et al.*, 1999). Red palm oil has been reported to have beneficial effects on arterial thrombosis and hypertension associated with oxidative stress (Edem, 2002; Narang *et al.*, 2004). Many studies have demonstrated the protective effects of RPO in ischemia/reperfusion in animal model against oxidative stress (Esterhuyse *et al.*, 2005; Bester *et al.*, 2006; Engelbrecht *et al.*, 2006; Kruger *et al.*, 2007) and modulation of the serum lipid profile in rats (Karaji-Bani *et al.*, 2006). Other scientific evidence have highlighted the antithrombotic properties of RPO: inhibition of blood clotting (production of prostacyclin/inhibition of thromboxane), reduction of restenosis in carotid atherosclerosis patients (action of palm oil tocotrienols). Wilson and colleagues (2005) reported that palm oil preparations reduce plasma cholesterol concentrations and aortic cholesterol accumulation in hypercholesterolemic hamsters. A research work by Bayorh *et al.* (2005) investigated the effect of palm oil on blood pressure, endothelial function and oxidative stress. The outcome of the research reveals that supplementation with palm oil attenuates endothelial dysfunction, oxidative stress and reduce the mortality associated with hypertensive rats. Thus, palm oil can be seen as a natural tool against vascular resistance and remodeling in hypertension but also as a natural tool to improve endothelium dependent relaxation. Other studies have also highlighted the cardioprotective effects of supplementation with red palm oil in hyperlipidemic rats (Esterhuyse *et al.*, 2006). Moreover, other studies on RPO indicated that RPO has a protective effect in hypercholesterolemia (Hariharan *et al.*, 1996). This study indicated that RPO protective effect in hypercholesterolemia is due mainly to the presence of tocotrienols, tocopherol (Hariharan *et al.*, 1996).

Many additional studies on red palm oil and oxidative stress related condition and health disorders are being investigated. For instance, Boateng and co-workers (2006) showed how palm oil displays an increase protection against various cancers. Hence, potential health benefits attributed to red palm oil dietary supplementation, as previously mentioned in CVD, vitamin A deficiency, cancers, and diabetes mellitus, still need further exploration. A plausible explanation for RPO positive health impact might simply rely on the synergistic action of each component of its nutritious composition. Nevertheless, the challenge to elucidate exactly the complex relationships between palm oil nutrients taken all together and human CVD is not yet totally clarified. This might generally be due to the fact that many studies omit to synchronize with one another, do not analyze synergistically all RPO dietary components at the same time, and also due to the existence of external neglected socio-cultural and environmental factors such as age, gender, and daily cholesterol ingestion. Consequently, a need of a multidisciplinary approach appears essential to confirm this hypothesis and research towards palm oil supplementation still needed.

Conclusions

With the recent explosive expansion of the tropical crop *Elaeis guineensis* in Southeast Asia, intensive researches have been conducted and oil palm knowledge has been brought to a new dimension. Current knowledge have shown that red palm oil (RPO) obtained from the tropical plant *Elaesis guineensis* is rich in nutritional fatty acids and antioxidant vitamins such as vitamin A and E. Moreover, increasing data suggest increase intake of fruit and vegetable including RPO as a long-term, sustainable, and safe approach to increase serum and tissue level of antioxidants and benefit health issues such as CVD, vitamin A deficiency, vision, cancers. In this review, we have shown how palm oil could decrease onset of cardiovascular event by looking separately at each of its main components (dietary fat and antioxidant content). Since each single component bears a potential health benefits, we support the hypotheses that palm oil have a great potential as a preventive and/or therapeutic tool in the management of chronic diseases such as cardiovascular disease. At present, different evidence of protective antioxidant power of RPO are still being gathered as a probable dietary approach to overcome the risk of CVD and other non communicable health conditions. Nevertheless, many challenges to elucidate the exact relationships between all RPO dietary components in single studies provide limited information and further studies to investigate the effects of palm oil supplementation are still needed.

References

Akusu, M.O., Achinewhu, S.C., and Mitchell, J. (2000). Quality attributes and storage stability of locally and mechanically extracted crude palm oils in selected communities in Rivers and Bayelsa states, Nigeria. *Plant Foods Hum Nutr.*, **55(2):** 119-26.

Aladedunye, F.A., and Przybylsk, R. (2009). Protecting oil during frying: a comparative study. *Eur. J. Lipid Sci. Technol.*, **111**: 893-901.

Allard, J.P., Aghdassi, E., Chau, J., Tam, C., Kovacs, C.M., Salit, *I.E.*, and Walmsley, S.L. (1998). Effects of vitamin E and C supplementation on oxidative stress and viral load in HIV-infected subjects. *AIDS*, **12(13)**: 1653-9.

Al-Saqer, J.M., Sidhu, J.S., Al-Hooti, S.N., Al-Amiri, H.A., Al-Othman, A., Al-Haji, L., Ahmed, N., Mansour, I.B., and Minal, J. (2004). Developing functional foods using red palm oil. IV. Tocopherols and tocotrienols. *Food Chem.*, **85(4):** 579-583.

Arbonés-Mainar, J.M., Navarro, M.A., Carnicer, R., Guillén, N., Surra, J.C., Acín, S., Guzmán, M.A., Sarría, A.J., Arnal, C., Aguilera, M.P., Jiménez, A., Beltrán, G., Uceda, M., and Osada, J. (2007). Accelerated atherosclerosis in apolipoprotein E-deficient mice fed Western diets containing palm oil compared with extra virgin olive oils: a role for small, dense high-density lipoproteins. *Atherosclerosis*, **194(2):** 372-82.

Banks, R., Speakman, J.R., and Selman, C. (2010). Vitamin E supplementation and mammalian lifespan. *Mol Nutr Food Res.*, **54(5):** 719-25.

Bayorh, M.A., Abukhalaf, I.K., and Ganafa, A.A. (2005). Effect of palm oil on blood pressure, endothelial function and oxidative stress. *Asia Pac J Clin Nutr.*, **14(4):** 325-339.

Berger, K.G. (2007). Trans-free fats with the products of the oil palm– a selective review. *Czech J. Food Sci.*, **25(4):** 174 -181.

Bergman, C.J., and Xu, Z. (2003). Genotype and environment effects on tocopherol, tocotrienol, and γ-oryzanol contents of Southern US rice. *Cereal Chemistry*, **80 (4):** 446-449.

Bester, D.J., Van Rooyen, J., Du Toit, E. F., and Esterhuyse, A. J. (2006). Red palm oil protects against the consequences of oxidative stress when supplemented with dislipidaemic diets. *Medical Technology South Africa*, **20 (1):** 3-10.

Boateng, J.,Verghese, M., Chawan, C.B., Shackelford, L., Walker, L.T., Khatiwada, J., and Williams, D.S. (2006). Red pal oil suppresses the formation of azoxymethane (AOM) induced aberrant crypt foci (ACF) in Fisher 344 male rats. *Food Chem. Toxicol.*, **44(10):** 1667-1673.

Bora, P.S., Rocha, R.V., Narain, N., Moreira-Monteiro, A.C., and Moreira, R.A. (2003). Characterization of principal nutritional components of Brazilian oil palm (*Eliaes guineensis*) fruits. *Bioresour Technol.*, **87(1):** 1-5.

Brown, C.R.(2005 0. Antioxidants in potato. *Am. J. Potato Res.*, **82(2):** 163-172.

Burton, G.W., and Ingold, K.U. (1981). Autoxidation of biological molecules. The antioxidant activity of vitamin E and related chain-breaking phenolic antioxidants *in vitro*. *J. Am. Chem. Soc.*, **103**: 6472-6477.

Canfield, L.M., and Kaminsky, R.G. (2000). Red palm oil in the maternal diet improves the vitamin A status of lactating mothers and their infants. *Food Nutr Bull.*, **21(2):** 144-148.

Canfield, L.M., Kaminsky, R.G., Taren, D.L., Shaw, E., and Sander, J.K. (2001). Red palm oil in the maternal diet increases provitamin A carotenoids in breastmilk and serum of the mother-infant dyad. *Eur J Nutr.*, **40:** 30-38.

Cao, G., Sofic, E., and Prior R.L. (1996). Antioxidant capacity of tea and common vegetables. *J. Agric. Food Chem.*, **44 (11):** 3426–3431.

Chan, K.M., and Decker, E.A. (1994). Endogenous skeletal muscle antioxidants. *Crit Rev Food Sci Nutr.*, **34(4)**: 403-26.

Chen, B.H., and Yang, S.H. (1992). An improved analytical method for the determination of carotenes and xanthophylls in dried plant materials and mixed feeds. *Food Chem.*, **44(1)**: 61-66.

Chiu, M.C., Coutinho, C.M., and Gonçalves, L.A.G. (2009). Carotenoids concentration of palm oil using membrane technology. *Desalination*, **245**: 783-786.

Chopra, V.L. (ed.)., Peter, K.V. (ed.). (2005). Handbook of industrial crops. Binghamton, N.Y: Food products and The Haworth reference.

Cristol,J.P., Bosc, J.Y., Badiou, S., Leblanc, M., Lorrho, R., Descomps, B., and Canaud, B. (1997). Erythropoietin and oxidative stress in haemodialysis: beneficial effects of vitamin E supplementation. *Nephrol Dial Transplant.*,**12(11)**: 2312-7

Crook, M.A. (2000). Lipid clearance and total parenteral nutrition: the importance of monitoring plasma lipids. *Nutrition*, **16(9):** 774-5.

Ebong, P. E., Owu, D. U., and Isong, E. U. (1999). Influence of palm oil (*Elaesis guineensis*) on health. *Plant Foods Hum Nutr.*, **53 (3):** 209-22.

Edem, D.O. (2002). Palm oil: biochemical, physiological, nutritional, hematological, and toxicological aspects: a review. *Plant Foods Hum Nutr.*, **57(3-4):** 319-41.

Ellison, D., and Ellison, A. (2001).Cultivated palms of the world. Pretoria: Briza.

Engelbrecht, A., Esterhuyse, J., du Toit, E. F., Lochner, A. and van Rooyen, J. (2006). p38 -MAPK and PKB/Akt, possible role players in red palm oil-induced protection of the isolated perfused rat heart? *J. Nutr. Biochem.*, **17 (4):** 265-71.

Esterhuyse, A. J., Du Toit, E. F., Benade, A. J., and Van Rooyen, J. (2005). Dietary red palm oil improves reperfusion cardiac function in the isolated perfused rat heart of animals fed a high cholesterol diet. Prostaglandins Leukot. *Essent. Fatty Acids*, **72:** 153-61.

Esterhuyse, J.S., van Rooyen, J., Strijdom, H., Bester, D., and du Toit, E.F. (2006). Proposed mechanisms for red palm oil induced cardioprotection in a model of hyperlipidaemia in the rat. Prostaglandins Leukot. *Essent. Fatty Acids*, **75**: 375-384.

Faber, M., and van Jaarsveld, P.J. (2007). The production of provitamin A-rich vegetables in home-gardens as a means of addressing vitamin A deficiency in rural African communities. *J. Sci. Food Agric.*, **87(3):** 366-377.

Farombi, E.O., and Britton, G. (1999). Antioxidant activity of palm oil carotenes in organic solution: effects of structure and chemical reactivity. *Food Chem.*, **64(3):** 315-321.

Feng, Z., Liu, Z., Li, X., Jia, H., Sun, L., Tian, C., Jia, L., and Liu, J. (2010). Alpha-tocopherol is an effective phase II enzyme inducer: protective effects on acrolein-induced oxidative stress and mitochondrial dysfunction in human retinal pigment epithelial cells. *J Nutr Biochem.*, **10:** 1016.

Frei, B. (ed). (1994). Natural antioxidant in human health and disease.London: Academic press.

Goh, S.H., Hew, N.F., Norhanom, A.W., and Yadav, M. (1994). Inhibition of tumour promotion by various palm-oil tocotrienols. *Int J Cancer*, **57(4):** 529-31.

Gumustekin, K., Taysi, S., Alp, H.H., Aktas, O., Oztasan, N., Akcay, F., Suleyman, H., Akar, S., Dane, S., and Gul, M. (2010). Vitamin E and *Hippophea rhamnoides* L. extract reduce nicotine-induced oxidative stress in rat heart. *Cell Biochem Funct.*, **28(4):** 329-33.

Guo, J., Luo, Y., Lua, A.C., Chi, R., Chen, Y., Bao, X., and Xiang, S. (2007). Adsorption of hydrogen sulphide (H2S) by activated carbons derived from oil-palm shell. *Carbon*, **45(2):** 330-336.

Grundy, S.M., and Denke, M.A. (1990). Dietary influences on serum lipids and lipoproteins. *J Lipid Res.*, **31(7):** 1149-72.

Han, J.R., Deng, B., Sun, J., Chen, C.G., Corkey, B.E., Kirkland, J.L., Ma, J., and Guo, W. (2007). Effects of dietary medium-chain triglyceride on weight loss and insulin sensitivity in a group of moderately overweight free-living type 2 diabetic Chinese subjects. *Metabolism*, **56(7):** 985-991.

Han, S.N., Leka, L.S., Lichtenstein, A.H., Ausman, L.M., Schaefer, E.J., and Meydani, S.N. (2002). Effect of hydrogenated and saturated, relative to polyunsaturated, fat on immune and inflammatory responses of adults with moderate hypercholesterolemia. *J Lipid Res.*, **43(3):** 445-52.

Hariharan, K., Purushothama, S., and Raina, P.L. (1996). Studies on red palm oil: Effect of partial supplementation of saturated fats upon lipids and lipoproteins. *Nutr Res.*, **16(8):** 1381-1392.

Henderson, J., and Osborne, D.J. (20000. The oil palm in all our lives: how this came about. *Endeavour*, **24(2):** 63-8.

Hu, W., Wells, J.H., Shin, T.S., and Godber, J.S. (1996). Comparison of isopropanol and hexane for extraction of vitamin E and oryzanols from stabilized rice bran. *J Am Oil Chem Soc.*, **73(12):** 1653-1656.

Hu, C., and Kitts, D.D. (2000). Studies on the antioxidant activity of *Echinacea* root extract. *J Agric Food Chem.*, **48(5):** 1466-72.

Hunter, R.F., and Krakenberger, R.M. (1946). Palm oil carotenoids. *Biochem J.*, **40:** 492-493.

Jalani, B.S., Yusof, B., Ariffin, D., Chan, K.W., and Rajanaidu, N. (2002). Prospects of elevating national oil palm productivity: a Malaysian perspective. *Oil palm industry economic journal*, **2(2):** 1-9.

Jitputti, J., Kitiyanan, B., Rangsunvigit, P., Bunyakiat, K., Attanatho, L., and Jenvanitpanjakul, P. (2006).Transesterification of crude palm kernel oil and crude coconut oil by different solid catalysts. *Chem Eng J.*, **116**: 61-66.

Karaji-Bani, M., Montazeri, F., and Hashemi, M. (2006). Effect of palm oil on serum lipid profile in rats. *Pak J Nutr.*, **5(3):** 234-36.

Knekt, P., Kumpulainenm, J., Järvinen, R., Rissanen, H., Heliövaara, M., Reunanen, A., Hakulinen, T., and Aromaa, A. (2002). Flavonoid intake and risk of chronic diseases. *Am J Clin Nutr.*, **76(3):** 560-8.

Kooyenga, D.K., Geller, M., Watkins, T.R., Gapor, A., Diakoumakis, E., and Bierenbaum, M.L. (1997). Palm oil antioxidant effects in patients with hyperlipidaemia and carotid stenosis-2 year experience.*Asia Pacific J Clin Nutr.*, **6(1):** 72-75.

Krinsky, N.I. (1993). Actions of carotenoids in biological systems.*Annu Rev Nutr.*, **13:** 561-87.

Kruger, M. J., Engelbrecht, A., Esterhuyse, J., du Toit, E. F., and van Rooyen, J. (2007). Dietary red palm oil reduces ischaemia –reperfusion injury in rats fed hypercholesterolaemic diet. *Br. J. Nutr.*, **97 (4):** 653-60.

Kurilich, A.C., and Juvik, J.A. (1999). Quantification of carotenoid and tocopherol antioxidants in Zea mays. *J. Agric. Food Chem.*, **47 (5):** 1948–1955.

Ladeia, A.M., Costa-Matos, E., Barata-Passos, R., and Costa, A. (2008). A palm oil-rich diet may reduce serum lipids in healthy young individuals. *Nutrition*, **24 (1):** 11-15.

Leng, T.Y., Mohamed, A.R., and Bhatia, S. (1999). Catalytic conversion of palm oil to fuels and chemicals. *Canadian Journal of Chemical Engineering*, **77(1): 15**6-162.

Leong, X.F., Aishah, A., Nor Aini, U., Das, S., and Jaarin, K. (2008).Heated palm oil causes rise in blood pressure and cardiac changes in heart muscle in experimental rats. *Arch. Med. Res.*, **39(6):** 567-572.

Lichtenstein, A.H., Ausman, L.M., Jalbert, S.M., and Schaefer, E.J. (1999). Effects of different forms of dietary hydrogenated fats on serum lipoprotein cholesterol levels. *N Engl J Med.*, **340(25):** 1933-40. Erratum in: *N Engl J Med.*, **341(11)**: 856.

Lietz, G., Henry, C.J.K., Mulokozi, G., Mugyabuso, J.K.L., Ballart, A., Ndossi, G.D., Lorri, W., and Tomkins, A. (2001). Comparison of the effects of supplemental red palm oil and sunflower oil on maternal vitamin A status. *Am. J. Clin. Nutr.*, **74(4):** 501-509.

Liu, H.K., Wang, Q., Li, Y., Sun, W.G., Liu, J.R., Yang, Y.M., Xu, W.L., Sun, X.R., and Chen, B.Q. (2010). Inhibitory effects of [gamma]-tocotrienol on invasion and metastasis of human gastric adenocarcinoma SGC-7901 cells. *J. Nutr. Biochem.*, **21(3):** 206-213.

Manorama, R., and Rukmini, C. (1992). Nutritional evaluation of crude palm oil in rats. *Am. J. Clin. Nutr.*, **53:** 1031S-1033S.

Manorama, R., Chinnasamy, N., and Rukmini, C.(1993). Effect of red palm oil on some hepatic drug-metabolizing enzymes in rats. *Food Chem. Toxicol.*, **31(8):** 583-588.

Marnewick, J.L., Gelderblom, W.C.A., and Joubert, E. (2000). An investigation on the antimutagenic properties of South African herbal teas. *Mutat. Res.*, **471:** 157-166.

Matthan, N.R., Dillard, A., Lecker, J.L., Ip, B., and Lichtenstein, A.H. (2009). Effects of dietary palmitoleic acid on plasma lipoprotein profile and aortic cholesterol accumulation are similar to those of other unsaturated fatty acids in the F1B golden Syrian hamster. *J Nutr.*, **139(2):** 215-21.

Mattson, F.H., and Grundy, S.M. (1985). Comparison of effects of dietary saturated, monounsaturated, and polyunsaturated fatty acids on plasma lipids and lipoproteins in man. *J. Lipid Res.*, **26:** 194-202.

Mensink, R.P., Zock, P.L., Katan, M.B., and Hornstra, G. (1992). Effect of dietary cis and trans fatty acids on serum lipoprotein[a] levels in humans. *J Lipid Res.*, **33(10):** 1493-501.

Milionis, H.J., Winder, A.F., and Mikhailidis, D.P. (2000). Lipoprotein (a) and stroke. *J Clin Pathol.*, **53(7):** 487-96.

Muharis, S.P., Top, A.G., Murugan, D., and Mustafa, M.R. (2010). Palm oil tocotrienol fractions restore endothelium dependent relaxation in aortic rings of streptozotocin-induced diabetic and spontaneously hypertensive rats. *Nutr Res.*, **30(3):** 209-16.

Murphy, D.J. (2007). Future prospects for oil palm in the 21st century: Biological and related challenges. *Eur J Lipid Sci Technol.*, **109(4):** 296-306.

Narang, D., Sood, S., Thomas, M. K., Dinda, A. K., and Maulik, S. K. (2004). Effect of dietary palm olein oil on oxidative stress associated with ischemic-reperfusion injury in isolated rat heart. *BMC Pharmacology*, **4:** 29.

Nicolle, C., Cardinault, N., Aprikian, O., Busserolles, J., Grolier, P., Rock, E., Demigné, C., Mazur, A., Scalbert, A., Amouroux, P., and Rémésy, C. (2003). Effect of carrot intake on cholesterol metabolism and on antioxidant status in cholesterol-fed rat. *Eur J Nutr.*, **42(5):** 254-61.

Nomanbhay, S.M., and Palanisamy, K. (2005). Removal of heavy metal from industrial wastewater using chitosan coated oil palm shell charcoal. *Electron. J. Biotechnol.*, **8(1):** 43-53.

Nwoko, C.O., and Ogunyemi, S. (2010). Evaluation of palm oil mill effluent to maize (*Zea mays.* L) crop: Yields, tissue nutrient content and residual soil chemical properties. *AJCS.* **(1):** 16-22.

Ogunlesi, M., Okiei, W., Azeez, L., Obakachi, V., Osunsanmi, M., and Nkenchor, G. (2010). Vitamin C contents of tropical vegetables and foods determined by voltammetric and titrimetric methods and their relevance to the medicinal uses of the plants. *Int J Electrochem Sc.*, **5:** 105-115.

Oguntibeju, O.O., Esterhuyse, A.J.,and Truter, E.J. (2009). Cardiovascular disease and the potential protective role of antioxidants. *Afr. J. Biotechnol.*, **8(14):** 3107-3117.

Ong, A.S., and Goh, S.H. (2002). Palm oil: a healthful and cost-effective dietary component. *Food Nutr Bull.*, **23(1):** 11-22.

Ong, K.K., Fakhru'l-Raz,i A., Baharin, B.S., and Hassan, M.A. (1999). Degumming of crude palm oil by membrane filtration. *Artif Cells Blood Substit Immobil Biotechnol.*, **27(5-6):** 381-5.

Onwudike, O.C. (1986). Palm kernel meal as a feed for poultry. 3. Replacement of groundnut cake by palm kernel meal in broiler diets. *Animal Feed Science and Technology*, **16(3):** 195-202.

Ooi, Y.S., Zakaria, R., Mohamed, A.R., and Bhatia, S. (2004). Catalytic conversion of palm oil-based fatty acid mixture to liquid fuel. *Biomass and Bioenergy*, **27:** 477-484.

Popkin, B.M. (2003). The nutrition transition in the developing world. *Development Policy Review*, **21(5-6):** 581-597.

Popkin, B.M. (2006). Global nutrition dynamics: the world is shifting rapidly toward a diet linked with noncommunicable diseases. *Am J Clin Nutr.*, **84(2):** 289-98.

Poppitt, S.D., Strik, C.M., MacGibbon, A.K., McArdle, B.H., Budgett, S.C., and McGill, A.T. (2010). Fatty acid chain length, postprandial satiety and food intake in lean men. *Physiol Behav.*, **101(1):** 161-7.

Price, Z., Mayes, S., Billotte, N., Hafeez, F., Dumortier, F., and MacDonald, D. (2007). Palm oil. *Genome Mapping and Molecular Breeding in Plants*, **6:** 93-108.

Rao, B.S.N. (2000). Potential use of red palm oil in combating vitamin A deficiency in India. *Food Nutr Bull.*, **21(2):** 202-211.

Roob, J.M., Khoschsorur, G., Tiran, A., Horina, J.H., Holzer, H., and Winklhofer-Roob, B.M. (2000). Vitamin E attenuates oxidative stress induced by intravenous iron in patients on hemodialysis. *J Am Soc Nephrol.*, **11(3):** 539-49.

Roynette, C.E., Rudkowska, I., Nakhasi, D.K., and Jones, P.J. (2008) Structured medium and long chain triglycerides show short-term increases in fat oxidation, but no changes in adiposity in men. *Nutr Metab Cardiovasc Dis.*, **18(4):** 298-305.

Samant, G.V., Wali, V.B., and Sylvester, P.W. (2010). Anti-proliferative effects of gamma-tocotrienol on mammary tumour cells are associated with suppression of cell cycle progression. *Cell Prolif.*, **43(1):** 77-83.

Schwartz, H., Ollilainen, V., Piironen, V., and Lampi, A.M. (2008). Tocopherol, tocotrienol and plant sterol contents of vegetable oils and industrial fats. *Journal of Food Composition and Analysis*, **21(2):** 152-161.

Scrimshaw, N.S. (2000). Nutritional potential of red palm oil for combating vitamin A deficiency. *Food Nutr Bull.*, **21(2):** 195-201.

Seppanen, C.M., Song, Q., and Csallany, A. S. (2010). The antioxidant functions of tocopherol and tocotrienol homologues in oils, fats, and food systems. *J Am Oil Chem Soc.*, **87(5):** 469-481.

Shyu, S.L., Hau, L.B., and Hwang, L.S. (1997). Effect of vacuum frying on the oxidative stability of oils. *J Am Oil Chem Soc.*, **75(10):** 1393-1398.

Sreekala, M.S., George, J., Kumaran, M.G., and Thomas, S. (2002). The mechanical performance of hybrid phenol-formaldehyde-based composites reinforced with glass and oil palm fibres. *Composites Science and Technology*, **62**: 339–353.

Sundu, B., Kumar, A., and Dingle, J. (2006). Palm kernel meal in broiler diets: effect on chicken performance and health. *World's Poultry Science Journal*, **62:** 316-325.

Sweeney, M.I., Kalt, W., MacKinnon, S.L., Ashby, J., and Gottschall-Pass, K.T. (2002). Feeding rats diets enriched in lowbush blueberries for six weeks decreases ischemia-induced brain damage. *Nutr Neurosci.*, **5(6):** 427-31.

Tan, B., and Chu, F.L. (1991). Effects of palm carotenoids in rat hepatic cytochrome P450-mediated benzo (a) pyrene metabolism. *Am. J. Clin. Nutr.*, **53 (4):** 1071S-1075S.

Tang, G., Qin, J., Hu, S., Hao, L., Xu, Q., Gu, X-F., Fjeld, C.R., Gao, X., Yin, S.A., and Russell, R.M. (2000). Protection of vitamin A status in Chinese children by a dietary intervention with vegetables. *Food Nutr Bull.*, **21(2):** 161-164.

Tappeiner, C., Meyenberg, A., Goldblum, D., Mojon, D., Zingg, J.M., Nesaretnam, K., Kilchenmann, M., and Frueh, B.E. (2010). Antifibrotic effects of tocotrienols on human Tenon's fibroblasts. *Graefes Arch Clin Exp Ophthalmol.*, **248(1):** 65-71.

Tay, J.H., and Show, K.Y. (1995). Use of ash derived from oil-palm waste incineration as a cement replacement material. *Resources, Conservation and Recycling*, **13:** 27-36.

Tosun, I., and Inkaya, A.N. (2010). Resveratrol as a health and disease benefit agent. *Food Rev Int.*, **26(1):** 85 - 101

Uto-Kondo, H., Ohmori, R., Kiyose, C., Kishimoto, Y., Saito, H., Igarashi, O., and Kondo, K. (2009). Tocotrienol suppresses adipocyte differentiation and Akt phosphorylation in 3T3-L1 preadipocytes. *J Nutr.*, **139(1):** 51-7.

Van Rooyen, J., Esterhuyse, A. J., Engelbrecht, A., and du Toit, E. F. (2008). Health benefits of a natural carotenoid rich oil: a proposed mechanism of protection against ischaemia/reperfusion injury. *Asia Pacific Journal of Clinical Nutrition*, **17:** 316-19.

van Stuijvenberg, M.E., and Benadé, A.J.S. (2000). South African experience with the use of red palm oil to improve the vitamin A status of primary school children. *Food Nutr Bull.*, **21(2):** 210-218.

Varoglu, E., Seven, B., Gumustekin, K., Aktas, O., and Sahin, A. (2010). The effects of vitamin E and selenium on blood flow to experimental skin burns in rats using the 133 Xe clearance technique. *Cent.Eur.J.Med.*, **5(2):** 219-223.

Vega-López, S., Ausman, L.M., Jalbert, S.M., Erkkilä, A.T., and Lichtenstein, A.H. (2006). Palm and partially hydrogenated soybean oils adversely alter lipoprotein profiles compared with soybean and canola oils in moderately hyperlipidemic subjects. *Am J Clin Nutr.*, **84(1):** 54-62.

Velioglu, Y.S., Mazza, G., Gao, L., and Oomah, B.D. (1998). Antioxidant activity and total phenolics in selected fruits, vegetables, and grain products. *J. Agric. Food Chem.*, **46 (10):** 4113-4117.

Wahid, M.B., Weng, C.K., May, C.Y., and Chin, C.M. (2006). The need to reduce national greenhouse gases emissions: oil palm industry's role. *Journal of Oilpalm Research*, 1-123.

Wang, H., Cao, G., and Prior, R.L. (1996). Total antioxidant capacity of fruits. *J. Agric. Food Chem.*, **44 (3):** 701-705.

Watanabe, M. (1998). Catechins as antioxidants from buckwheat (*Fagopyrum esculentum* Moench) groats. *J. Agric. Food Chem.*, **46(3):** 839-845.

Witt, E.H., Reznick, A.Z., Packer, L. (1991). Protective effects of tocopherol and tocotrienol supplementation against exercise-induced oxidative protein damage. Proc 6th ACN: 426-431.

Yusoff, S. (2006). Renewable energy from palm oil - innovation on effective utilization of waste. *Journal of Cleaner Production*, **14(1):** 87-93.

Zhang, D., and Hamauzu, Y. (2004). Phenolics, ascorbic acid, carotenoids and antioxidant activity of broccoli and their changes during conventional and microwave cooking. *Food Chem.*, **88(4):** 503-509.

Zevenbergen, H, de Bree, A., Zeelenberg, M., Laitinen, K., van Duijn. G., Flöter, E. (2009). Foods with a high fat quality are essential for healthy diets. *Ann Nutr Metab.*, **54 Suppl 1**: 15-24.

Medicinal Plants: Phytochemistry, Pharmacology and Therapeutics Vol. 2 (2012) *Pages* 369–378
Editor-in-Chief: V.K. Gupta
Published by: DAYA PUBLISHING HOUSE, NEW DELHI

22

Antibacterial Properties of Some Essential Oils against Selective Human Pathogenic Bacteria

S. Gochhait[1], Chandi C. Rath[1*] and U.B. Mohapatra[1]

ABSTRACT

Seven essential oils (Amomum aromatica, Syzygium aromaticum, Alpinia malaccensis, Ocimum basilicum, Mentha arvensis, Mentha citrata, Eucalyptus citriodora) were investigated against thirteen human pathogenic bacteria. The oils were active even at a concentration of 2.5µl/disc when studied through disc diffusion method. The minimum inhibitory concentration (MIC) of the oils varied between 0.79 µl/ml to 125 µl/ml and the activities reported to be bactericidal. The minimum killing time (MKT) of the oils varied up to 24hours, whereas, in many instances immediate killing of the pathogens was reported. Antibacterial activity of the oils was retained even after boiling and autoclaving.

Keywords: Antibacterial activity, Essential oils, Minimum Inhibitory Concentration (MIC), Minimum Killing Time (MKT), Phenol coefficient index.

Introduction

The use of antibiotics is very vast now a days. Instead of controlling diseases, antibiotics are also used in feeding young farm stocks to encourage growth, employed as food preservatives. These antibiotics have direct toxic effect, hypersensitive and production of antibiotic resistant pathogenic organisms transmissible to human beings (Taylor *et al.*, 2006). In contrast to these, natural products of plant origin proves to be safe without any side effect and is biodegradable. Foremost, among these are the

1 Department of Botany, North Orissa University, Takhatpur, Baripada – 757 003, India.

* *Corresponding author*: E-mail: chandicharanrath@yahoo.com

medicinal plants. In recent years this interest, to evaluate plant possessing antibacterial activity is growing day by day (Clark and Hufford, 1993). The antibacterial activity of the plants is due to the presence of a wide variety of secondary metabolites. One of such groups of secondary metabolites complexed to a liquid formulation and deposited in plants is the essential oils. Essential oils are concentrated, hydrophobic liquid containing volatile aromatic compounds commonly used in urology, dermatology, sleep and nervous disorders, laxatives, erosive gastritis, cardiac and vascular system, immune modulating drugs, cold and cough. Therefore, the present investigation was aimed on (*i*) assessment of antibacterial activity against some common human pathogenic bacteria, (*ii*) determination of Minimum Inhibitory Concentration (MIC), (*iii*) determination of Minimum Killing Time (MKT), (*iv*) effect of high temperature and pressure on antibacterial activity of the oils, (*v*) determination of antibiogram pattern of the pathogens and comparison of the antibacterial activity of the oils with standard antibiotics, and (*vi*) determination of phenol coefficient value of the oils.

Materials and Methods

Test Pathogens

Thirteen common human pathogenic bacteria investigated in this study *viz.*, Enteropathogenic *E. coli*, Enterotoxigenic *E. coli*, *E. coli* 0157:H_7, *Shigella sonnei*, *S. dysenteriae*, *S. boyedii*, *S. flexneri*, *Salmonella typhimurium*, *Staphylococcus aureus*, *Vibrio cholerae* (0139), *Vibrio cholerae* (Inaba), *Vibrio cholerae* (Ogawa) and *Bacillus subtilis* were procured from National Institute of Cholerae and Enteric Diseases(NICED), Kolkata and Regional Medical Research Centre(RMRC, ICMR), Bhubaneswar, India.

Essential Oils

The essential oils *viz.*, *Amomum aromatica*, *Alpinia malaccensis* investigated in this study were obtained from Bangladesh Council of Scientific and Industrial Research (BCSIR), Chittagong, *Ocimum basilicum*, *Mentha citrata* and *Syzygium aromaticum* from DLR College, Gollalimamidada, A.P, India, and *Mentha arvensis* from College of Agriculture, Acharya, N.G. Ranga University, Hydrabad, A.P., and *Eucalyptus citriodora* from Forest Research Institute (FRI), Deradhun.

Methods

Bioactivity of the essential oils was preliminarily studied by disc diffusion method described by Bauer *et al.* (1966) with slight modifications (Rath *et al.*, 1999).

The Minimum Inhibitory Concentration (MIC) of the oils were determined by tube dilution technique described elsewhere (Rath *et al.*, 1999). Further, bactericidal nature of the oils was determined by subculturing one loop of the pathogen from MIC dilution tubes on to nutrient agar plates and observing their growth after over night incubation at 37°C (Rath *et al.*, 2005).

Minimum Killing Time (MKT) of the oils was evaluated by adding 20μl of overnight broth culture of the pathogen in to two separate tubes containing 1ml of nutrient and tween-20 broth. Further, the tubes were supplemented with MIC level of oils separately, one tube was incubated at 37°C and the other at 4°C. From each tube one loop of the sample was subcultured on to nutrient agar plates at time intervals of 0min, 5min, 10min, 15min, 30min, 45min, 1hr, 2hr, 3hr, 4hr, 5hr, 6hr, and after 24hrs and the plates were incubated. The plate exhibiting no growth, at a corresponding time interval was regarded as MKT of the oil.

Effect of temperature and pressure on antibacterial activity of oils was determined by treating the oils at 100°C and autoclaving separately. Antibacterial activity of the treated oils were studied by disc diffusion method loading MIC level of the oils on to sterile filter discs, as described earlier (Rath *et al.*, 2005; 2007).

The antibiogram pattern of the test pathogens was studied through the method of Bauer *et al.* (1966) and multiple antibiotic resistance (MAR per cent) index was determined (Mohapatra *et al.*,2006). Phenol coefficient of the oils and phenol coefficient index percentage was determined to compare and analyze the bioactivity of the oils against the pathogens, following the method of Rath *et al.*(2008).

Results and Discussion

Antibacterial activity of the oils by disc diffusion method is represented in Table 22.1. From the bioactivity evaluation, essential oils such as*Ocimum basilicum, Mentha arvensis* and *Eucalyptus citriodora* showed strong antibacterial activity. Amongst all, *Ocimum basilicum* oil was most active against all the test pathogens exhibiting inhibition zone size of 30mm and effective even at its lower concentration (2.5 µl/disc). *Eucalyptus citriodora* oil showed better activity against all *Shigella* species, *Vibrio cholerae* (Inaba), *Bacillus subtilis* and *E. coli* 0157:H7 at a concentration of 2.5 µl/disc, with inhibition zone size of 30mm. *Mentha arvensis* oil showed better activity against all the *E. coli* strains studied followed by *Bacillus subtilis* and *Salmonella typhimurium* representing a zone size of 30mm. Among the other five essential oils studied *Sygigium aromaticum* was most active showing an average zone size of 10mm at 2.5 µl/disc and the zone size increased with increased oil concentration.*Mentha citrata*, *Amomum aromatica* and *Alpinia malaccenisis* oils showed activity against all the test pathogens. However, a degree of variability was observed in terms of zones of inhibition. A remarkable increase in the zone of inhibition was observed among these oils with increase concentrations against all the test pathogens. From this preliminary study the degree of bioactivity of the essential oils studied follow the pattern*Ocimum bacilicum* > *Eucalyptus citriodora* > *Mentha arvensis* > *Syzygium aromaticum*> *Mentha citrate* > *Amomum aromatica* > *Alpinia malaccensis*. In contrast to our findings Das (2008) and Das *et al.* (2009) reported that both Enterotoxigenic *E. coli* and *V. cholerae* (Inaba) showed resistance towards *Ocimum basilicum* seed essential oil. Whereas, other pathogens used in this study were susceptible to *Ocimum basilicum* seed oil, corroborates with our findings. Based on the bioactivity it may be conclude that the essential oils of Indian origin (*Syzygium aromaticum, Ocimum basilicum, Mentha arvensis, Mentha citrata, Eucalyptus citriodora*) showed better activity than that of the Bangladesh origin (*Amomum aromatic, Alpinia malaccensis*). Therefore, the five essential oils of Indian origin were used in further experiments in this investigation.

The MIC values of the oils ranged between 0.79 – 125µl/ml (Table 22.2). Lowest MIC value of 0.79µl/ml was reported in case of *Mentha arvensis* oil against *Sh. dysenteriae*, *V. cholerae* (Inaba) and *E. coli* 0157:H7. *Eucalyptus citriodora* oil showed minimum MIC

Table 22.1. Preliminary screening for antibacterial activity of essential oils by Disc Diffusion Method*.

Pathogen	*Amomum aromatica*			*Syzygium aromaticum*			*Alpinia malaccensis*			*Ocimum basilicum*			*Mentha arvensis*			*Mentha citrata*			*Eucalyptus citriodora*		
	2.5μl	*5μl*	*10μl*	*2.5μl*	*5μl*	*10μl*	*2.5μl*	*5μl*	*10μl*	*2.5μl*	*5μl*	*10μl*	*2.5μl*	*5μl*	*10μl*	*2.5μl*	*5μl*	*10μl*	*2.5μl*	*5μl*	*10μl*
Sh. dysenteriae	5	7	10	7	13	18	8	8	10	30	30	30	8	10	12	6	8	9	30	30	30
Sh. boyedii	5	6	9	8	15	20	5	6	9	30	30	30	7	14	20	6	7	10	30	30	30
Sh. flexneri	4	6	10	9	14	16	8	10	11	30	30	30	10	17	22	8	8	11	30	30	30
Sh. sonnei	6	6	9	8	12	16	7	8	10	30	30	30	12	22	28	7	8	10	30	30	30
V. chlolerae (Ogawa)	5	7	9	8	16	18	7	8	9	30	30	30	11	30	30	8	10	15	30	30	30
V. cholerae (0139)	4	6	9	11	16	21	4	6	7	30	30	30	10	15	30	7	7	8	11	25	30
V. cholerae (Inaba)	6	7	9	16	17	20	7	8	9	30	30	30	9	9	10	6	7	9	30	30	30
Enteropathogenic *E. coli*	5	6	10	11	16	17	6	7	9	30	30	30	30	30	30	6	10	10	18	30	30
Enterotoxigenic *E. coli*	6	9	11	10	11	19	7	9	9	30	30	30	30	30	30	7	8	10	11	20	30
S. typhimurium	6	7	11	10	16	16	5	6	9	30	30	30	30	30	30	7	8	10	9	16	26
S. aureus	7	10	12	13	14	15	5	6	7	30	30	30	5	7	9	6	8	9	12	15	20
B. subtilis	8	11	13	9	13	13	8	8	10	30	30	30	30	30	30	7	9	11	30	30	30
E. coli 0157:H7	5	9	12	11	11	18	7	8	9	30	30	30	30	30	30	14	16	18	30	30	30

* Oils were loaded in different aliquots(2.5, 5.0 and 10ul) per disc. Values represented are the zones of inhibition in mm.

value 0.19µl/ml against *E. coli* 0157:H7. Surprisingly *Ocimum basilicum* flower oil that showed better zone of inhibition against the test pathogens during disc diffusion method represented a higher MIC value (3.9 – 7.8µl/ml) in comparison to *Eucalyptus citriodora* and *Mentha arvensis* oil. Maximum MIC value was exhibited by *Syzygium aromaticum* against Enteropathogenic *E. coli* (125µl/ml). Higher MIC values 31.25µl/ml, 15.62µl/ml of *Ocimum basilicum* was recorded against *Sh. dysenteriae* and *V. cholerae* (Inaba) strains respectively by Das *et al.* (2009) in comparison to our findings. While studying the vibriocidal activity of aniseed and coriander oils Rath*et al.*(2007), reported a MIC value of 7.8µl/ml and 1.5µl/ml respectively against *V. cholerae* (Inaba) that corresponds to our findings in case of *Ocimum basilicum* and *Eucalyptus citriodora* oil. Also a lower MIC value was observed in case of *Mentha arvensis* and *Mentha citrata* in contrast to their findings against *V. cholerae*. Pattnaik *et al.* (1996) also reported higher MIC values of *Eucalyptus citriodora* and *Mentha citrata* oils against these pathogens that properly corroborates with our observations. The results obtained regarding the MIC values in this study proportionately correlated with our preliminary study *i.e.* a higher zone size observed against a pathogen by oil showed lower MIC values, except *O. basilicum*. Further, recording of very low MIC value of these oils against the test pathogens is suggestive of presence of very effective antibacterial compounds or secondary metabolites in these oils.

Table 22.2. Minimum Inhibitory Concentration (MIC) of the oils.

Pathogen	*MIC (Minimum Inhibitory Concentration) in µl/ml.*				
	Oils				
	Syzigium aromaticum	*Ocimum baislicum*	*Mentha arvensis*	*Mentha citrata*	*Eucalyptus citriodra*
Sh. dysenteriae	7.8	3.9	0.79	0.79	1.562
V. cholerae (Inaba)	3.9	7.8	0.79	0.395	1.562
B. subtilis	31.25	3.9	1.56	0.395	0.79
S. aureus	3.9	3.9	1.56	0.79	0.395
E. coli 0157:H7	62.5	7.8	0.79	1.56	0.197
Enteropathogenic *E. coli*	125	7.8	1.56	3.125	1.56

The activity of all the five essential oils were observed to be bactericidal, as no growth was observed when subcultured on to nutrient agar plates from MIC tubes. Bactericidal activity of various essential oils is also well documented in literature (Pattnaik *et al.*, 1996; Gupta *et al.*, 2004; Baswa *et al.*, 2001; Rath *et al.*, 1999, 2001, 2002, 2005; Das *et al.*, 2009).

While studying the Minimum Killing Time (MKT) of the oils at two different temperatures *i.e.* 37°C and 4°C, it was observed that in most cases the oils kill the organisms immediately. However, a variation in MKT values was also recorded (Table 22.3). In many cases the pathogens were killed immediately, which implies that the oils result in an irreversible damage when come in contact with the bacterial cells.

Table 22.3. Minimum Killing Time (MKT) of oils.

Pathogen	*Minimum Killing Time (MKT) in minutes*									
	Syzygium aromaticum		*Ocimun baislicum*		*Mentha arvensis*		*Mentha citrata*		*Eucalyptus citiodra*	
	4°C	*37°C*	*4°C*	*37°C*	*4°C*	*37°C*	*4°C*	*37°C*	*4°C*	*37°C*
Sh. dysenteriae	45	45	60	45	60	10	15	10	0	0
V. cholerae (Inaba)	10	10	0	0	5	10	0	0	0	0
B. subtilis	0	0	0	0	0	0	3 hrs	24hrs	15	10
S. aureus	5	0	0	0	5	0	45	60	0	0
E. coli 0157:H7	15	10	0	0	10	10	60	30	10	10
Enteropathogenic *E. coli*	0	0	45	10	60	15	6 hrs	10	0	0

Further, the oils were heated in a boiling water bath (100°C for 1hr.) and were also autoclaved separately, and were tested for their antibacterial activities by Disc Diffusion Method (loading MIC level of oils on discs). Significant increase in activity in terms of increased zone of inhibition was observed in case of *Syzygium aromaticum* against all the test pathogens. Surprisingly, all the oils showed increased antibacterial activity against *S. aureus*, Entropathogenic *E. coli*, and *E.coli* 0157:H7, when tested with heat treated and autoclaved oils (Table 22.4). In certain cases (*Eucalyptus citriodora* and *Mentha arvensis* oils), smaller zone of inhibition was also recorded in comparison to preliminary screening. This could be attributable to the application of less amount of oils on to the discs, as the MIC level of the oils reported to very less, except *Syzygium aromaticum*. Gupta *et al.* (2004) have reported the persistence of antibacterial activity of carrot (*Daucus carota*) and celery (*Apium graveolens*) seed essential oils against both Gram-positive and Gram-negative pathogens after heat treatment and autoclaving, indicating the presence of heat stable components in these essential oils as reported in our investigation. Similar results were also reported by Rath *et al.* (2005) while studying the antibacterial activity of lime (*Citrus lemoncum*) and Juniper (*Juniperus communis*) oils against Methicillin resistant *Staphylococcus aureus*, in proper agreement to our findings.

From antibiogram pattern it was reported that all the organisms were sensitive to Chloramphenicol, Ciprofloxacin, Norfloxacin, Tetracycline, and Polymyxin except Enteropathogenic *E.coli*, which was resistant to Polymyxin. On the other hand all the organisms were resistant to Bacitracin, Ampicillin, Trimethoprim and Sulfadiazine. Except *V. cholerae* (Inaba), all other pathogens were resistant to Nalidixic acid. A high degree of MAR percentage (30-60 per cent) was recorded (Figure 22.1). It is significant to mention that the degree of inhibition (in terms of zone size) by these essential oils could be well compared with standard antibiotics. In some cases the zones of inhibition were smaller in comparison to antibiotics studied which could be attributable to the crudeness of the oils or active antibacterial compounds.

Phenol coefficient value of the oils ranged between 0.125 to 1.0 (Table 22.5; Figure 22.2). Highest phenol coefficient value was observed for *Mentha citrata i.e.* 1.0 followed by *Syzygium aromaticum* and *Eucalyptus citriodora* oil *i.e.* 0.5. Lowest phenol coefficient

Table 22.4. Antibacterial activity of the oils at higher temperature and pressure.

Pathogen	*Zone of Inhibition in mm**									
	Syzygium aromaticum		*Ocimum baislicum*		*Mentha arvensis*		*Mentha citrata*		*Eucalyptus citiodora*	
	100°C	*Autoclaving*	*100°C*	*Autoclaving*	*100°C*	*Autoclaving*	*100°C*	*Autoclaving*	*100°C*	*Autoclaving*
Sh. dysenteriae	21	22	10	15	4	5	9	9	6	6
V. cholerae (Inaba)	13	11	18	17	7	7	11	11	9	9
B. subtilis	30	30	50	50	9	9	9	7	7	7
S. aureus	28	28	44	44	40	40	48	50	5	5
E. coli 0157:H7	46	46	18	14	8	7	20	15	50	40
Enteropathogenic *E. coli*	38	37	25	22	9	9	10	10	9	8

* MIC level of heat treated and autoclaved oils were loaded on the discs.

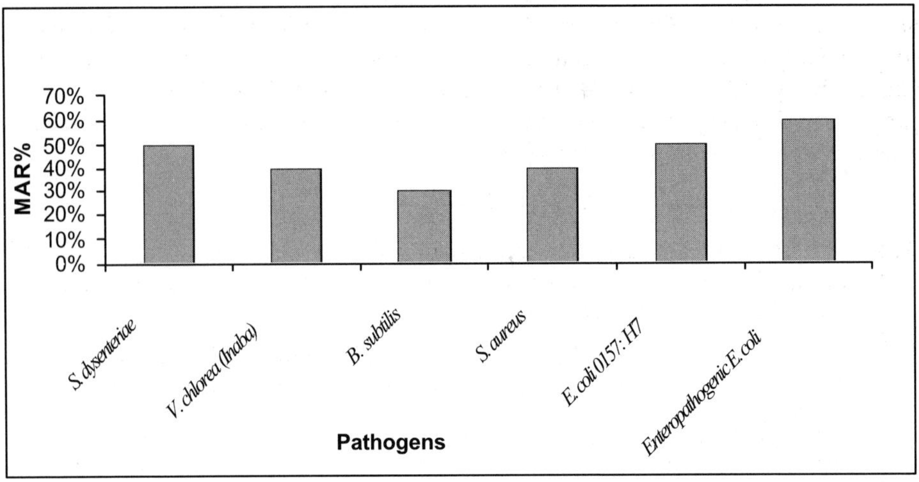

Figure 22.1. Multiple antibiotics resistance index percentage of the pathogens.

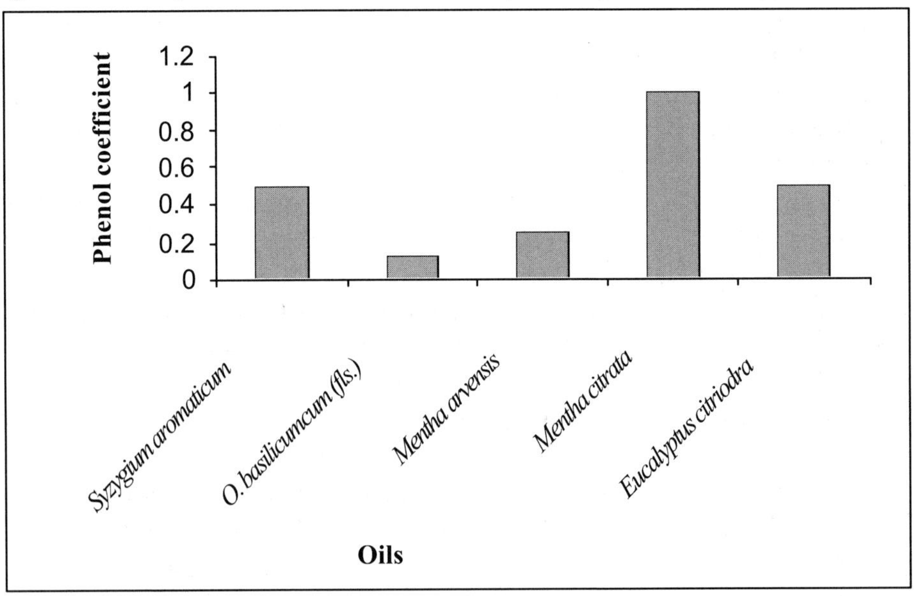

Figure 22.2. Phenol coefficient value of oils.

value was observed for *O. basilicum* oil *i.e.* 0.125. The phenol coefficient values observed to be statistically significant, $P<0.05$. The findings of phenol coefficient experiment directly corroborates with our earlier findings during this investigation *i.e.* oils representing lower MIC value showed better phenol coefficient, index.

Table 22.5. Phenol coefficient value of the oils.

Oils	*Phenol Co-efficient Value*
Syzygium aromaticum	0.5
*O. basilicum*cum	0.125
Mentha arvensis	0.25
Mentha citrata	1.0
Eucalyptus citriodra	0.5

Thus in this present investigation we have reported the antibacterial activity of *Syzygium aromaticum, Ocimum basilicum, Mentha arvensis,Mentha citrata and Eucalyptus citriodora* oils against human pathogens in a great detail. Encouraged results were obtained when the activities were compared with standard antibiotics and phenol, is suggestive of their possible use in pharmaceuticals, and cosmetic industries, as an alternate against costly and harmful chemotherapeutic agents.

References

Baswa, M., Rath, C.C., Dash, S.K. and Mishra, R.K.(2001). Antibacterial activity of Karanj (*Pongamia pinnata*) and Neem (*Azadirachta indica*) seed oil: A preliminary report. *Microbios,* **105**: 183-189.

Bauer, A.W., Kirby, W.H.M., Sherric, J.C., Truckm. (1966). Antibiotics susceptibility testing by standard disc diffusion method. *Am. J. Clin. Pathol.,* **45**: 493-496.

Clark, A.M., Hufford, C.D. (1993). In: Human Medical Agents form Plant. American Chemical Society (ACS Symposium series 534), Washington, D.C., pp: 228-241.

Das, I.(2008). *In vitro* antibacterial potential assessment of essential oils of three *Ocimum* spp. M.Phil Thesis, North Orissa University, India, pp: 1-60.

Das, I., Tayung, K., Rath, C.C., Mohapatra, U.B.(2009). Antibacterial Assessment of Essential oils of three *Ocimum* spp. Against food borne pathogens. *Pl. Sci.,* **31(1 and 2):** 60-65.

Gupta, R, Rath, C. C., Dash S., Mishra, R. K.(2004). *In vitro* antibacterial potential assessment of carrot and celery seed essential oils against twenty one bacteria. *J. Essent. Oil Bearing Pl.,* **7(1):** 79-86.

Mohapatra, S., Rath, C.C., Das, S.K., Mishra, R.K. (2006). Microbial evaluation of wounds and their susceptibility to antibiotics and essential oils. *J. Microbial World,* **8(1):** 101-109.

Pattanaik, S., Subramanyam, V. R. and Kole, C.(1996). Effect of essential oils on the viability and morphology of *E. coli. Microbios,* **86:** 237-246.

Rath C. C., Mishra, S., Dash, S. K., and Mishra, R. K.(2005). Anti *Staphylococcal* activity of lime and juniper essential oils against MRSA. *Ind. Drugs,* **42(12)**: 797-801.

Rath, C.C., Das, S. K., Mishra, R. K., Charyulu, J.K., Ramachandraiah,O.S.,and Azeemoddim, G.(1999). A note on the characterization of Turmeric (*Curcuma longa*) leaf oil against *Shigella* spp. *Ind. Drugs,* **36(2):** 133-136.

Rath, C. C., Das, S. K., Mishra, R. K., and Charyulu, J.K.(2001). Anti *E. coli* activity of Turmeric essential oil. *Ind. Perf.,* **43(4)** : 172-178.

Rath, C.C., Das, S. K., and Mishra, R.K.(2002). Antibacterial efficacy of six Indian essential oils individually and in combination. *J.Essent. Oil Bearing Pl.,* **5(2):**99-107.

Rath, C.C., Singh, S., Dash, S.K., Mishra, R.K. (2007). *In vitro* vibriocidal activity of coriander (*Coriandrum sativum*) and aniseed (*Pimpinella anisum* L.) essential oils. *Food,* **1(2):** 216-219.

Rath, C.C., Devi, S., Das, S.K., Mishra, R.K.(2008). Antibacterial potential assessment of Jasmine essential oil against *E. coli. Ind. J. Pharm. Sci.,* **70(2):** 238-241.

Taylor, D.J., Green, N.P.O., Stout, G.W. (2006). In: Biological Science, Cambridge University Press, NY, USA, pp: 519-520.

Medicinal Plants: Phytochemistry, Pharmacology and Therapeutics Vol. 2 (2012) *Pages* **379–386**
Editor-in-Chief: **V.K. Gupta**
Published by: **DAYA PUBLISHING HOUSE, NEW DELHI**

23

Hypoglycemic Effect of *Allium porrum* L. Leaves in Healthy and Streptozotocin-Induced Diabetic Mice

Maryam Eidi[1]*, Akram Eidi[2], Alireza Sadeghipour[3], Fatemeh Soleimani[4] and Samira Ebrahimi[4]

ABSTRACT

The goal was to investigate hypoglycemic effect of the ethanolic extract of Allium porrum L. (Leek) leaves on both healthy and streptozotocin-induced diabetic mice. Diabetes was induced using streptozotocin (175 mg/kg, i.p.). The ethanolic extract at doses 100, 200, 250 and 300 mg/kg were administered for 14 days intraperitoneally. The saline was administered to the control group. Blood samples were obtained from heart after 14 days. The results illustrated that ethanolic extract of leek significantly reduced the serum glucose levels in streptozotocin-induced diabetic but not in healthy mice. Moreover, the ethanolic extract increased serum insulin levels in diabetic mice. The present data indicates that extract of leek has hypoglycemic effect on diabetic animals by releasing insulin from pancreas. Subsequently, this plant should be considered in future therapeutic studies.

Keywords: *Allium porrum,* Hypoglycaemia, Leek, Mice, Streptozotocin, Diabetes.

1 Department of Biology, Varamin Branch, Islamic Azad University, Varamin, Iran.

2 Department of Biology, Science and Research Branch, Islamic Azad University, Tehran, Iran.

3 Oncopathology Research Center, Tehran University of Medical Sciences, Tehran, Iran.

4 Young Researchers Club, Varamin Branch, Islamic Azad University, Varamin, Iran.

* *Corresponding author*: E-mail: eidi@iauvaramin.ac.ir

Introduction

Intensive efforts for developing novel and improved agents for controlling serum glucose has led to discovery of a large number of natural and synthetic hypoglycemic agents. The available literature shows that there are more than 400 plant species showing hypoglycemic activity (Mukherjee, 1981; Oliver-Bever, 1986; Ivorra *et al.*, 1989; Atta Ur-Rahman and Zaman, 1989; Rai, 1995) and presently several laboratories have focused on isolating new herbal oral hypoglycemic agents.

Among the naturally occurring plants, garlic, onion, fenugreek have received special attention (Eidi *et al.*, 2007; Eidi *et al.*, 2006; Alarcon-Aguilar *et al.*, 2002). *Allium porrum* L. or leek (Liliaceae family), is one of the most important of 75 species of Iranian *Allium* species cultivated in several areas of the country (Mozaffarian, 1996). The Leek originates from the wild species *Allium ampeloprasum* that occurs from Portugal and North Africa eastwards to Turkey, Iran and Tajikistan. *Allium porrum* L. (Leek) is a green leaf vegetable, whole dried or fresh leaves of the plant, like other *Allium* species, have been widely used in Persian foods as a flavor component and in Iranian folk medicine for treatment of gastrointestinal and infectious complaints (Harris *et al.*, 2001; Nafisy, 1999). Effects on digestive disorders, arteriosclerosis, joint pain, respiratory inflammation and kidney stone have been reported (Zargari, 1997). In some regions of Iran, leek is claimed to be especially effective in prevention of hyperglycaemia. In this study, to determine the hypoglycemic effect of *Allium porrum* leaves, we evaluated the effects of *Allium porrum* ethanolic extract leaves on serum glucose and insulin levels in healthy and streptozotocin-induced diabetic mice.

Materials and Methods

Plant Material

Leek leaves were collected from local supermarket in summer and ascertained in the department of botany of Varamin branch, Islamic Azad University. The plant was cleaned, shed dried at 25°C. The dried leaves of the plant were ground with a blender, and the powder was kept in nylon bags in a deep freezer until the time of experiments.

Extraction of Ethanolic Plant Material

Dried and ground leaves (about 60 g) were submitted to extraction with 300 ml ethanol (80 per cent) in a Soxhlet apparatus for 72 h. After extraction, the solvents were filtered and then evaporated by Rotavapor.

Animals

Mice weighing 20-25 g were housed in clean cages with temperature (22-24 °C), 12-h light/12-h dark cycle and relative air humidity 40-60 per cent. Animals had continuous access to food and to tap water. Permission for the study was obtained from the official authorities.

Preparation of Diabetic Mice

Mice were injected (i.p.) with streptozotocin 175 mg/kg. Five days after injection, the animals with fasting serum glucose higher than 180 mg/dl were used for experiments.

Experimental Design

In the present experiment, 110 mice (60 diabetic and 50 healthy mice) were used. The mice were divided into 11 groups. Ten mice were used in each group.

- Group 1: Normal control mice were administrated 1 ml saline for 14 days.
- Groups 2–5: Normal mice were administrated leek alcoholic extract (100, 200, 250 and 300 mg/kg body wt.) intraperitoneally for 14 days.
- Group 6: Diabetic control mice were administrated 1 ml saline for 14 days.
- Groups 7–10: Diabetic mice were administrated garlic alcoholic extract (100, 200, 250 and 300 mg/kg body wt.) intraperitoneally for 14 days.

Blood Sampling

The ethanolic extract of leek was administered for 14 days in different doses intraperitoneally. After administration period, the animals were anesthetized by ether and blood samplings from heart were performed. Serum glucose level was measured by enzymatic method of glucose oxidase. The serum insulin level was measured by using the radioimmunoassay kit (Diasorin, Italy).

Preliminary LD_{50} Test

To find LD_{50} of The plant extract, it was administered as i.p. single shots at doses of 2000, 3000, 3500 and 5000 mg/kg to the each group (n=10), animal subjects were monitored for the next 72 h after each injection (Bodi and Nodine, 1964).

Statistical Analysis

All data were expressed as mean ± S.D. Differences between groups were considered to be significant at $p<0.05$ using one-way ANOVA.

Results

Effect of Ethanolic Extract of Leek on Serum Glucose in Healthy Fasted Mice

It has been observed that the i.p. administration of leek ethanolic extract at doses 100, 200, 250 and 300 mg/kg did not produce significant hypoglycemic effect on healthy animals (Figure 23.1).

Effect of Ethanolic Extract of Leek on Serum Glucose in Streptozotocin-Induced Diabetic Fasted Mice

The results have shown that the i.p. administration of leek ethanolic extract at doses 100, 200, 250 and 300 mg/kg ($p<0.001$) decreased serum glucose in streptozotocin-induced diabetic mice (Figure 23.2).

Effect of Ethanolic Extract of Leek on Serum Insulin in Streptozotocin-Induced Diabetic Mice

Also, the administration of leek ethanolic extract at dose of 250 mg/kg ($p<0.01$), as significant dose, increased insulin serum in streptozotocin-induced diabetic mice (Figure 22.3).

LD_{50}

The leek ethanolic extract was injected at doses 2000, 3000, 3500 and 5000 mg/kg. The LD_{50} for leek leaves was determined 3500 mg/kg (i.p.) (Table 23.1).

Table 23.1. Mortality and LD50 values of *Allium porrum* ethanolic extract leaves within 72 h after i.p. administration.

Dose g/kg	*Number of Animal Deaths at*						
	0.5 h	*5 h*	*8 h*	*24 h*	*48 h*	*72 h*	*Total*
2000	0	0	0	0	0	0	0
3000	1	1	1	0	0	0	3
3500	2	2	1	0	0	0	5
5000	7	3	0	0	0	0	10
LD50 (i.p. treatment)							5

N=10 in each groups.

Discussion

Currently, available therapeutic choices for diabetes mellitus such as dietary modification, oral hypoglycemic agents and insulin have limitations of their own (Vats *et al.*, 2002). Streptozotocin as an antibiotic and anticancer agent has been

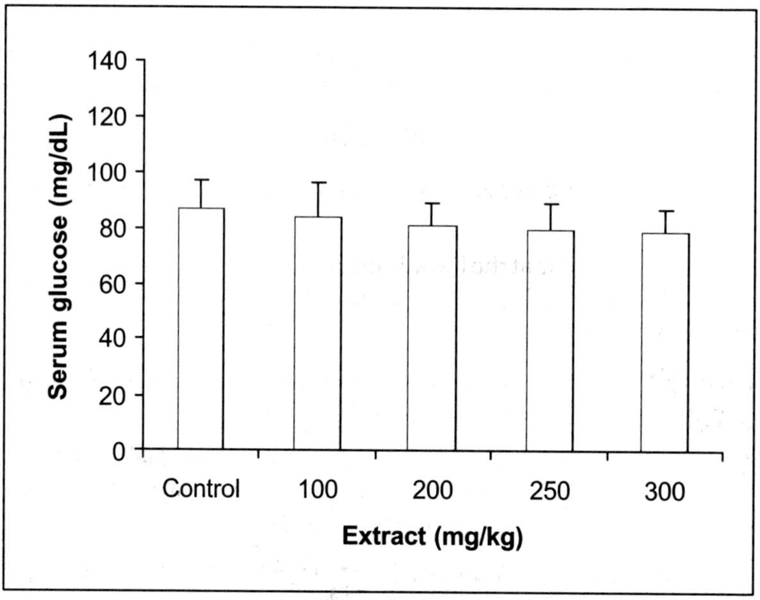

Figure 23.1. Effect of intraperitoneally administration of ethanolic extract of leek at doses of 100, 200, 250 and 300 mg/kg body weight on serum glucose in healthy fasted mice for 14 days. Each point represents mean ± S.D. for 10 mice. Control group was administered with saline as vehicle.

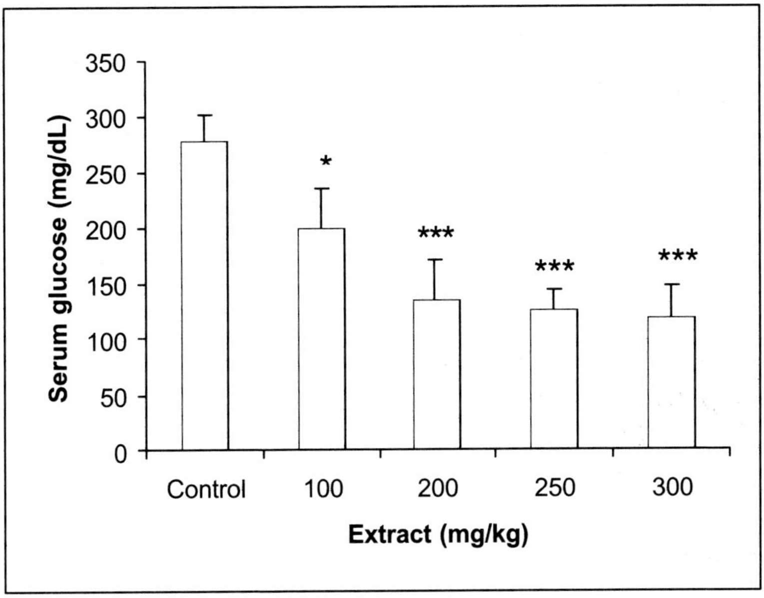

Figure 23.2. Effect of intraperitoneally administration of ethanolic extract of leek at doses of 100, 200, 250 and 300 mg/kg body weight on serum glucose in streptozotocin-induced diabetic fasted mice for 14 days. Each point represents mean ± S.D. for 10 mice. * $p<0.05$, *** $p<0.001$ different from control group. Control group was administered with saline as vehicle.

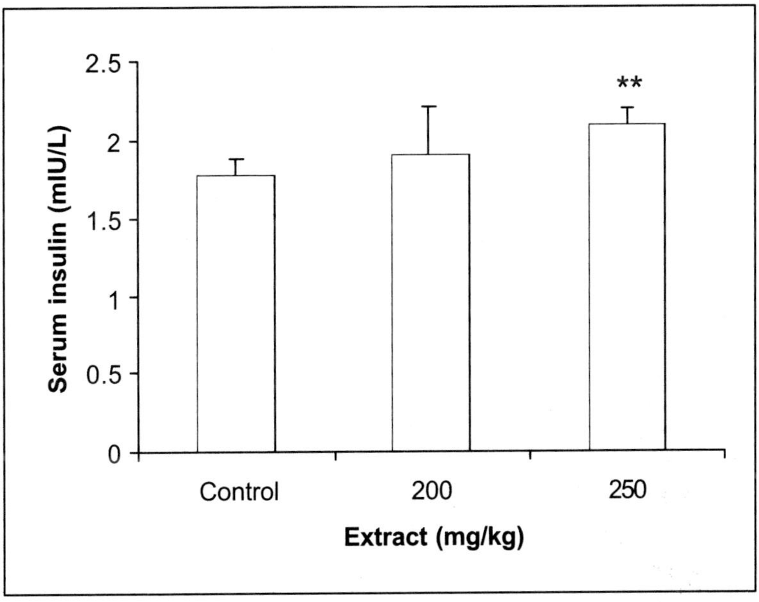

Figure 23.3. Effect of intraperitoneally administration of ethanolic extract of leek at doses of 200 and 250 mg/kg body weight on serum insulin in streptozotocin-induced diabetic fasted mice for 14 days. Each point represents mean ± S.D. for 10 mice. ** $p<0.01$ different from control group. Control group was administered with saline as vehicle.

widely used for inducing diabetes in a variety of animals by affecting degeneration and necrosis of pancreatic β-cells (Merzouk *et al.*, 2000).

Allium porrum L. is an herbaceous plant from the Liliaceae family and has been widely used in Persian foods as a flavor component and in Iranian traditional medicine as an anti-atherogenic remedy. Some of investigations are available on the hypolipidemic effects of leaves of *Allium porrum* (Movahedian *et al.*, 2004, 2006). The leaves of *Allium porrum* have maltase, dextrinase, enortase and emolsion enzymes.

In the present study, the serum glucose data clearly indicated that the i.p. administration of leek ethanolic extract produce significant hypoglycemic effect in streptozotocin-induced fasted diabetic but not in normal fasted mice.

It is suggested that the hypoglycemic effects of plants are related to existence of saponins and flavonoids compounds. The presence of these compounds in*A. Porrum* may play a role in observed hypoglycemic effect. An investigation of the extracts from bulbs of *Allium porrum* L. has led to the isolation of four spirostanol saponins. Two of them are new compounds and have been identified as (25R)-5α-spirostan-3β, 6 β-diol 3-*O*-{*O*- β-D-glucopyranosyl-(1→2)-*O*-[β-D-xylopyranosyl-(1→3)]-*O*-β-D-glucopyranosyl-(1→4)- β-D-galactopyranoside} (Carotenuto *et al.*, 1999) and (25*R*)-5a-spirostan-3 β,6 β-diol 3-*O*-{*O*- β-D-glucopyranosyl-(1→3)-*O*- β-D-glucopyranosyl-(1→2)-*O*-[β-D-xylopyranosyl-(1→3)]-*O*-β-D-glucopyranosyl-(1→4)-β-D-galactopyranoside}. The isolated compounds were evaluated for their antifungal activity (Carotenuto *et al.*, 1997), but their antidiabetic effect has not known yet.

A phytochemical investigation of the extracts obtained from bulbs of leek,*Allium porrum* L. has led to the isolation of five flavonoid glycosides based on the kaempferol aglycone. Two of them are new compounds and have been identified as kaempferol 3-*O*-[2-*O*-(*trans*-3-methoxy-4-hydroxycinnamoyl)- β-D-galactopyranosyl]-(1→4)-*O*- β-D-glucopyranoside, and kaempferol 3-*O*-[2-*O*-(*trans*-3-methoxy-4-hydroxycinnamoyl)-β-D-glucopyranosyl]-(1→6)-*O*- β-D-glucopyranoside, on the basis of spectroscopic methods, including 2D NMR (Fattorusso *et al.*, 2001). Other research showed that the garlic alcoholic extract significantly decreased serum glucose and increased serum insulin levels in treated diabetic rats compared with control diabetic rats (Eidi *et al.*, 2006).

Also, the extract of plant increased insulin releasing from the pancreas in diabetic mice. So, the mechanism of hypoglycemic action probably involves direct or indirect stimulation of insulin secretion. Further experiments are needed to identify the active components of the plant to determine their mechanism in lowering serum glucose in diabetic mice. The hypoglycemic action of leek leaves may be due to increasing insulin releasing from pancreatic beta cells.

In conclusion, our results have shown that ethanolic extract of *Allium porrum* L. leaves possess a hypoglycemic effect on streptozotocin-induced diabetic mice. Further work would be necessary to evaluate the activity of the active constituents and their mechanisms. However, the findings of the present work indicate that this plant may be useful for the treatment of hyperglycaemia.

Acknowledgements

We would like to thank deputy research of the Young Researcher's Club, Varamin Branch, Islamic Azad University for financial support of the project.

References

Alarcon-Aguilar, F. J., Roman-Ramos, R., Flores-Saenz, J.L., and Aguirre- Garcia, F. (2002). Investigation on the hypoglycemic effects of extracts of four Mexican medicinal plants in normal and Alloxan-diabetic mice. *Phytotherapy Research,* **16**: 383– 6.

Atta Ur-Rahman, K., and Zaman, K. (1989). Medicinal plants with hypoglycemic activity. *Journal of Ethnopharmacology,* **26**: 1-55.

Bodi, T., and Nodine, J.H. (1964). Clinical techniques for evaluation of antianxiety drugs. In: Nodine, J.H., Siegler, P.E. (Eds.), Animal and Clinical Pharmacologic Techniques in Drug Evaluation, first ed. Yearbook Medical, USA, pp. 325–329.

Carotenuto, A., Fattorusso, E., Lanzotti, V., and Magno, S. (1999). Spirostanol saponins of *Allium porrum* L. *Phytochemistry,* **51**: 1077-1082.

Carotenuto, A., Fattorusso, E., Lanzotti, V., Magno, S., Carnuccio, R., and D'Acquisto, F. (1997). 12-Keto-porrigenin and the unique 2, 3-seco-porrigenin, new antiproliferative sapogenins from *Allium porrum*. *Tetrahedron,* **53**: 3401-3406.

Eidi, A., Eidi, M., and Sokhteh, M. (2007). Effect of fenugreek (*Trigonella foenum-graecum* L.) seeds on serum parameters in normal and streptozotocin-induced diabetic rats. *Nutrition Research,* **27**: 728–733.

Eidi, A., Eidi, M., and Esmaeili, E. (2006). Antidiabetic effect of Garlic (*Allium sativum* L.) in normal and streptozotocin-induced diabetic rats. *Phytomedicine,* **13**: 624-629.

Fattorusso, E., Lanzotti, V., Taglialatela-Scafati, O., and Cicala, C. (2001). The flavonoids of leek, *Allium porrum,* **57**: 565-569.

Harris, J.C., Cottrell, S.L., Plummer, S., and Lloyd, D. (2001). Antimicrobial properties of *Allium sativum* (garlic). *Applied Microbiology Biotechnology,* **57**: 282-286.

Ivorra, M.D., Paya, M., and Villar, A. (1989). Review of natural products and plants as potent antidiabetic drugs. *Journal of Ethnopharmacology,* **27**: 243-276.

Merzouk, H., Madani, S., and Chabane, D. (2000). Time course of changes in serum glucose, insulin, lipids and tissue lipase activities in macrosomic offspring of rats with streptozotocin-induced diabetes. *Clinical Science,* **98**: 21-30.

Movahedian, A., Sadeghi, H., Ghannadi, A., Gharavi, M., and Azarpajooh, S. (2006). Hypolipidemic activity of *Allium porrum* L. in cholesterol-fed rabbits. *Journal of Food Medicine,* **9**: 98-101.

Movahedian, A., Ghannadi, A., Sadeghi, H., Gharavi, M., and Azarpajhoh, S. (2004). Study of leek (*Allium porrum* L.) extract on cholesterol plasma levels in hyperlipidemic animals. *Asia Pacific Journal of Clinical Nutrition,* **13** (Suppl): S103.

Mozaffarian, V. (1996). A Dictionary of Iranian Plant Names, Farhang Mo'aser, Tehran, Iran, pp. 27-31.

Mukherjee, S.K. (1981). Indigenous drugs in Diabetes mellitus. *Journal of the Diabetes Association Ind.*, **21**: 97-106.

Nafisy, A. (1999). Medicinal Foods and Drinks, Isfahan University Publications, Isfahan, Iran, pp. 287-289.

Oliver-Bever, B. (1986). Oral hypoglycemic action. Medicinal plants in Tropical West Africal, Cambridge University Press, London; 1986, p. 245-267.

Rai, M.K. (1995). A review on some antidiabetic plants of India. *Ancient Science of Life*, **14**: 42-54.

Vats, V., Grover, J.K., and Rathi, S.S. (2002). Evaluation of anti-hyperglycemic and hypoglycemic effect of *Trigonella foenum-graecum* Linn, *Ocimum sanctum* Linn and *Pterocarpus marsupium* Linn in normal and alloxanized diabetic rats. *Journal of Ethnopharmacology*, **79**: 95-100.

Zargari, A. (1997). Medicinal Plant. Vol. 4. Tehran University Press, Iran, pp. 59-64.

Medicinal Plants: Phytochemistry, Pharmacology and Therapeutics Vol. 2 (2012) *Pages* **387–403**
Editor-in-Chief: **V.K. Gupta**
Published by: **DAYA PUBLISHING HOUSE, NEW DELHI**

24

Head Lice, Pediculocides and Anti-Head Lice Efficacy of *Annona squamosa* Linn.

Wandee Gritsanapan[1]*, Peeranuch Mangmeesri[2] and Peerachatra Mangmeesri[3]

ABSTRACT

Human head louse, a small insect, creates a public health problem all over the world, especially in unsanitary condition. Patients with head louse infestation always have scalp pruritus, rash, or viral infection. Many chemical compounds in pyrethroid and non-pyrethroid insecticides, which were popularly used to kill head lice in the past, have been reported to be toxic and harmful to humans. They can cause burning sensation, skin irritation, hyper activity, increasing susceptibility to infections, acute hallucination, and also disruption of immune system. Thus, the effective and safe natural products that have been supported by in vitro data and adequate clinical trials would be desirable to replace synthetic pediculocides on the market in the near future. Some plant products from neem and tea tree oils offer promising anti-head lice activity. Annona squamosa Linn. or custard apple, a medicinal plant in the family Annonaceae, has long been used to kill head lice in many countries. Organic solvent extracts of the leaves and seeds dissolved in coconut oil could kill head lice both in vitro and in louse infested in female students. However, the seed extract alone showed higher potency. The active component in the seed extract was found to be a triglyceride with one oleate ester. The cream preparation (20 per cent w/w) prepared from the petroleum ether extract of A. squamosa seeds could kill 95 per cent of head lice after exposing to the hair of the female students for 3 hours

1 Department of Pharmacognosy, Faculty of Pharmacy, Mahidol University, 447 Sri-Ayudthaya Road, Ratchatewi, Bangkok 10400, Thailand.

2 Faculty of Medicine Ramathibodi Hospital, Mahidol University, Rama VI Road, Ratchatewi, Bangkok 10400, Thailand

3. Ban Kruat Hospital, Ban Kruat District, Buri Ram 31180, Thailand

* *Corresponding author*: E-mail: pywgs@mahidol.ac.th

but the preparation could not nullify their eggs. The head louse eggs hatch into young head lice in approximately 7-10 days. Therefore, A. squamosa seed cream should be applied once a week for 3 consecutive weeks to kill all young and mature head lice. The toxicity test on rabbits' eyes and ears, the petroleum ether extract of A. squamosa seeds in propyleneglycol (1:10 w/v) caused conjunctival redness, rugged cornea, skin erythema and oedema. Thus, the treatment with the cream prepared from A. squamosa seeds to treat head lice in human should be carefully done to avoid eye contact. Since the preparation from the seed extract of A. squamosa exhibited high efficacy against head lice at low cost, it could potentially be commercialized instead of synthetic pediculocides such as gamma benzene hexachloride, which had been reported to produce acute and chronic nervous toxicity, and cause hepatic cancer. Furthermore, A. squamosa seeds are byproduct from consuming ripe fruits. By taking its pharmaceutical advantage, we could produce a cheaper herbal preparation to treat head lice infestations in our societies in the near future.

Keywords: *Annona squamosa,* Annonaceae, Anti-head lice, Custard apple, Head lice, Pediculocide, Pediculosis, *Pediculus humanus capitis*.

Introduction

Head lice (*Pediculus humanus* var. *capitis*) are small wingless insects that have been an obligate parasite of humans since 8,000 BC. (Heukelbach *et al.*, 2006). These lice have evolved with mankind and thus, were distributed all over the world and caused a public health problem in all socio-economic classes especially in unsanitary communities (Puapatanakul, 1980). Head lice infestation, which is a worldwide public health concern, may become a severe health problem (called pediculosis), namely severe inflammation and super-infection of the skin. The lice that infest human beings are always blood-sucking lice that live in close association with the host and lay their eggs on hair shaffs. Head louse infestation occurs among affluent sub-urban school and also inner-city school students (Ko and Elston, 2004).

Pediculosis generally occurred in children, primarily girls, aged 3-12 years. Transmission happened through head-to head close contact and sharing of personal items such as hats, brushes, combs, and other hair accessories that can spread head lice (Limchalearn, 2001). Females seem to be infected more often than males, due to a more frequent head to head contact. One of the reasons why head lice spread easily is the increase of globalization, leading to closer contact between many individuals. Such a contact offered the chance for a fed and gravid female louse to transmit from one head to another one (Takano-Lee *et al.*, 2005; Abdel-Ghaffar *et al.*, 2010). Another reason for the recent constant spreading of head lice was the lowered efficacy of available anti-louse compounds since many of them had been repeatedly used, consequently contributed to the development of resistance (Picollo *et al.*, 1998; 2000; Vassena *et al.*, 2003; Mogabure *et al.*, 2008; Yang *et al.*, 2004). Patients with louse infestation could be asymptomatic but scalp pruritis was common. Their presence cause itching and loss of sleep (Leung *et al.*, 2005). The louse saliva and feces may sensitize people with their bites, thereby, promoting the irritation, mild fever, muscular aches and, occasionally, swelling of the cervical glands. Excessive scratching increased the chance of secondary infections (Abdel-Ghaffar and Semmler, 2007). Head lice infestation may result in considerable discomfort, parental anxiety and embarrassment to the child.

Life Cycle of Head Louse (Figure 24.1)

Head lice belong to Phylum Arthropoda, Class Insecta, Order Phthiraptera, Suborder Anoplura, Family Pediculidae or Pthiridae (Limchalearn, 2001). They are wingless, flattened dorsoventrally and elongated. They have short antennae, and 3 pairs of clawed legs that are adapted to grasping hairs. They cannot fly or jump but can climb and crawl very fast to avoid light. The size of head louse is nearly equal to a sesame seed, 1-3 mm in length. Louse egg cases, called nits, are firmly cemented to human hair and difficult to remove. The warmth and moisture of the scalp assist in the egg incubation. Within one week, young lice hatch and pass through 3 nymphal instar stages, growing larger and maturing to adults in about 10 days. Their life cycles last about 30 days after hatching until death. A fertilized female louse lays 6-10 eggs a day for the next 16 days until it dies. They obtain their nutrients from blood by feeding once or more in a day. Lice have evolved, developing positive phototropism that urges them to run just after feeding to the end of the hair strand and to wait for a hair-to-hair contact with another host (Martini, 1946). If the contact does not occur, the females return to the warm scalp's surface and start another blood meal there while gluing eggs at the basis of the hair (Abdel-Ghaffar *et al.*, 2010).

Treatment of Head Lice

Chemical treatments for head lice are known as pediculocides. Those that kill adult and nymphal lice are sometime called lousicides, while those that kill the developing embryo with the eggs are called ovicides. The ideal topical anti-head lice products should kill 100 per cent of lice and embryo, removing all eggs from hair shafts and preventing reinfection. Until now, the ideal product has not yet been developed. Researches on topical treatment for head lice have focused on 100 per cent insecticidal and ovicidal effects. Insecticidal effect has been achieved with many chemicals and natural products but ovicidal effect could not be achieved (Heukelbach *et al.*, 2006).

History of Pediculosis Treatment

Several options are available to cope with infestation ranging from physically removing head lice with a special fine-toothed comb to chemical treatments with pesticides. In the twentieth century, treatments of pediculosis were based on chemical insecticides, composing of several natural and synthetic compounds. DDT was discovered in 1939 and used to control lice until the end of World War II (Buxton, 1945). Four active ingredients were licensed to be used against head lice *i.e.*, permethrin and phenothrin, active principles in pyrethroid insecticides, and carbaryl and malathion in non-pyrethroid insecticides. These compounds were designed to kill lice and their eggs. On the other hand, they were harmful to humans especially when they were applied to the scalp where it was particularly permeable. Moreover, children had weaker immune systems and underdeveloped detoxification mechanisms. Therefore, they were more susceptible and sensitive to the toxic effects of pesticides

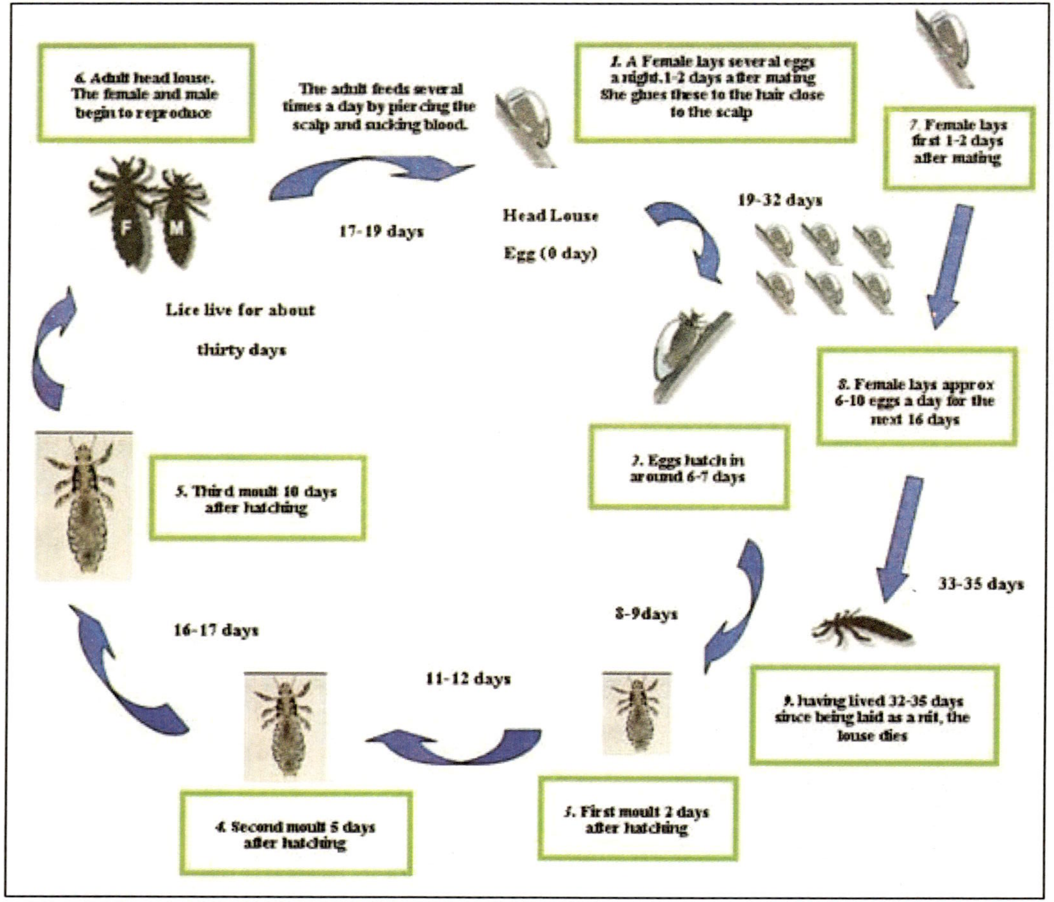

Figure 24.1. Life cycle of head louse (modified from Heukelbach *et al.,* 2006; Lice Advisory Bureau, 2006).

(Abdel-Ghaffar and Semmler, 2007). Symptoms reported include burning sensations, skin irritation, headaches, dizziness, hyperactivity and increased susceptibility to infections. Moreover, malathion, an organophosphate insecticide acting as a cholinesterase inhibitor, was reported to produce acute hallucination and could disrupt the immune system (Swadener,1992).

Hexachlorocyclohexane (HCH) was a widely used insecticide employed to control insect infestations on livestock, pets, humans, and agricultural products. It was a mixture of isomers, of which the α and γ-isomers were central nervous system stimulants, while the β- and δ-isomers were central nervous system depressants. Of all the isomers, γ-isomer (lindane) had the highest acute toxicity in humans (Boyd and Chen,1968; Hayes,1982; Gosselin *et al.,* 1984; Hall and Hall, 1999).

In late 1940, lindane, an organochlorine, was found to be more effective pediculocide than DDT. Lindane gradually replaced DDT in many countries and had been used until today in some countries despite of its reported neurotoxic and carcinogenic effects (Busvine, 1948). A severely poisoned patient experienced neurological and psychiatric symptoms (Hall and Hall, 1999). Lindane could be absorbed through skin, inhaled when in vapor form, or consumed orally and the contact could cause internal and external damages to the organ. It could possibly be cumulatively carcinogenic and mutagenic agent, having teratogenic, immunotoxic, and neurotoxic properties (Hayes,1982; Hall and Hall,1999). Lindane and other organochlorine insecticides had been shown to produce hepatic, neuronal, renal, and testicular damage, as well as bone marrow disorders, peripheral paresthesias and neuropathies, muscular weakness,impaired coordination, aplastic anemia, and agranulocytopenia if exposed repetitively (Gosselin *et al.*,1984; Hall and Hall, 1999). Damaging of developing fetuses and might decrease fertility in females is also reported (Boyd and Chen,1968; Hayes,1982; Gosselin *et al.,* 1984; Hall and Hall,1999). The average lethal dose in humans of lindane is 125 mg/perkg (Hayes,1982; Gosselin *et al.,* 1984). Lindane had been banned in many countries and was severely restricted in the others. However, a variety of generic brands of lindane are still available (Hall and Hall, 1999). Lindane-containing lotions and shampoos are available by a variety of brand names. The FDA's recommended that lindane-containing products should only be used after patients have either failed to respond to adequate doses of other treatments or have been shown to be intolerantto other approved therapies for scabies and mites (Hall and Hall, 1999).

As resistance to DDT emerged a decade later in the United Kingdom and in Israel, organophosphates such as malathion were used as alternatives. Carbamates and other chemicals in this group were found to be highly effective against lice. Carbaryl, a carbamate, was initially sold over the counter in the United Kingdom, but was subsequently restricted to doctor's prescription to limit resistance (Scowen, 1995). However, resistance to carbaryl had been found in the same places in the United Kingdom (Downs *et al.,* 2002). DDT had been banned in many countries due to their high toxicity (Mehlhorn, 2008; Mehlhorn and Mehlhorn, 2009; Mumcuoglu *et al.,* 2009). In November 1995, the UK Government's Committee on carcinogenicity concluded that Carbaryl was a potential human carcinogen. Some synthetic pyrethroids such as permethrin were classified by the US Environmental Protection

Agency as Class C possible human carcinogens (US Environmental Protection Agency, 1997). Moreover, the exposures to permethrin and phenothrin might potentially be linked to leukemia, lymphoid cancer and multiple chemical sensitivity (Pesticides News, 1995) and there were reports about corneal damage after their treatments. Pollack *et al.* (1999) reported resistance of pyrethroid insecticides by some head lice. In some developing countries, especially in rural areas, people are accustomed to treating pediculosis with inexpensive home remedies like kerosene and gasoline despite of it being flammable (Abdel-Ghaffar and Semmler, 2007). In Thailand, 25 per cent benzyl benzoate in form of emulsion has been used to control head lice in school children while hexin™, a commercial preparation (1 per cent w/w gamma benzene hexachloride) is still available on the market as a drug for anti-head lice.

Nowadays, the awareness of the hazardous impacts of pesticides on human health is increasing rapidly. The problem is to find substances/preparations that are not immunogenic and nontoxic, but are active against all developmental stages of the louse including ovicidal activity. The safe and effective alternatives, especially from natural sources, are required.

Herbal Insecticides against Head Lice

Plants and phytochemicals have been used in traditional medicines to treat pediculosis. Hundred percent effective topical treatments of motile head lice can kill less than 50 per cent of the embryo in eggs. One reason is that the most effective insecticides are neurotoxins and the nervous system of young embryo is too immature to be affected. Thus, the insecticides cannot kill very young developmental stages of the eggs. Another reason is that insecticides cannot penetrate into the egg shell that is mostly composed of waxy substances. An altered skin barrier will enhance the resorption of topically applied insecticides. Plant-based pediculocides containing a mixture of essential oils and/or short-chain fatty acids may solve this problem. Since most products cannot claim a 100 per cent ovicidal action, the second treatment should be applied seven days after the first to kill young lice, which have hatched over the intervening days (Heukelbach *et al.*, 2006). Yang *et al.* (2005) reported that the essential oils from cinnamon bark could be useful as a fumigant and an ovicide for lice. Ovicidal effects from a direct contact bioassay were measured by reduced hatching. It was found that after 24 hours of exposure, cinnamon oil reduced hatching to 3 per cent at 0.25mg/cm^2.

The extracts from Chrysanthemum flowers (*Chrysanthemum cinerariaefolium* Trev. Bocc.), which the active compound pyrethrin was identified, have been used as insecticides since 1940. Six natural pyrethrins were reported and they are still popularly used nowadays despite several synthetic analogues on the market. Natural pyrethrins have many advantages over other insecticides for their active effect, lower toxicity to mammalians, biodegradability, and rapidly disable an insect. The mode of action of pyrethrins is similar to that of organochlorines in that they interfere with the permeability of sodium ion channels across nerve membranes. However, a large number of synthetic pyrethrins have popularly replaced natural pyrethrins since they are more active than natural pyrethrum and less toxic to mammals (Heukelbach *et al.*, 2006).

The etheric oils*e.g.* cocos oil, anise oil, and eucalyptus oil were used as insecticides but they were not completely successful due to the induction of unwanted immune reactions, leading to allergic skin problem by several components of etheric oil (Heukelbach *et al.,* 2006). The insecticidal qualities of terpenoid compounds that were commonly found in essential oils were well known (Weston *et al.,* 1997). The most comprehensive *in vitro* study of natural products comprised 54 essential oils against adult female head lice collected from children in South Korea. It was found that 16 of the 54 essential oils had efficacy equal to or greater than pyrethrum. The most active essential oils had a fumigant activity due to its volatility as well as a contact activity on head lice, whereas pyrethrum and phenothrin possessed only contact activity (Yang *et al.,* 2004; Heukelbach *et al.,* 2006). The most active oil was the oil from *Eucalyptus globulus* Labilla. leaves, followed by oils from *Mentha pulegium* L., marjoram (*Origanum majorana* L.) and rosemary (*Rosmarinus officinalis* L.). The Cinnamon oil caused 86 per cent mortality of body lice and was shown to be effective against head lice (Yang *et al.,* 2005). All oils reduced transmission to a treated hair by 33-65 per cent due to its slippery nature. This can explain why head lice are more prevalent in clean hair heads than in greasy hair heads. Besides being a flavor, lavender, which is a common ingredient in head lice preventative preparations, is also useful in limiting blood feeding for head lice (Heukelbach *et al.,* 2006).

Tea tree oil is obtained from steam distillation of the leaves of *Melaleuca alternifolia* Cheel prepared in form of 1 per cent o/w emulsion showed 94 per cent mortality against body lice (Veal, 1996). *In vitro* study on head lice showed that 1 per cent tea tree oil caused no mortality after 2 hours while 10 per cent resulted in 86 per cent mortality (Downs *et al.,* 2000). Five percent tea tree oil in 20 per cent ethanol exhibited 97 per cent mortality of head lice after a 4-hour treatment but more than 50 per cent mortality with concentrations of 1 per cent and 2 per cent of the oil (Heukelbach *et al.,* 2006). Four compounds from tea tree oil showed obvious different efficacies against head lice *in vitro* (Downs *et al.,* 2000). The most active compounds were terpinen-4-ol, terralin and α-terpeninol which were each 100 per cent effective at 10 per cent concentration. 1,8-Cineole and terpinen-4-ol in tea tree oil showed an inhibitory effect on acetylcholinesterase, which is an enzyme targeted by the organophosphate insecticides (Mills *et al.,* 2004). A mixture of tea tree oil and cinnamon leaf oil (*Cinnamomum zeylanicum* Nees) (1:1) at 1 per cent in 40 per cent ethanol had 100 per cent efficacy against adult body lice after 17 hours exposure to the oil mixture (Veal, 1996). Tea tree oil was almost used in combination with other essential oils in products for pediculosis. However, it could be used alone. Higher doses of tea tree oil could cause skin irritation while allergic contact dermatitis might be observed after the use. The topical application of tea tree oil could be considered as safe (Hartford and Zug, 2005; Hammer *et al.,* 2006; Willcox, 2005; Crawford *et al.,* 2004; Khanna *et al.,* 2000; Bruynzeel, 1999; Rubel *et al.,* 1998; Apted, 1991). Tea tree oil was shown to be the superior repellant and anti-feedant. Over half of head lice transferring to a tea tree-treated head would be expected to transfer out as soon as possible and would be less inclined to survive since blood meals would be inhibited (Canyon and Speare, 2007).

Neem (*Azadirachta indica* A. Juss. var. *indica*) extract was reported to kill head lice slowly *in vitro* but less effective than malathion, permethrin and benzyl benzoate

(Morsy *et al.*, 2000). In contrast, a shampoo prepared from neem seed extract was highly effective against all stages of head lice after exposure in male and female children for 10, 15 and 30 min with no side effect. It was recommended to apply for 10-15 min once a week for two successive weeks (Abdel-Ghaffar and Semmler, 2007). Formulations containing neem had long been used in Indian traditional medicines due to its repellant, insecticidal and pesticidal activities. Neem-based products used in agriculture are biodegradable and less toxic to mammalians, but they are toxic to fish and aquatic invertebrates. The therapeutic topical used of neem products on human could be considered as safe as well (Brahmachari, 2004). Recently, a shampoo product containing extracts of grapefruits was tested against head lice in children for 10 and 20 minutes of exposure. It was found that the product could kill larvae and adult head lice quickly and efficiently with high skin safety profile, pleasant odor, and no side effects. The second treatment 8-10 days later was recommended to kill all young head lice hatched from the eggs (Abdel-Ghaffar *et al.*, 2010).

Annona squamosa Linn. is a medium-sized tree that has many local names *i.e.* custard apple, sugar apple, sweet sop and noi naa. Belonging to the family Annonaceae, it is native to West Indies and tropical America and is widely grown throughout the tropical regions. The fruit is a compound fruit, nearly round, separating when the fruit is ripe and revealing the mass of creamy-white, glistening, delightfully fragrant, juicy, sweet, and delicious. Many of the segments enclose a single oblong-cylindric, black or dark-brown seed, totally of 20-38 seeds in each fruit (Morton, 1987). Custard apple tree is cultivated for fruits in Mexico, Florida and California of the United States, Peru, Brazil and other tropical Asian countries such as The Philippines, Ceylon, India, Malaysia and Thailand. In Thailand, they are widely cultivated in the central and north-eastern parts of the country.

Traditional Uses of Annona squamosa

The leaves, young fruits and seeds of *A. squamosa* are insecticidal. The leaf juice can kill lice. The bark contains anonaine while the root bark yields 3 alkaloids *i.e.*, anonaine, liriodenine and reticuline (Morton, 1987). In Thailand, several parts of *A. squamosa* are claimed to be ethnomedicines (Farnsworth and Bunyapraphatsara, 1992):

Leaves are used for treatment of ringworm, tinea versicolor and skin diseases, as an anthelmintic, pediculocide, scabicide and is anti-inflammatory.

Stem bark is used for wounds and periodontitis, as an antisnake venom, antidiarrhea and astringent.

Roots are used as a laxative, emetic and antisnake venom.

Fruits are used for treatment of neck abscesses, ringworm, tinea versicolor, herpes virus, as an antisnake venom, and anthelmintic.

Seeds are used as a pediculocide and antiedema.

Chemical Constituents

Stem bark contains anonaine, borneol, camphor, corydine, isocorydine, β-sitosterol (Reyes and Santos, 1931; Rao *et al.*, 1978).

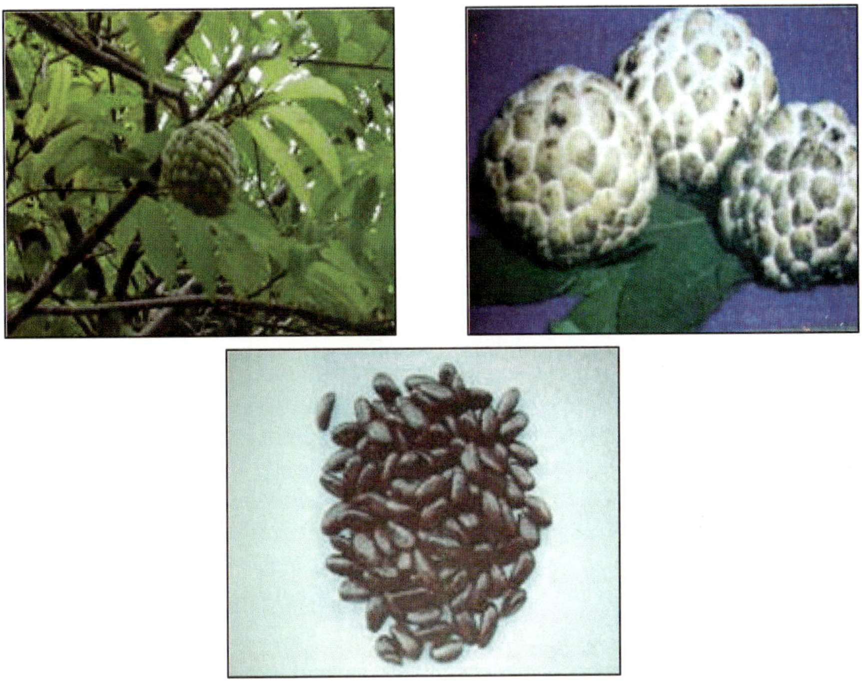

Figure 24.2. Leaves, fruits and seeds of *Annona squamosa* Linn.

Leaves contain anonaine, benzyltetrahydro-isoquinoline, borneol, camphene, carvone, β-caryophylline, eugenol, farnesol, geraniol, hesperoside, isocorydine, and stigmasterol (Farnsworth and Bunyapraphatsara, 1992).

Seeds contain acetylcholine, annonacins, annonastatin, annonin, anonaine, fatty acids, linoleic acid, oleic acid, palmitic acid, and β-sitosterol (Farnsworth and Bunyapraphatsara, 1992).

Anti-head Lice Activity of Annona squamosa

In Thailand, fresh leaves and seeds of *A. squamosa* have been used for killing head lice. Traditional recipes as a pediculocide are as followed (Farnsworth and Bunyapraphatsara, 1992):

1. Seven or eight fresh leaves are pounded with water and the water extract is applied on the hair, left for 15 min, and then rinsed out.
2. Three or four fresh leaves are pounded with arrack, then the extract is applied on the hair and left for 10 minutes, and then rinsed out.

Several scientific researches underwent to investigate the anti-head lice activity of *A. squamosa* leaves and seeds. The solution made from blended and crushed seeds with coconut oils at a concentration of 1:2 could kill 98 per cent of head lice in 72 students within 2 hours while the leaf extract showed less potency (Puapatanakul,

1980). Later, our research group studied paraciticidal activity *in vitro* of various organic solvent extracts from the leaves and seeds of this plant dissolved in coconut oil against head lice and male ticks from dogs. The results showed that the petroleum ether extracts of the leaves and seeds in coconut oil at the ratio of 1:1 gave the 90 per cent efficacy (LT_{90}) against head lice in 53 and 26 min, respectively. The less potent extracts were the chloroform leaf extract and the ethanol seed extract in coconut oil 1:1 and 1:2, respectively with the same LT_{90} at 67 min. In contrast, all the extracts showed no activity against male ticks (Gritsanapan *et al.*, 1996). Areekul and Chaikledkaew (1994) compared anti-head lice activity of the oil in water cream preparation of different concentrations*i.e.* 20, 30 and 50 per cent w/w prepared from the petroleum ether extract of *A. squamosa* seeds (Areekul and Chaikledkaew,1994; Gritsanapan *et al.*, 1998). The 50 per cent cream was able to eliminate 100 per cent of the lice when tested *in vitro* on pig skin within 32 minutes while 30 per cent and 20 per cent creams took 48 and 62 min, respectively. Twenty and fifty percent creams were tested clinically against head lice in female students. The 20 per cent cream was the optimal formula and killed 93 per cent head lice within 3 hour after application. In the same experiment, the 50 per cent cream and the commercial preparations, 1 per cent gamma benzene hexachloride and 25 per cent benzyl benzoate, were able to eliminate 96, 81 and 11 per cent of head lice, respectively.

Ariyadejvanich and Kongjaroan (1995) reported anti-head lice activity of the 20 per cent cream of *A. squamosa* seed extract in human subjects. The amounts used of 10 and 20 g of the 20 per cent cream preparation could kill 56.7 and 92.4 per cent of the lice within 3 hours of exposure, respectively. No test subject was found to be irritated during the treatment. Boonsuk and Athikomkulchai (1996) compared the effectiveness for killing head lice at different concentrations (5, 10, 15 and 20 per cent w/w) of *Annona squamosa* cream preparation both *in vitro* and *in vivo*. In *in vitro* test, all head lice were killed by the 20 per cent freshly prepared cream within 15 min. The creams with lower concentrations needed a longer period of exposure to eliminate lice. Thirty grams of each cream preparation (5, 10, 15 and 20 per cent w/w) were tested in female students and the outcome showed that the 5, 10 and 15 per cent creams had killing effect less than the 20 per cent preparation. The 20 per cent w/w freshly prepared cream could kill 56.8, 88.1 and 95.7 per cent of head lice after 1, 2 and 3 hours of application, respectively. The 3 month old *A. squamosa* seed preparations were tested for their physical stabilities at 15-45° C and tested for anti-head lice activity *in vitro*. The 20 per cent creams kept at 15°C and at room temperature (28-30° C) were physically stable and could kill head lice within 2 hours. Other cream preparations kept at 45° C were not physically stable (Kongklaeo and Suthichaloenporn, 1996). The 20 per cent cream kept at room temperature (28.30°C) and kept in a refrigerator for (4°C) 7 months exhibited 72.0 and 79.5 per cent of head lice after applying 30 g of the creams for 3 hours in school girls, respectively (Klinniyom and Yukare, 1997; Gritsanapan *et al.*, 1998). Whereas, both creams showed no efficacy against louse eggs.

Later, Tiangda *et al.* (2000) reported the anti-head lice efficacy and stability of 20 per cent w/w oil in water cream prepared from the petroleum ether extract of the seeds of *A. squamosa* in school girls. After 3 hours-hair exposure to 20 g of the freshly prepared cream, 95.34 per cent of head lice were killed, while only 60.09 per cent of killing rate was found in the commercial preparation *i.e.* 25 per cent benzyl benzoate emulsion. For 6 and 12 month-storaged preparations in a refrigerator (4° C) and 12 month-storaged at room temperature (28-32°C), the anti-head lice efficacy were found to be 99.19, 97.55 and 89.47 per cent, respectively, which were not significantly different from that of the freshly prepared cream. The custard apple seed creams did not cause any irritation on the scalp or neck skin while benzyl benzoate emulsion produced burning sensation and redness. These results demonstrate that the petroleum ether extract of *A. squamosa* seeds prepared as a cream is biologically stable for at least 12 months. In 2006, Intaranongpai *et al.*(2006) reported the two major components oleic acid (13.25 per cent) and triglyceride with one oleate ester (7.74 per cent) of the hexane seed extract of *A. squamosa*. The compounds were tested *in vitro* against head lice and compared to the crude extract from the seeds. The triglyceride with one oleate ester and the crude hexane extract, diluted with coconut oil (1:1), and oleic acid, could kill all tested head lice in 11, 30 and 49 minutes, respectively. From the results, the triglyceride ester can be used as a marker for quantitative analysis of the active compound for quality control of *A. squamosa* raw materials, seeds and its extract. Also, it can be used for quality assessment and chemical stability evaluation of the anti-head lice preparations from this plant (Intaranongpai *et al.*, 2006; Gritsanapan *et al.*, 2006). In 2007, our research group tested the efficacy of freshly prepared 20 per cent w/w cream of custard apple seeds against human head lice and their eggs in school girls. The results demonstrate that single treatment of the 20 per cent w/w of *A. squamosa* seed cream could kill 92 per cent of head lice, but could not kill their eggs. The cream should be applied once a week for 3 consecutive weeks to kill all adults and new young head lice developed from the eggs (Gritsanapan *et al.*, 2007).

Toxicity of Annona squamosa

The bark of *A. squamosa* contains 0.12 per cent anonaine. Injection of the bark extract caused paralysis in a rear limb of an experimental toad. The sap from cut

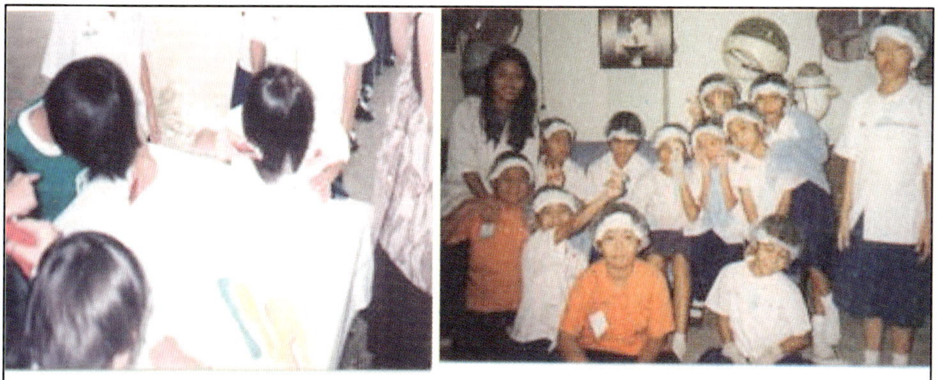

A B

Figure 24.3. A: Head lice were separated from school girls hair using a special fine-toothed comb; B: School girls were treated with *A. squamosa* seed cream.

branches irritated and severely injured the eyes (Morton, 1987). The leaves and seeds of *A. squamosa* extracted with water or coconut oil (1:1 w/v) produced no toxicity to rabbit's eyes (Paupatanakul, 1980). Sookvanichsilp *et al.* (1994) reported the toxicity to eye and ear skins of rabbits of the 4 organic solvents (petroleum ether, ether, chloroform, and ethanol) extracts from *A. squamosa* leaves and seeds dissolved in propylene glycol (1:10 w/v). The results revealed that the organic solvent extracts producing adverse effects on rabbit eyes were in order of severity of ether>petroleum ether> chloroform> ethanol, while those on rabbit ear skin were found to be petroleum ether> ether> chloroform> ethanol. The petroleum ether extract of the leaves and the ether and chloroform extracts of the leaves and seeds produced an acute and immediate redness on eyes, while the effect on chemosis seemed to be delayed. The petroleum ether and ether extracts from the seeds may be considered to produce the highest toxic effect to the eyes due to the ability to cause rugged cornea. Ether and chloroform extracts of the seeds produced more toxicity to rabbit ear skin than extracts from the leaves. This result agreed with the former report (Puapatanakul, 1980), indicating that extracts from the seeds of *A. squamosa* caused more irritation to rabbit skin than extracts from the leaves. The leaf extract in coconut oil (1:2 w/v) applied to the whole body surface (except the head) of the patients with scabies for 12 hours produced no irritation, no allergic reaction and other adverse reactions to skin (Kullavanijaya *et al.*, 1992). In contrast, the petroleum ether extracts from the leaves and seeds of this plant exhibited an opposite results and they were considered to cause toxicity to rabbit ear skin while ethanol extracts of the leaves and seeds seemed to produce the mildest toxicity to rabbit eyes and not toxic to rabbit ear skin (Sookvanichsilp *et al.*, 1994). The toxicities to the rabbit eyes of the extracts from the leaves and seeds of *A. squamosa,* suggested that the preparations prepared from this plant extracts should be cautiously used and without eye contact.

Conclusions

Although ideal products against head lice are expected to kill 100 per cent of lice and embryo and remove all eggs from hair shafts and repelled lice, this kind of product could not been developed. Research on topical treatment of head lice has focused on insecticidal and ovicidal effects. Since most products cannot claim a 100 per cent ovicidal action, the second treatment should be applied 7 days after the first to kill young lice, which have hatched over the intervening days (Heukelbach *et al.*, 2006).

Louse eggs are laid at the base of hairs close to the scalp and are attached firmly. Hatching takes approximately 6-10 days and empty egg shells (nits) and dead eggs remain attached to the hair for 6-12 months. Since human hair grows at a rate of about 1 cm per month, nits are more visible due to the hair growth. The presence of nits commonly results in misdiagnosis and social disturbance. The common method to remove lice eggs is to use fine toothed nit combs. Wetting the hair or applying a slicking agent such as vegetable oils, hair conditioners, acid shampoos, or 5 per cent acetic acid can facilitate the removal of eggs from the hair. However, there are no chemical or natural remedies for nit removal that have been clinically evaluated. (Heukelbach *et al.*, 2006).

A large number of compounds and products from plants such as Chrysanthemum flowers, tea tree oil, neem leaves, and custard apple seeds exhibit a preferable ability to kill head lice *in vitro* and *in vivo*. Moreover, they showed only mild toxicity compared to other synthetic drugs. Therefore, they should be developed and promoted as pediculocidal products on the market instead of harmful and toxic synthetic organophosphates and organochlorines that have decreasing susceptibility worldwide (Shaalan *et al.*, 2005). Particularly, *A. squamosa* seeds, which are a byproduct from consuming the ripe fruits, offered high potency against head lice in clinical trials. Not only can it be produced into commercial and pharmaceutical products against head lice, another benefit is the increase in value of the custard apple seeds that would otherwise be negligible wastes. The remarkable results of custard apple seeds and leaves to kill head lice prove that traditional herbs are still useful and beneficial, and are better and safer alternative to synthetic chemicals.

References

Abdel-Ghaffar, F., and Semmler, M. (2007). Efficacy of neem seed extract shampoo on head lice of naturally infected humans in Egypt. *Parasitology Research*, **100**: 329-332.

Abdel-Ghaffar, F.; Semmler, M.; Al-Rasheid, K.; Klimpel, S., and Mehlhorn, H. (2010). Efficacy of a grapefruit extract on head lice: a clinical trial. *Parasitology Research*, **106:** 445-449.

Apted, J.H. (1991). Contact dermatitis associated with the use of tea-tree oil. *Australasian Journal of Dermatology*, **32:** 177.

Areekul, M., and Chaikledkaew, U. (1994). Antiparasitic cream from *Annona squamosa* Linn. A Special Project of the Faculty of Pharmacy. Mahidol University, Bangkok.

Ariyadejvanich, L., and Kongjaroen, W. (1995). A study on anti-head lice activity of a cream of *Annona squamosa* seeds. A Special Project of the Faculty of Pharmacy, Mahidol University. Bangkok.

Boonsuk, J., and Athikomkulchai, S. (1996). Evaluation of an effectiveness of intensive hair masks from *Annona squamosa* Linn. seed extract on head lice. A Special Project of the Faculty of Pharmacy, Mahidol University. Bangkok.

Boyd, E. M., and Chen, C.P. (1968). Lindane toxicity and protein-deficient diet. *Archives of Environmental Health*, **17**: 156–163.

Brahmachari, G. (2004). Neem-An omnipotent plant: A retrospection. *Chem BioChem*, **5:** 408-421.

Bruynzeel, D.P. (1999). Contact dermatitis due to tea tree oil. *Tropical Medicine and International Health*, **4**: 630.

Busvine, J.R. (1948). The head and body races of *Pediculus humanus* L. *Parasitology*, **39**: 1–16.

Buxton, P.A. (1945). The use of new insecticide DDT in relation to the problems of tropical medicine. *Transactions of the Royal Society of Tropical Medicine and Hygiene*, **38:** 367–393.

Canyon, D.V. and Speare, R. (2007). A comparison of botanical and synthetic substances commonly used to prevent head lice (*Pediculus humanus* var. *capitus*) infestation. *International Journal of Dermatology*, **45**: 543–546.

Crawford, G.H., Sciacca, J.R., and James, W.D. (2004). Tea tree oil: cutaneous effects of the extracted oil of *Melaleuca alternifolia*. *Dermatitis*, **15:** 59-66.

Downs, A.M.; Stafford, K.A., and Coles, G.C. (2000). Monoterpenoids and tetralin as pediculocides, *Acta Dermato-Venereologica*, **80:** 69-70.

Downs, A.M.R., Stafford, K.A., Hunt, L.P., Ravenscroft, J.C., and Coles, G.C. (2002). Widespread insecticide resistance in head lice to the over-the-counter pediculocides in England, and the emergence of carbaryl resistance. *British Journal of Dermatology*, **146:** 88-93.

Farnsworth, N.R., and Bunyapraphatsara, N. (1992). Thai Medicinal Plants. Medicinal Plant Information Center, Faculty of Pharmacy, Mahidol University, Bangkok.

Gosselin, R.E., Smith, R.P., and Hodge, H. (1984). Clinical Toxicology of Commercial Products, 5th Edition. Williams and Wilkins, Baltimore.

Gritsanapan, W., Somanabandhu, A., Titirungruang, C., and Lertchaiporn, M. (1996). A study on the antiparasitic activities and chemical constituents of extracts from the leaves and seeds of custard apple (*Annona squamosa* Linn.). Proceeding of The Third NRCT-JSPS Joint Seminar, 1996, Bangkok, pp. 209-215.

Gritsanapan, W., Pithayanukul, P., Klinniyom, A., and Yukase, I. (1998). Studies of stability and effectiveness of intensive hair masks from *Annona squamosa* seed extract. The 50th IPC and 17th FAPA Congress. Mumbai.

Gritsanapan, W., Intaranongpai, J., and Chavasiri, W. (2006). Active anti-head lice component from custard apple seed. *Planta Medica*, **72**: 966.

Gritsanapan, W., Klaymongkol, C., and Wannasawage, C. (2007). Antiparasitic activity against head lice and head louse nits of *Annona squamosa* seed preparation. *Planta Medica*, **73**: 851.

Hall, R.C.W., and Hall, R.C.W. (1999). Long-term psychological and neurological complications of lindane poisoning. *Psychosomatics*, **40:** 513-517.

Hammer, K.A., Carson,C.F., Riley, T.V., and Nielsen, J.B. (2006). A Review of the toxicity of *Melaleuca alternifolia* (tea tree) oil. *Food and Chemical Toxicology*, **44:** 616-625.

Hartford, O., and Zug, K.A. (2005). Tea tree oil. *Cutis*, **76:** 178-180.

Hayes, W.J. (1982). Pesticides Studied in Man. Williams and Wilkins, Baltimore.

Heukelbach, J., Speare, R., and Canyon, D. (2006). Natural products and their application to the control of head lice: An evidence-based review. *In:* Chemistry of Natural Products: Recent Trends and Developments, Ed.By Brahmachari, G., Research Signpost, India, pp. 1-26.

Intaranongpai, J., Chavasiri, W., and Gritsanapan, W. (2006). Anti-head lice effect of *Annona squamasa* seeds. *Southeast Asian Journal of Tropical Medicine and Public Health*, **37**: 532-535.

Khanna, M., Qasem, K., and Sasseville, D. (2000). Allergic contact dermatitis to tea tree oil with erythema multiforme-like id reaction. *American Journal of Contact Dermatitis,* **11:** 238-242.

Klinniyam, A. and Tukase, I. (1997). Studies of stability and effectiveness of intensive hair masks form *Annona squamosa* seed extraction. A Special Project of the Faculty of Pharmacy. Mohidal University, Bangkok.

Ko, C.J., and Elston, D.M. (2004). Pediculosis. *Journal of The American Academy of Dermatology,* **50**: 1-12.

Kongklaeo, P., and Suthichaloenporn, P. (1996). Formulation of intensive hair masks from *Annona squamosa* Linn. seed extraction. A Special Project of the Faculty of Pharmacy, Mahidol University. Bangkok.

Kullavanijaya, P., Pakoonvanich, V., Sudsukh, N., and Chongsathien, S. (1992). Treatment of scabies with solution made from custard apple's leaves in coconut oil. *Bulletin of the Department of Medical Services* (Thai), **17**: 31-34.

Leung, A.K.C., Fong, J.H.S., and Pinto-Rojas, A. (2005). *Pediculus capitis. Journal of Pediatric Health Care,* **19**: 369-373.

Lice Advisory Bureau. Life cycle of head louse. www.headliceadvice.net/images/lice-cycle.gif (accessed April 27, 2006).

Limchalearn, P. (2001). Anti-head lice activity of *Annona squamosa* seed cream in school girls and its irritation tests in rabbits. A Master Thesis, Faculty of Pharmacy, Mahidol University, Bangkok, Thailand.

Martini, G. (1946). Medizinische Entomologie. G. Fischer, Jena.

Mehlhorn, H. (Ed.) (2008). Encyclopedia of parasitology. 3rd edition. Springer, New York.

Mehlhorn, B., and Mehlhorn, H. (2009). Louse alarm. Dusseldorf University Press, Dusseldorf.

Mills, C., Cleary, B., Gilmer, J.F., and Walsh, J.J. (2004). Inhibition of acetylcholinesterase by Tea Tree oil. *Journal of Pharmacy and Pharmacology,* **56:** 375-379.

Mogabure, C.G., Zerba, E., and Picollo, M.I. (2008). Evidence of pyrethroid resistance in eggs of *Pediculus humanus capitis* (Phthiraptera: Pediculidae) from Argentina. *Journal of Medical Entomology,* **45:** 693-697.

Morsy, T.A., el-Ela, R.G.; Nasser, M.M., Khalaf, S.A., and Mazyad, S.A. (2000). Evaluation of the *in vitro* pediculicidal action of four knock insecticides and three medicinal plant extracts. *Journal of the Egyptian Society of Parasitology,* **30:** 699-708.

Morton, J.F. (1987). Custard apple. *In:* Fruits of Warm climates, Ed. By Morton, J.F., Miami, FL. pp. 80-83. Available from: http://www.hort.purdue.edu/newcrop/morton/sugar_apple.html (accessed 2005, March 31).

Mumcuoglu, K., Gilead, L., and Ingber, A. (2009). New insights in pediculosis and scabies. *Expert Review Dermatology*, **4:** 285-302.

Pesticides News. (1995). Household spray cancer link. *Pesticide News*, **28**: June.

Picollo, M.I. (2003). Prevalence and levels of permethrin resistance in*Pediculus humanus capitis* De Geer (Anoplura; Pediculidae) from Buenos Aires, Argentina. *Journal of Medical Entomology*, **40:** 447-450.

Picollo, M.I.; Vassena, C.; Casadio, A.; Massimo, J. and Zerba, E. (1998). Laboratory studies of susceptibility and resistance to insecticides in *Pediculus capitis* (Anoplura; Pediculidae). *Journal of Medical Entomology*, **35:** 814-.817.

Picollo, M.I., Vassena, C.; Mougabure, C.G., Vernitti, M., and Zerba, E. (2000). Resistance to insecticides and effect of synergists on permethrin toxicity in *Pediculus capitis* (Anoplura; Pediculidae) from Buenos Aires. *Journal of Medical Entomology*, **37:** 721-725.

Pollack, R.J., Kiszewski, A; Armstrong, P.; Hahn, C., Wolfe, N., Rahman, H.A., Laserson, K., Telford III, S. R., and Spielman, A. (1999). Differential permethrin susceptibility of head lice sample in the US and Borneo. *Archives of Pediatrics and Adolescent Medicine*, **153**: 969-973.

Puapatanakul, O. (1980). Clinical studies of *Annona squamosa* seeds and leaves for the treatment of head lice. 37 pp. (in Thai), Bangkok.

Rao, R., Krishna, V., Murty, N., and Seshagiri, R.J.V.L.N. (1978). Occurrence of borneol and camphor and a new terpine in *Annona squamosa*. *Indian Journal of Pharmaceutical Sciences*, **40**: 170-171.

Reyes, F.R.,and Santos, A.C. (1931). Isolation of anonaine from *Annona squamosa. Philippine Journal of Science*, **44:** 409.

Rubel, D.M., Freeman, S., and Southwell, I.A. (1998). Tea tree oil allergy: what is the offending agent? Report of three cases of tea tree oil allergy and review of the literature. *Australasian Journal of Dermatology*, **39:** 244-247.

Scowen, P. (1995). Government restricts the use of carbaryl for head lice. *Professional Care of Mother and Child*, **5:** 163-165.

Shaalan, E.A., Canyon, D., Younes, M.W., bdel-Wahab, H., and Mansour, A.H. (2005). A review of botanical phytochemicals with mosquitocidal potential. *Environment International*, **31:** 1149-1166.

Sookvanichsilp, N., Gritsanapan, W., Somanabandhu, A., Lekcheroen, K., and Tiankrop, P. (1994). Toxicity testing of organic solvent extracts from *Annona squamosa* : Effect on rabbit eyes and ear skin. *Phytotherapy Research*, **8**: 365-368.

Swadener, C. (1992). Low doses of malathion disrupt immune system function. *Journal of Pesticide Reform*, **12:** 25.

Takano-Lee, M., Edman, J., Mullens, B., and Clark, M. (2005). Transmission potential of the human head louse, *Pediculus capitis* (Anoplura: Pediculidae). *International Journal of Dermatology*, **44**: 811-816.

Tiangda, Ch., Gritsanapan, W., Sookvanichsilp, N., and Limchalearn, A.(2000). Anti-head lice activity of *Annona squamosa* seed extract. *Southeast Asian Journal of Tropical Medicine and Public Health,* **31**: 174-177.

US Environmental Protection Agency. (1997). Office of Pesticide Programs. List of chemicals evaluated for carcinogenic potential. Memo from W.L. Burnman, HED, to HED branch chiefs. Washington D.C. (Feb.19).

Veal, L. (1996). The potential effectiveness of essential oils as a treatment for head lice, *Pediculus humanus capitis. Complementary Therapies in Nursing and Midwifery,* **2**: 97- 101.

Weston, S.E., Burgess, I., and Williamson, E.M. (1997). Oils against head lice in development in pharmacognosy. *The Pharmaceutical Journal,* **259:** 482.

Willcox, M. (2005). An evaluation of tea tree oil as an alternative microbicide. *Nursing Times,* **101:** 32-33.

Yang, Y.C., Lee, H.S., Clark, J.M., and Ahn, Y.J. (2004). Insecticidal activity of plant essential oils against *Pediculus humanus capitis* (Anoplura; Pediculidae). *Journal of Medical Entomology,* **41**: 699-704.

Yang, Y.C., Lee, H.S., Lee, S.H., Clark, J.M., and Ahn, Y.J. (2005). Ovicidal and adulticidal activities of *Cinnamomum zeylanicum* bark essential oil compounds and related compounds against *Pediculus humanus capitis* (Anoplura: Pediculicidae). *International Journal for Parasitology,* **35,** 1595-1600.

Medicinal Plants: Phytochemistry, Pharmacology and Therapeutics Vol. 2 (2012) *Pages* **405–412**
Editor-in-Chief: **V.K. Gupta**
Published by: **DAYA PUBLISHING HOUSE, NEW DELHI**

25

Orthosiphon stamineus Modulates Acetaminophen-Induced Changes in Serum Hepatic Markers, Hepatocytes Viability and Glutathione-S-Transferase Activity in Rats

J.H. Chin[1]*, A.H. Hussin[2] and S. Ismail[2]

ABSTRACT

Orthosiphon stamineus (Family: Lamiaceae) is widely used for the treatment of diabetes mellitus, hypertension and various kidney problems. The first objective of the present study is to examine the hepatoprotective effect of methanol leave extract of O. stamineus in acetaminophen-induced liver toxicity rats. The second objective is to evaluate the effect of O. stamineus on the phase II hepatic drug metabolising enzymes. Healthy female Sprague Dawley (SD) rats weighing 160 ± 20 g were used throughout the experiment. Based on the results obtained, pre-treatment with 500 mg/kg (P<0.05) of O. staminues reduced the liver damages induced by acetaminophen as evident by the reduction in serum hepatic liver markers and associated with the increment of percentage of hepatocytes viability and glutathione-s-transferase (GST) catalytic activity. In conclusion, O. stamineus extract demonstrated a potent hepatoprotective activity against acetaminophen-induced hepatic damages in rats by inducing the hepatic phase II GST catalytic activity.

Keywords: Acetaminophen, Glutathione-s-transferase, Hepatocytes, *Orthosiphon stamineus*, Serum enzymes, Silymarin.

1 Faculty of Pharmaceutical Sciences, UCSI University, UCSI Heights, No.1, Jalan Menara Gading, 56000. Cheras, Kuala Lumpur, Malaysia.

2 Centre for Drug Research, Universiti Sains Malaysia, 11800. Minden, Pulau Pinang, Malaysia

* *Corresponding author*: E-mail: jhchin@ucsi.edu.my;Tel: +603-91018880

Introduction

Orthosiphon stamineus (Family: Lamiaceae) has attracted increasing attention in the past several decades for its great medicinal values. The decoction of the leave is traditionally used in Malaysia and Indonesia for the treatment of arteriosclerosis, gout, rheumatism, bladder and kidney discomfort.

Antidiabetic, anti-hyperuricemia, anti-inflammatory, analgesic and diuretic properties of *O. stamineus* have been studied scientifically (Sriplang *et al.*, 2007; Arafat *et al.*, 2008; Yam *et al.*, 2008). Acute and sub-chronic oral toxicity studies of methanol leave extract of *O. stamineus* in rats have been reported. The plant was observed safe to be consumed and the LD_{50} was reported to be greater than 5 g/kg (Abdullah *et al.*, 2009; Chin *et al.*, 2008). Associated with that, we have continued our effort to study on the antioxidant property of this plant. Methanol leave extract of *O. stamineus* was able to induce the activity of several antioxidative enzymes, *i.e.* glutathione peroxidase, catalase and superoxide dismutase in rats (Chin *et al.*, 2008). Phytochemical analyses have identified the antioxidant property of *O. stamineus* is mainly contributed by the phenolic compounds. These phenolic compounds are including rosmarinic acid, eupatorin and sinensitin.

Liver disease is increasing rapidly and remains as one of the serious health problems in Asian countries. Hepatic injury is always associated with the metabolic disorder. The hepatoprotective effect of *O. stamineus* on the CCl_4-induced liver toxicity has been studied but the exact mechanism of protection is not well understood (Yam *et al.*, 2007). The objectives of the present study are to examine the protective effect of *O. stamineus* in acetaminophen-induced hepatotoxicity rats and to evaluate its protection from hepatic injuries by correlating to the phase II hepatic detoxification enzymes in rats. Two major phase II enzymes, known as glutathione-s-transferase and UDP-glucuronosyl transferase were chosen for the present study.

Materials and Methods

Chemicals

Acetaminophen, 1-chloro-2,4-dinitrobenzene, glutathione (reduced form), *p*-nitrophenol, potassium chloride, potassium dihydrogen phosphate, trypan blue was purchased from Sigma Aldrich Chemical Company Inc., St. Louis, MO, USA. The chemicals were of analytical grade.

Plant Material

Methanol extracts of *O. stamineus* were supplied by Professor Zhari Ismail from School of Pharmaceutical Sciences, USM. The leaves of the plant were collected in the late afternoon, from 30–45 days old white flowered plants. The leaves were chopped and dried at approximately 40°C for three days. Methanol extract of *O. stamineus* was prepared using a proportion of 10 g dried leaves in 100 mL of methanol by warming for four hours at 40°C. The solution was filtered through filter paper (Whatman No.1), concentrated and spray-dried to obtain the crude methanol extract.

Animal Selection

Healthy female Sprague Dawley (SD) rats weighing 160 ± 20g body weight bred in the Animal House Unit, Universiti Sains Malaysia were used throughout the experiment. All animals were freely access to tap water and standard food pallet *ad libitum*. Animals were kept in the standard condition, *i.e.* 12 hours dark/light cycle.

Hepatoprotective Study

All animals were randomly assigned into seven groups with six animals (n=6) per group. First group served as normal control group, orally treated with distilled water and second group served as acetaminophen (APAP) control treated with distilled water. Third group treated with standard drug, 20 mg/kg silymarin and group IV, V, VI and VII were served as treatment groups, orally treated with 5 mg/kg, 31.25 mg/kg, 125 mg/kg and 500 mg/kg of *O. stamineus* methanol leave extract, respectively. All animals were orally treated up to 14 days. 2g/kg of acetaminophen was orally fed to all animals except normal control group, 2 hours post-administration of last treatment at day-14. Blood samples were collected post 48 hours of 2g/kg acetaminophen administration. Collagenase perfusion technique was conducted to isolate the hepatocytes (Hussin and Skett, 1988). The hepatocytes were then counted using a haemocytometer and assayed for viability using inclusion method of trypan blue. Hepatocytes which excluded trypan blue were considered viable cells while hepatocytes with trypan blue stain were considered as damaged cells.

Study on the Phase II Hepatic Metabolising Enzymes

A total of 30 female rats were used to evaluate the effect of *O. stamineus* on the phase I and II hepatic drug metabolizing enzymes. First group served as control group treated with distilled water only. Group II, III and IV was orally treated with 5 mg/kg, 31.25 mg/kg, 125 mg/kg and 500 mg/kg of methanol leave extract of *O. stamineus* for 14 days.

Liver Samples Preparation for Phase II Enzyme Assay

All animals were sacrificed at day-15. Livers were removed from the sacrificed animals, washed with ice-cold KCl and then homogenized in 3 volumes of the same solution in a Potter-Elvehjem homogeniser using a Teflon pestle. The homogenates were centrifuged at 9000 x g for 20 min at 4° C. The supernatants (S9) were kept at –70° C until use for glutathione-s-transferase assay (Gibson and Skett, 1994).

Liver microsomes were prepared using calcium precipitation technique (Gibson and Skett, 1994). Part of the cytosolic fraction above was then used to prepare rat liver microsomes. Microsomal protein concentration was determined by the method of Lowry *et al.* (1951). The microsome was kept frozen at -80°C with 20 per cent (v/v) glycerol added. Protein concentration of the S9 fractions and liver microsomes was determined by Lowry's method using bovine serum albumin as standard (Lowry *et al.*, 1951).

Glutathione-S-transferase (GST) Assay

S-9 supernatant or known as S-9 liver fraction was used as an enzyme source for GST assay (Gibson and Skett, 1994). A convenient spectrophotometric method has been developed by Habig *et al.* (1974) for the analysis of GST activity based on the enzyme catalysed conjugation of glutathione with the model substrate, 1-choloro, 2,4-dinitrobenzene. The product formed (2,4-dinitrophenyl-glutathione) absorbs light at 340 nm with an extinction coefficient of 9.6 mM/cm, which facilitates the analysis of the enzyme activity based on product formation.

UDP-glucuronosyl transferase (UGT) Assay

UGT conjugation activity towards substrate, *p*-nitrophenol (*p*NP) was assayed following slight modifications of the method by Bock and Kohle (2004). Rat liver microsomes were used as a source of UGT enzyme. The absorbance was read at 405 nm using spectrophotometer.

Statistical Analysis

All results were presented as mean ± standard deviation and analysed using Dunnett's Test. $P<0.01$ and $P<0.05$ was considered as significant as compared with the control group.

Results and Discussion

Serum AST, ALT and GGT in APAP control group was significantly ($P<0.05$) higher than the normal control group (Table 25.1). All the serum liver parameters *i.e.* AST, ALT and GGT were significantly reduced in adult female SD rats after being treated with 20 mg/kg ($P<0.05$) body weight of silymarin. The serum levels of AST, ALT and GGT were significantly reduced in adult female SD rats fed with 125 mg/kg ($P<0.05$) and 500 mg/kg ($P<0.05$) body weight of methanol extract of *O. stamineus* when compared to APAP control group (Table 25.1).

Table 25.1. Effect of methanol extract of *O. stamineus* on serum hepatic markers and viability of hepatocytes in acetaminophen-induced hepatic injuries female rats.

Groups (mg/kg body weight)	*AST (U/L)*	*ALT (U/L)*	*GGT (U/L)*	*Viability of hepatocyte (per cent)*
Normal control	98.7±2.1	33.0±4.6	0.7±0.2	97.8±2.0
APAP control	1194.3±359.1#	1077.3±379.4#	8.7±1.5#	70.0±3.2#
Standard drug				
Silymarin (20)	394.7±160.8*	86.0±4.6*	4.3±2.1*	86.2±2.8*
Test group				
O. stamineus (5)	916.3±100.5	832.0±29.5	2.8±1.5*	79.0±5.1
O. stamineus (31.25)	710.0±273.9	621.5±213.5	2.8±1.0*	80.4±6.9
O. stamineus (125)	356.5±60.2*	449.3±49.2*	5.0±2.0*	81.9±2.1*
O. stamineus (500)	259.0±72.3*	149.3±30.5*	3.0±0.8*	90.0±1.5*

Results are analysed by using Dunnett Test; n=6; value = mean ± S.D.

*$P<0.05$ compared to APAP control group; # $P<0.05$ compared to normal control group.

A significant increase in percentage of hepatocytes viability was shown by the adult female SD rats fed with repeated doses of 20 mg/kg (P<0.05) body weight of silymarin as compared to APAP control group. Only the adult female SD rats repeatedly fed with 125 mg/kg (P<0.05) and 500 mg/kg (P<0.05) body weight of methanol extract of *O. stamineus* showed a significant increase in percentage of hepatocytes viability.

Table 25.2. Effect of methanol leave extract of *O. stamineus* on phase II drug metabolising enzymes in female SD rats.

Groups	*UDP-glucuronosyl transferase (nmol/min/mg protein)*	*Glutathione-s-transferase (µmol/min/mg protein)*
Control	26.80±6.58	20.82±0.48
5 mg/kg	27.61±5.50	20.74±0.01
31.25 mg/kg	32.23±6.1	20.84±0.05
125 mg/kg	24.52±1.02	20.84±0.06
500 mg/kg	31.61±8.61	24.10±0.07**

Results are analysed by using Dunnett Test; n=6; value = mean ± S.D.

**P<0.01 compared to control group.

In the study on phase II metabolising enzymes, a significant increase of the GST activity was observed in the female rats treated with 500 mg/kg (P<0.01) of *O. stamineus* when compared to the control group. UGT activity was not affected by the methanol leave extract of *O. stamineus*.

Acetaminophen is an antipyretic drug that is generally safe to be used up to 4g/day in humans (Hamm, 2000). However, overdosing of acetaminophen causes liver damages. This drug is commonly used in the anti-hepatotoxicity study for the induction of liver damages in experimental animals. In the present study, post 48-hour administration of 2 g/kg of acetaminophen to the adult female SD rats showed significant increase to approximately 11 fold in AST, 29 fold in ALT and 1 fold in ALP as compared to negative control group (Table 25.1). Post 24-hour was chosen as the checking time point because of previous results showing the highest level of liver toxicity in female SD rats. The elevated serum levels of AST, ALT and GGT are conventional indicators for hepatic injury. From serum biochemical analyses, it is demonstrated that adult female SD rats administered with 2 g/kg of acetaminophen was in the necrosis state (Zimmerman, 1998). The hepatoxicity induced by the over dose of acetaminophen is due to its active metabolite, *N*-acetyl-*p*-benzoquinoneimine (NAPQI) generated by a chtochrome P450 system (Wu *et al.*, 2008). NAPQI reacts rapidly with glutathione which depletes the intracellular pool of glutathione. This toxic metabolite is mainly eliminated by the conjugation with glutathione catalysed by glutathione-s-transferase.

Pretreatment of methanol extract of *O. stamineus* at dose 125 mg/kg and 500 mg/kg to adult female SD rats showed a significant decrease in serum AST, ALT and GGT levels. The liver protection produced by 125 mg/kg and 500 mg/kg of methanol extract of *O. stamineus* in adult female SD rats was further evident by an increase in the percentage of hepatocytes viability. To this end, the results have demonstrated that *O. stamineus* pretreatment suppresses the elevation of serum AST, ALT and GGT activity caused by overdosing of acetaminophen in rats. This reflects a functional improvement of hepatocytes due to the prevention of leakage intracellular enzymes by its membrane stabilizing activity.

Pretreatment of rats with standard drug, 20 mg/kg of silymarin reverted all the serum biochemical parameters and percentage of hepatocytes viability to the normal basal as compared to the negative control. Several studies have demonstrated the hepatoprotective effect of silymarin in relation to free radical trapping, reduction of lipoperoxidation of cell membrane and an amelioration of hepatic collagen accumulation (Farghali *et al.*, 2000).

Phase I and II xenobiotic metabolizing enzymes play a crucial role in the hepatic functions. Many of the hepatotoxins modulate the catalytic activity of phase I and II xenobiotic metabolising enzymes (Upadhyay *et al.*, 2007). Pretreatment of the adult female SD rats with methanol extract of *O. stamineus* especially at the high dose significantly induced the GST catalytic activity in female SD rat livers. GST is the major phase II metabolizing enzyme that responsible for the detoxification of toxins, free radical and xenobiotics. Increased of hepatic GST activity has been reported to be beneficial for liver protection against oxidative damage. Hence, it was suggestive that the liver protective effect exhibited by methanol extract of *O. stamineus* in the present study could be explained by its induction on GST activity to conjugate NAPQI to the glutathione. This reaction increases the conversion of active metabolites to harmless form in the hepatic system and prevents the binding of NAPQI with hepatocytes' DNA, RNA or proteins thus lead to serious hepatocyte damage (Murray, 2009). Therefore, the increased activity of GST induced by pretreatment of *O. stamineus* extract reduced the acute acetaminophen-induced hepatotixicity in rats.

The present results have correlated the induction effect of methanol extract of *O. stamineus* on GST catalytic activity in SD rats in protecting acetaminophen-induced hepatic damages. 500 mg/kg of methanol extract of *O. stamineus* has demonstrated to be as potent as 20 mg/kg of silymarin in protecting hepatic functions. However, it is more meaningful to say that while using methanol extract of *O. stamineus* for other therapeutic purposes, at the same time, it could exert liver protection effect as well.

Conclusions

High doses of methanol leave extract of *O. stamineus* demonstrated potent liver protection effect against acetaminophen-induced hepatotoxicity. 500 mg/kg of methanol leave extract of *O. stamineus* was exhibited the highest liver protective activity associated with the induction on the GST activity in rat livers.

Acknowledgements

Authors would like to thank the financial support of the Intensified Research in Priority Areas (IRPA) grant from the Malaysian Ministry of Science, Technology and Innovative and also Prof. Zhari Ismail for supplying methanol extract of *O. stamineus*.

References

Abdullah, N.R., Ismail, Z., and Ismail, Z. (2009). Acute toxicity of *Orthosiphon stamineus* Benth standardised extract in Sprague Dawley rats. *Phytomedicine*, **16(2-3):** 222-226.

Adam, Y., Somchit, M.N., Sulaiman, M.R., Nasaruddin, A.A., Zuraini, A., Bustamam, A.A., and Zakaria, Z.A. (2009). Diuretic properties of *Orthosiphon stamineus* Benth. *Journal of Ethno-pharmacology*, **124(1):** 154-158.

Arafat, O.M., Tham, S.Y., Sadikun, A., Zhari, I., Haughton, P.J., and Asmawi, M.Z. (2008). Studies on diuretic and hypouricemic effects of *Orthosiphon stamineus* methanol extracts in rats. *Journal of Ethno-pharmacology*, **118(3):** 354-360.

Bock, K.W., and Kohle, C. (2004). Coordinate regulation of drug metabolism by xenobiotic nuclear receptors: UGTs acting together with CYPs and glucuronide transporters. *Drug Metabolism Review*, **36 (3-4):** 595-615.

Chin, J.H., Akowuah, G.A., Hussin, A., Ismail, Z., Fei, Y.M., and Ismail, S. (2008). Toxicity and *In-vivo* antioxidant effect of *Orthosiphon stamineus* leaf extracts in rats. *In:* Recent Progress in Medicinal Plants Vol. 21, Ed. By Singh, V.K., Govil, J.N. Studium Press LLC, USA, pp. 137-146.

Farghali, H., Kameniková, L., Hynie, S., and Kmonicková, E. (2000). Silymarin effects on intracellular calcium and cytotoxicity: A study in perfused rat hepatocytes after oxidative stress injury. *Pharmacological Research*, **41(2):** 231-237.

Gibson, G.G., and Skett, P. (1994). Introduction to drug metabolism. Blackie Academic and Professional, Glasgow.

Habig, W.H., Pabst, M.J., Jakoby, W.B. (1974). Glutathione-S-transferase. The first enzymatic step in mercapturic acid formation. *Journal of Biological Chem*istry, **249 (22):** 7140-7147.

Hamm, J. (2000). Acute acetaminophen overdose in adolescents and adults. *Toxicology*, **20** (3): 1-6.

Hussin, A.H., and Skett, P. (1988). Lack of effect of insulin in hepatocytes isolated from streptozotocin-diabetic male rats. *Biochemical Pharmacology*, **37(9):** 1683-1686.

Lowry, O.H., Rosebrough, N.J., Farr, A.L., and Randall, R.J. (1951). Protein measurement with the folin phenol reagent. *Journal of Biological Chemistry*, **193:** 265-275.

Murray, R.K. (2009). Metabolism of xenobiotics. *In:* Harper's Illustrated Biochemistry. 28th Ed. By Murray, R.K., Bender, D.A., and Kennelly, P.J., Rodwell, V.W., and Weil, P.A. Mc.Graw-Hill, New York, pp.609-615.

Sriplang, K., Adisakwattana, S., Rungsipipat, A., and Yibchok-Anun, S. (2007). Effect of *Orthosiphon stamineus* aqueos extract on plasma glucose concentration and lipid concentration in normal and streptozotocin-induced diabetic rats. *Journal of Ethno-pharmacology*, **109(3):** 510-514.

Upadhyay, G., Kumar, A., and Singh, M.P. (2007). Effect of silymarin on pyrogallol- and rifampicin-induced hepatotoxicity in mouse. *European Journal of Pharmacology*, **565:** 190-201.

Wiart, C. (2002). *Orthosiphon stamineus* Benth. *In:* Medicinal plants of Southeast Asia, Ed. By Wong, F.K. Prentice Hall, Kuala Lumpur, pp. 265.

Wu, Y., Piao, D., Han, X., and Nan, J. (2008). Protective effects of salidroside against acetaminophen-induced toxicity in mice. *Biological and Pharmaceutical Bulletin*, **31(8):** 1523-1529.

Yam, M.F., Basir, R., Asmawi, M.Z., and Ismail, Z. (2007). Antioxidant and hepatoprotective activity of *Orthosiphon stamineus* Benth standardized extract. *American Journal of Chinese Medicine*, **35(1):** 115-126.

Yam, M.F., Asmawi, M.Z., and Basir, R. (2008). An investigation of the anti-inflammation and analgesic effects of *Orthosiphon stamineus* leaf extract. *Journal of Medicinal Food*, **11(2):** 362-368.

Zimmerman, H.J. (1998) Drug-induced hepatic disease. *In:* Toxicology of the Liver, Ed. By Plaa, G.L., and Hewitt, W.R. Taylor and Francis: Washington, pp. 3-60.

Previous Volume

— Volume 1 —

2010, xiii+464p., col. plts., figs., tabls., ind., 25 cm **Rs. 1800**

ISBN 978-81-7035-627-1

Index

B

H

J

K

L

M

N

O

P